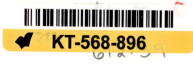

Energy-Yielding Macronutrients and Energy Metabolism in Sports Nutrition

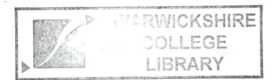

edited by

Judy A. Driskell
Ira Wolinsky

CRC Press

Boca Raton   London   New York   Washington, D.C.

NUTRITION in EXERCISE and SPORT

Edited by Ira Wolinsky and James F. Hickson, Jr.

Published Titles

Exercise and Disease,
Ronald R. Watson and Marianne Eisinger

Nutrients as Ergogenic Aids for Sports and Exercise,
Luke Bucci

Nutrition in Exercise and Sport, Second Edition,
Ira Wolinsky and James F. Hickson, Jr.

Nutrition Applied to Injury Rehabilitation and Sports Medicine,
Luke Bucci

Nutrition for the Recreational Athlete,
Catherine G.R. Jackson

NUTRITION in EXERCISE and SPORT

Edited by Ira Wolinsky

Published Titles

Sports Nutrition: Minerals and Electrolytes,
Constance V. Kies and Judy A. Driskell

Nutrition, Physical Activity, and Health in Early Life:

Studies in Preschool Children,
Jana Parizkova

Exercise and Immune Function,
Laurie Hoffman-Goetz

Body Fluid Balance: Exercise and Sport,
E.R. Buskirk and S. Puhl

Nutrition and the Female Athlete,
Jaime S. Ruud

Sports Nutrition: Vitamins and Trace Elements,
Ira Wolinsky and Judy A. Driskell

Amino Acids and Proteins for the Athlete—The Anabolic Edge,
Mauro G. DiPasquale

Nutrition in Exercise and Sport, Third Edition,
Ira Wolinsky

Published Titles Continued

Gender Differences in Metabolism: Practical and Nutritional Implications, Mark Tarnopolsky

Macroelements, Water, and Electrolytes in Sports Nutrition,
Judy A. Driskell and Ira Wolinsky

Sports Nutrition,
Judy A. Driskell

Energy-Yielding Macronutrients and Energy Metabolism in Sports Nutrition,
Judy A. Driskell and Ira Wolinsky

NUTRITION in EXERCISE and SPORT
Edited by Ira Wolinsky

Forthcoming Titles

High Performance Nutrition: Diets and Supplements for the Competitive Athlete, Mauro DiPasquale

Nutrition and the Strength Athlete,
Catherine R. Jackson

Sports Drinks: Basic Science and Practical Aspects,
Ron Maughan

Nutrition and Exercise Immunology,
David C. Nieman

Nutritional Applications in Exercise and Sport,
Ira Wolinsky

Nutrients as Ergogenic Aids for Sports and Exercise, Second Edition,
Luke R. Bucci

| Project Editor: | Sylvia Wood |
| Cover design: | Dawn Boyd |

Library of Congress Cataloging-in-Publication Data

Energy-yielding macronutrients and energy metabolism in sports
nutrition / edited by Judy A. Driskell, Ira Wolinsky.
        p.   cm.--Nutrition in exercise and sport
   Includes bibliographical references and index.
   ISBN 0-8493-0755-4 (alk. paper)
   1. Energy metabolism. 2. Athletes--nutrition. 3. Dietary
supplements. 4. Nutrition. I. Driskell, Judy A (Judy Anne). II. Wolinsky, Ira. III. Series.
QP176.E546 1999
612.3′ 9′ 088796—dc21
                                                     99–32452
                                                       CIP

No claim to original U.S. Government works
International Standard Book Number 0-8493-0755-4 Library of Congress Card Number 99-32452
Printed in the United States of America   2 3 4 5 6 7 8 9 0
Printed on acid-free paper

Series Preface

The CRC series **Nutrition in Exercise and Sport** provides a setting for in-depth exploration of the many and varied aspects of nutrition and exercise, including sports. The topic of exercise and sports nutrition has been a focus of research among scientists since the 1960s, and the healthful benefits of good nutrition and exercise have been appreciated. As our knowledge expands, it will be necessary to remember that there must be a range of diets and exercise regimes that will support excellent physical condition and performance. There is not a single diet–exercise treatment that can be the common denominator, or the single formula for health, or panacea for performance.

This series is dedicated to providing a stage upon which to explore these issues. Each volume provides a detailed and scholarly examination of some aspect of the topic. Contributors from a bona fide area of nutrition and physical activity, including sports and the controversial, are welcome.

Ira Wolinsky, Ph.D.
Series Editor

Preface

This volume is part of a special miniseries within the CRC series on **Nutrition in Exercise and Sport**. It is a mature series that contains some of the best books in the field. The subject matter covered in this particular volume focuses on energy-yielding macronutrients and energy metabolism. Its first section discusses the energy-yielding nutrients, followed by a section on the use of energy-yielding supplements with ergogenic value. The book concludes with a section that reviews gender and age differences that may be related to energy metabolism, and the important issues of weight gain and weight loss in the athlete. Each chapter has been written by experienced and highly accredited researchers and experts in the field. Where possible, practical applications and recommendations are made. Students, teachers, researchers, and health practitioners, as well as the educated layman, will find this book interesting and informative.

Companions to this book are three other volumes we edited: *Sports Nutrition: Vitamins and Trace Elements*, 1997, *Macroelements, Water, and Electrolytes in Sports Nutrition*, 1999, and *Nutritional Applications in Exercise and Sport*, to be published soon.

Ira Wolinsky, Ph.D.

Judy A. Driskell, Ph.D., R.D.

Dedication

To our significant others for their patience and support.

The Editors

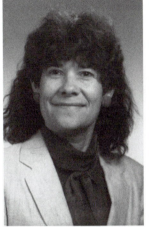

Judy Anne Driskell, Ph.D., R.D. is professor of Nutritional Science and Dietetics at the University of Nebraska. She received her B.S. degree in biology from the University of Southern Mississippi in Hattiesburg, and M.S. and Ph.D. degrees from Purdue University. Dr. Driskell has served in research and teaching positions at Auburn University, Florida State University, Virginia Polytechnic Institute and State University, and the University of Nebraska, as the Nutrition Scientist for the U.S. Department of Agriculture/Cooperative State Research Service and as a professor of Nutrition and Food Science at Gadjah Mada and Bogor universities in Indonesia.

Dr. Driskell is a member of numerous professional organizations, including the American Society of Nutritional Sciences, the Institute of Food Technologists, and the American Dietetic Association. In 1993 she received the Professional Scientist Award of the Food Science and Human Nutrition Section of the Southern Association of Agricultural Scientists. In addition, she received the Borden Award for Research in Applied Fundamental Knowledge of Human Nutrition in 1987. She is listed as an expert in B-complex vitamins by the Vitamin Nutrition Information Service.

Dr. Driskell recently co-edited CRC Press books *Sports Nutrition: Minerals and Electrolytes* with the late Constance V. Kies; and *Sports Nutrition: Vitamins and Trace Elements,* and *Macroelements, Water, and Electrolytes,* both with Ira Wolinsky. She has published about 100 refereed research articles and 10 book chapters, as well as several publications intended for lay audiences, and has given numerous professional and lay presentations. Her current research interests center around vitamin metabolism and requirements, including the interrelationships between exercise and water-soluble vitamin requirements.

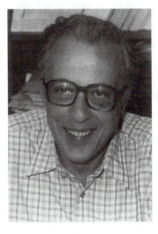

Ira Wolinsky, Ph.D., is professor of Nutrition at the University of Houston. He received his B.S. degree in chemistry from City College of New York and his M.S. and Ph.D. degrees in biochemistry from the University of Kansas. He has served in research and teaching positions at Hebrew University (both medical school and faculty of agriculture), the University of Missouri, and Pennsylvania State University. He has also conducted basic research in NASA life sciences facilities.

Dr. Wolinsky is a member of the American Society of Nutritional Sciences among other honorary and scientific organizations. He has contributed numerous nutrition research papers in the open literature. His current major research interests relate to the nutrition of bone and calcium and to sports nutrition. He has received research grants from both public and private sources as well as several international research fellowships, including a Fulbright Senior Scholar Fellowship. These have included research and teaching experiences in India, Russia, Bulgaria, Hungary, and Greece.

Dr. Wolinsky co-wrote a book on the history of the science of nutrition, *Nutrition and Nutritional Diseases.* He is the editor of *Nutrition in Exercise and Sport* and co-editor of *Sports Nutrition: Vitamins and Trace Elements,* and *Macroelements, Water, and Electrolytes* with Judy A. Driskell and *Nutritional Concerns of Women* with Dorothy Klimis-Tavantzis. He is also the editor for the CRC *Series on Nutrition in Exercise and Sport*, the CRC *Series on Modern Nutrition*, the CRC *Series on Exercise Physiology*, and the CRC *Series on Methods in Nutrition Research*.

Contributors

John J.B. Anderson, Ph.D.
Department of Nutrition
University of North Carolina
Chapel Hill, NC

Jenna Anding, Ph.D., R.D.
Department of Human Development
University of Houston
Houston, TX

Luke R. Bucci, Ph.D., R.D., C.C.N.
Weider Nutrition International
Salt Lake City, UT

Timothy P. Carr, Ph.D.
Department of Nutritional Science
  and Dietetics
University of Nebraska
Lincoln, NE

Russell L. Cowles, M.S.
Department of Nutritional Science
  and Dietetics
University of Nebraska
Lincoln, NE

Stephen F. Crouse, Ph.D.,
F.A.C.S.M., F.A.W.H.P.
Department of Health and Kinesiology
Texas A&M University
College Station, TX

Mauro G. Di Pasquale
M.D., M.R.O., M.S.F.
University of Toronto
Toronto, Ontario
Canada

J. Andrew Doyle, Ph.D.
Department of Kinesiology and Health
Georgia State University
Atlanta, GA

Judy A. Driskell, Ph.D., R.D.
Department of Nutritional Science
  and Dietetics
University of Nebraska
Lincoln, NE

J. Larry Durstine, Ph.D.,
F.A.C.S.M., F.A.A.C.V.P.R.
Department of Exercise Science
University of South Carolina
Columbia, SC

Daniel D. Gallaher, Ph.D.
Department of Food Science
  and Nutrition
University of Minnesota
St. Paul, MN

Jean E. Guest, B.S., R.D.
Department of Nutritional Science
  and Dietetics
University of Nebraska
Lincoln, NE

Catherine G. R. Jackson, Ph.D.,
F.A.C.S.M.
Department of Kinesiology
California State University at Fresno
Fresno, CA

Satya S. Jonnalagadda, Ph.D.
Department of Nutrition
Georgia State University
Atlanta, GA

Richard B. Kreider, Ph.D.
Department of Human Movement Sciences
  and Education
University of Memphis
Memphis, TN

Nancy M. Lewis, Ph.D., R.D.,
F.A.D.A.
Department of Nutritional Science
  and Dietetics
University of Nebraska
Lincoln, NE

Melinda M. Manore, Ph.D., R.D.,
F.A.C.S.M.
Department of Family Resources
  and Human Development
Arizona State University
Tempe, AZ

Robert J. Moffatt, Ph.D.
Department of Nutrition, Food
  and Exercise Sciences
Florida State University
Tallahassee, FL

Charilaos Papadopoulos, M.S.
Department of Kinesiology
  and Health
Georgia State University
Atlanta, GA

Alan J. Ryan, Ph.D.
Department of Internal Medicine
University of Iowa School of Medicine
Iowa City, IA

**Mark Tarnopolsky, M.D., Ph.D.,
F.R.C.P.E.**
Departments of Medicine and Kinesiology
McMaster University Medical Center
Hamilton, Ontario
Canada

Janice L. Thompson, Ph.D.
Department of Pediatrics
University of New Mexico
  School of Medicine
Albuquerque, NM

Lisa M. Unlu, B.S.
Weider Nutrition International
Salt Lake City, UT

Ira Wolinsky, Ph.D.
Department of Human Development
University of Houston
Houston, TX

Contents

Physiological Aspects of Energy Metabolism

Introduction

CHAPTER 1

Introduction to Energy-Yielding Macronutrient Needs of Athletes

John J.B. Anderson

CONTENTS

0-8493-0755-4/00/$0.00+$.50

1.1 INTRODUCTION

Energy is a critical nutrient variable that must be consumed in amounts that approximately equal the energy in kilocalories (kcal) required for activities in sports, dance, or other physically demanding activities, including work. Energy extracted from food macronutrients in body tissues supports not only the major energy systems operating during physical activities, but also mental functions and concentration. The brain, therefore, must be able to extract its share of glucose and possibly other macronutrients so that individuals can function mentally as well as physically; the optimal functioning of the brain may help prevent injuries, and the full capacity of the other organ systems permits an individual to reach his or her personal best physical performance.

Of course, the energy-yielding macronutrients from the diet must be complemented by adequate intakes of water and the many micronutrients needed to keep the body running smoothly, especially for highly competitive athletes (see Driskell and Wolinsky, Eds., *Macroelements, Water, and Electrolytes in Sports Nutrition*, 1999).

This introductory chapter provides glimpses of several topics relating to macronutrient intakes that are covered in this volume and a few that are not.

1.1.1 Concept of Linking Nutrient Intakes to Energy Consumption

The energy-yielding macronutrients from foods, as opposed to macronutrient supplements, serve also as the vehicles for the consumption of micronutrients. Therefore, the consumption of foods for their energy value has an added benefit because of the micronutrients that coexist in these same foods — not to mention the many non-nutrient phytochemical molecules in plant foods. Foods rich in complex carbohydrates (for energy), i.e., plant foods of many types, have the advantage of providing other essential nutrients as well as phytochemicals, many of which are antioxidants that protect against cell damage from reactive oxygen species.

1.1.2 Macronutrient Recommendations—Old Recommended Dietary Allowances and New Dietary Reference Intakes

The macronutrient recommendations currently used are the Recommended Dietary Allowances (RDAs)[1] rather than the Dietary Reference Intakes (DRIs),[2] both published by the Food and Nutrition Board. New DRIs for energy and protein consumption across the life cycle and across genders will be published in the next year or two.[3] The Recommended Energy Intake or Average Energy Allowance for healthy young adult males has not yet been set, but the old energy RDA is 2900 kcal per day and 2200 kcal per day for healthy young adult women. These recommendations will probably not change much when the new DRIs are released. Energy is not a nutrient *per se*, but rather it is a nutrient variable (based on a physical concept) derived from the kilocalories generated by the combustion of carbohydrates, fats, and proteins in a bomb calorimeter under precise environmental conditions. Therefore, energy in whatever form the carbon-hydrogen bonds exist in hydrocarbon chains, i.e., saturated or unsaturated, is transformed from these macronutrients to cellular energy, such as adenosine triphosphate (ATP) and, in striated muscle, to creatine phosphate (CP).

The protein allowances (RDAs) are approximately 50 g per day for healthy young adult females and approximately 60 g per day for healthy young adult men.[1] The new DRIs for protein may increase these values somewhat, but the recommendations for protein have little influence on usual intakes by North Americans, who on average consume 150–175% of the RDAs recommended in 1989 for each gender. As is the case for energy, athletes' tissue needs more protein, especially to repair muscle damage from prolonged physical activities. Yet, the amounts of protein typically consumed by omnivorous athletes but not necessarily by vegetarian athletes, particularly females, are considered to be more than sufficient for tissue growth and tissue repair related to damage resulting from sports performance.

1.1.3 Potential Adverse Interactions from Excessive Intakes of Supplements

Some nutritional sports bars and other food products that are marketed as supplements for athletes may lead to potential adverse effects because of the rapid rise in glucose from the starches or sugars in these products. The hyperglycemic response of many of these quick-energy sources may contribute to declines in blood concentrations of chromium, zinc, and other essential micronutrients that are critical for the function of muscle and other tissues during physical performance. Not enough is known about the postulated adverse effects of these highly processed "food" supplements, but at least one recent publication cautions against using these carbohydrate-rich products,[4] mainly at concentrations of carbohydrates of 10% or higher, which have a high glycemic index and, therefore, an insulin-stimulatory effect. Low glycemic-index foods fed prior to cycling exercise (at 70% $V\dot{O}_2$ max) increased endurance by 20 minutes, presumably because of slower digestion, lower blood glucose, and more efficient glycogen storage.[5]

1.1.4 Water

Water, though not a macronutrient that provides energy, must be consumed in sufficient amounts to replace the amounts lost, i.e., maintain water balance. Needs for this nutrient are not efficiently signaled to the brain to increase water intake despite our "thirst-sensing" mechanism in the brain. Therefore, athletes should drink water or another water-based beverage before, often during, and after practices and events to replace losses or to maintain water sufficiency. Certain other beverages, such as alcohol, coffee, and even tea, have modest diuretic properties that increase water losses via the kidneys. Energy metabolism, it should be noted, requires a well-hydrated body to operate efficiently.

1.2 FACTORS THAT AFFECT THE NEEDS OF ESSENTIAL NUTRIENTS

Age, gender, climate, weather conditions, and other factors may affect athletes' requirements for macronutrients. The need for energy may be increased under certain conditions and reduced under others. Young athletes who are still growing — and there are many young aspiring athletes — need macronutrients to accommodate both growth and athletic participation. Often, the demands of a sport will be so great and the energy intakes somewhat inadequate that growth cannot be supported as long as a few months. This suspended growth can typically be corrected when the demands diminish, disappear, or nutritional intervention is initiated.

1.2.1 Estimates of Energy and Protein Balances

Caloric balances are almost impossible to conduct on most athletes who fully participate in a sport that requires routine training and periodic participation in competitive events. Therefore, surrogate measures are needed to provide reasonable estimates of energy needs. For mature adults, equations have been developed that permit good estimates of energy requirements, but it is much more difficult to estimate the needs of growing youngsters. In very athletic adults of healthy body weight, rough energy needs can be calculated by the following equation:

$$\text{Energy in kcal} = \text{REE} + 2.0 \times \text{Body Weight (kg)}$$

where REE means resting energy expenditure.

Also, the Harris-Benedict equations can be used to estimate energy needs,[6-7] but activity factors are also needed for active participants.

Protein balances also are extremely difficult to obtain on active individuals (outside of a metabolic unit), so alternative methods have been developed to estimate protein needs. Typically, the basic protein allowance is increased by a factor of 50 to 100% in very active individuals, depending on their sport or activity.

1.2.2   Exercise and Maintaining Nutrient Balances by Athletes

Estimating the needs of macronutrients for energy and protein balance, however, may not be practical for athletes who generally eat according to what they perceive as their needs. This aspect of sports nutrition is not as scientific as we might desire, but clearly well-trained athletes at mature ages neither gain nor lose much weight, except perhaps temporarily in an endurance event of considerable length of time. Endurance athletes, such as marathon runners and road cyclists, do better if they consume small amounts of energy drinks or similar sources of energy that contain only about 100 kcal per drink.

1.2.3   Summary

Energy and protein balance studies, though theoretically desirable, are generally too impractical to use to estimate energy and protein requirements because the intake requirements are based on complete records of food and drink consumption, plus complete collections of urine and feces (and sweat when feasible). Since this work calls for a special metabolic unit, it is next to impossible for an athlete to participate in most sports activities under these conditions. Alternative approaches, such as calculations based on body weight, may be used to estimate macronutrient requirements, but these calculations are rarely performed.

1.3 FOOD ISSUES THAT MAY IMPACT ATHLETES

Athletes, coaches, and trainers need to be aware of several food-related issues that are raised here. First, athletes — even more important than non-athletes — need to consume a variety of foods each day according to the Basic Food Guide or Pyramid[8] to maintain top physical conditioning. A Vegetarian Food Guide is also available.[9] Second, athletes should limit their consumption of fast foods to occasional meals and should limit packaged snacks to a few times a weeks (see above). Third, athletes probably need a daily supplement of micronutrients to complement their generally higher energy intakes; athletes who consume less than the recommended amount of kilocalories per day, especially females, should take a one-a-day type of vitamin. Fourth, athletes should avoid drinking alcohol or at least limit it to no more than two drinks a day for males and one drink a day for females.

1.3.1   Basic Food Guide Recommendations

A variety of foods, as opposed to a narrow list of food selections, is strongly recommended for athletes to assure that they consume sufficient amounts of all nutrients (and non-nutrient phytochemicals), not simply the macronutrients. The best way to do this is to follow the recommended minimum numbers of servings each day from the Food Guide Pyramid: 6–11 servings from the bread and grain group; 3–5 servings from vegetables; 2–4 servings from fruits; 2–3 servings from dairy foods (exclusive of butter); and 2–3 servings of the protein group (meats, fish, poultry, and legumes). Miscellaneous foods (desserts, sweets, fats, oils, butter, alcohol, soft drinks, and others) should be consumed only sparingly.

Typically athletes will need more than these minimal recommendations, and they should add servings from the food groups within the Pyramid, particularly the grain group for complex carbohydrates, rather than from the miscellaneous group of foods. This admonition is easy to give, but by far, most young athletes do not follow the Food Guide Pyramid and they eat a lot of high-calorie foods, sometimes referred to as "junk foods," and not enough nutrient-dense foods. One certainty is that these young athletes, especially those in college, eat relatively few servings of fruits and vegetables a day — fewer than the combined minimum "five a day" that are recommended. It is a generally held axiom among sports physiologists that a poor diet does not foster optimal physical performance.[10]

1.3.2 Fast Foods and Snack Foods

Highly processed foods of any type generally do not have many micronutrients, or non-nutrient phytochemicals. Many of the items classified as fast foods and snack foods are highly processed. This treatment by food processors does not diminish the energy or protein content of an item; rather, it generally increases the energy density of the item at the expense of dietary fiber and other phytochemicals. This elimination of many micronutrients in good quantities could have disastrous effects later in life. The possibility exists then that the typical intake patterns, are heavy on fast foods and snack foods, that many young athletes follow today may set these athletes up for later development of the chronic diseases so common in western nations (see Section I.C.).

1.3.3 Nutrient Supplements

Sports nutritionists, sports medicine physicians, and pediatricians are increasingly recommending nutrient supplements that contain a broad range of micronutrients, at levels that approximate the current DRIs for age-specific and gender-specific groups. No harm can result from low-dose micro-nutrient supplements (at DRI levels). And for some athletes who have poor diets (as stated above), the supplements may improve their health and prevent injuries. Most supplement studies of athletes have been inconclusive in being able to make positive statements about the benefits of one or more specific nutrient supplements. This may be because these studies often have had too few subjects to show any difference (Type II statistical error) and many have not lasted long enough. Studies of young athletes have frequently been complicated by the subjects' growth, both treatment and control.

This area of investigation has given plenty of examples of how difficult it is to conduct prospective trials of the effects of nutrient supplements on athletes' performance levels. Nevertheless, multinutrient supplement use has a place in the appropriate training regimens of athletes and others in the realm of physical performance. Female athletes have, perhaps, a unique need for supplements. And as far as can be determined in the U.S., very few sports programs strongly encourage athletes to take a daily supplement.

1.3.4 Alcohol

Alcohol consumption by young athletes, adult as well as those of high school age, appears to be increasing in the U.S. Excessive consumption, especially binge drinking to get drunk, has become for some a rite of adolescence, and it seems inconceivable that so many young athletes behave in this manner. Such drinking patterns have a few side effects, in addition to hangovers, that not only adversely affect performance but may also contribute to injuries. One effect is dehydration; the consumption of alcohol has a diuretic effect that cannot easily be overcome by a few nonalcoholic drinks following a bout of heavy drinking. Besides having an effect on physical performance, dehydration probably more seriously affects mental concentration — and poor concentration often leads to injuries.

1.3.5 Summary

It is not easy for athletes in today's world to eat right — the right foods in appropriate amounts. Athletes and others often perfer more "pleasant" choices, which typically are not the wholesome foods nutritionists recommend. These foods include fast foods, snack foods, and, increasingly alcohol. Athletes need nutrition education to get them on the right track if they wish to optimize their performances in athletics and related physical activities.

1.4 NUTRITIONAL PROBLEMS OF FEMALE ATHLETES

Female athletes have unique problems because of the reproductive role they play and the hormones that govern much of the reproductive tissues. It has become increasingly clear in recent years that women's participation in high-level competitive sports may affect reproductive performance, but not all the answers have yet been uncovered. The "female athlete triad" illustrates the interrelations of several important physiological changes in young athletic women that typically result from not taking in enough food-borne calories coupled with high performance, particularly in the running and endurance sports.

1.4.1 Female Athlete Triad

This disorder has three major components: disordered eating, sometimes referred to as anorexia athletica (but not anorexia nervosa); amenorrhea or oligomenorrhea; and osteopenia, which may lead to osteoporotic fracture(s).[10] The restrictive intakes of energy-yielding macronutrients and micronutrients generally lead to a gradual decline in body weight, a decrease in body fat content, and often dehydration. These athletes may overdo their activity routines and become overtired as well. Some individuals may develop a severe nutrient deficiency, such as iron deficiency anemia, because of the chronic nature of poor intakes.[10] Because of the diminishing estrogen concentrations circulating in blood, the rate of bone resorption may be increased and calcium will be lost in the urine in increasing amounts. Typically, women do not consume enough calcium, which means that body mineral stores cannot be maintained — all because of an inadequate intake of macronutrients (see the introduction to this chapter regarding this issue).

Although not so common, hairline fractures have been diagnosed in many female runners who have all three components of the triad. When this happens, the athletes must cease running, take supplements, gain weight, and allow the fractures you heal. Nutrition education toward the improvement of eating habits is essential, but too often it is inadequately provided or neglected by sports medicine personnel.

1.4.2 Effects of Estrogen Loss on Food Intake

Either the loss of estrogens, or possibly an increase in the stress hormone cortisol, may have a deleterious effect on the brain center controlling food ingestive behavior. Unfortunately, not enough is known about the control of food intake, even with recent discoveries of leptin and several brain peptides thought to be involved in the regulation of intake or satiety (inhibition of intake).

1.4.3 Summary

Studies of the "female athlete triad" have uncovered several physiological links among the three major components. Male athletes do not suffer from a similar set of dysfunctions. Therefore, special consideration of this triad must be made by sports personnel to try to prevent its occurrence and the potential for disordered reproductive function by these females after they stop participating in competitive sports.

1.5 CONCLUDING REMARKS

A few main conclusions can be drawn from the large literature in this field.

First, the diets of athletes today are generally not good; they do not contain enough complex carbohydrates, and they contain too much protein and animal fat. The sources of much of the macronutrients are fast foods and snack foods. They do not eat enough fruits and vegetables and, to a lesser extent, whole grains.

Second, as a consequence of their food selection a majority of athletes do not get enough micronutrients.

Third, athletes need to take a full array of micronutrients as supplementation, but few take multinutrient supplements daily.

Fourth, athletes need to be taught the importance of fluid replacement from water or other beverages, but not from alcoholic beverages. Dehydration can have injury-inducing effects because of declines in mental concentration. If possible, athletes need to drink small amounts of fluid frequently while playing sports.

Fifth, the level of general nutrition knowledge of athletes, at least college athletes, is woefully inadequate, and no programs are known to have been established to overcome this deficit.

REFERENCES

1. National Research Council, Subcommittee on the 10th Edition of the RDAs, Food and Nutrition Board, Commission on Life Sciences, *Recommended Dietary Allowances,* 10th ed., National Academy Press, Washington, D.C., 1989.
2. Institute of Medicine, Food and Nutrition Board, *Dietary Reference Intakes for Thiamin, Riboflavin, Niacin, Vitamin B_6, Folate, Vitamin B_{12}, Pantothenic Acid, Biotin, and Choline*, National Academy Press, Washington, D.C., 1998.
3. Yates, A.A., Schlicker, S.A., and Suitor, C.W., Dietary Reference Intakes: The new basis for recommendations for calcium and related nutrients, B vitamins, and choline, *J. Am. Diet. Assoc.,* 98, 699, 1998.
4. Davis, J.M., Burgess, W.A., Slentz, C.A., Bartoli, W.P., and Pate, R., Effects of ingesting 6% and 12% glucose/electrolyte beverages during prolonged intermittent cycling in the heat, *Eur. J. Appl. Physiol.,* 57, 563, 1988.
5. Thomas, D.E., Brotherhood, J.R. and Brand, J.C., Carbohydrate feeding before exercise: Effect of glycemic index, *Int. J. Sports Nutr.,* 12, 180, 1991.
6. Harris, J.A. and Benedict, F.G., *A Biometric Study of Basal Metabolism in Man*, Publ. No. 279, Carnegie Institution of Washington, Washington, D.C., 1919.

7. Mahan, L.K. and Escott-Stump, S., Eds., *Krause's Food, Nutrition, and Diet Therapy*, 9th ed., Saunders, Philadelphia, 1995, chap. 2 (Energy).
8. Cronin, F., Shaw, A., Krebs-Smith, S., Marsland, P., and Light, L., Developing a food guidance system to implement the dietary guidelines, *J. Nutr. Educ.*, 19, 281, 1987.
9. Whitten, C., Haddad, E., and Sabate, J., Developing a vegetarian food guide pyramid: A conceptual framework, *Vegetarian Nutr.*, 1, 25, 1997.
10. Hultman, E., Harris, R.C., and Spriet, L.L., Work and exercise, in *Modern Nutrition in Health and Disease*, 8th ed., Shils, M.E., Olsen, J.A., and Shike, M., Eds., Lea & Febiger, Philadelphia, 1994, chap. 42.
11. Anderson, J.J.B., Stender, M., Rondano, P., Bishop, L., and Duckett, A.B., Nutrition and bone in physical activity and sport, in *Nutrition in Exercise and Sport*, 3rd Ed., Wolinsky, I., Ed., CRC, Boca Raton, FL, 1998, chap. 9.

CHAPTER 2

Overview of Human Bioenergetics and Nutrition

Catherine G.R. Jackson

CONTENTS

2.1 BIOENERGETICS CONCEPTS

2.1.1   General

Within the human cell lies the capacity to convert potential chemical energy derived from food macronutrients into high-energy substances that can provide usable chemical energy for mechanical energy and work. The mechanisms by which this occurs are common throughout the life forms on earth. The way the human cell interconverts energy forms through different pathways to phosphorylate adenosine 5'-diphosphate (ADP) to form 5'-adenosine triphosphate (ATP), both a universal energy receiver and donor, is the object of continued study. General principles have been elucidated and refined in the past,[1] but much remains unclear.

Understanding bioenergetics, the study of the transfer of energy in chemical reactions of tissue, is crucial to determining appropriate exercise and dietary regimens. Determining whether an activity is nonaerobic, anaerobic, aerobic or some combination thereof enables one to choose the most supportive conditioning program and dietary practice with a minimum of wasted time and effort. For many years, researchers have recognized the specificity of conditioning practices as they relate to successful performance; however, only recently have they recognized the specificity of nutritional practice to support the different types of exercise.[2] The lack or misinterpretation of this knowledge has lead to considerable misinformation in the popular literature with respect to conditioning and nutritional regimens for activity. Many claims of enhanced performance cannot be supported by current knowledge of energy transfer.

In general, highly intense and short-term activities depend on stores of ATP immediately available in muscle. They can be characterized as nonoxidative or anaerobic because they do not rely on oxygen delivery to meet the immediate demand for energy delivery. These activities can also be described as "power" activities, as it takes only seconds to complete them. The shorter the time needed to complete the task, the more "powerful" an activity. When the stores of ATP immediately available can no longer sustain the activity as exercise progresses, ATP is supplied by another nonoxidative energy substrate that is glycolytic, glucose and glycogen. Activities of this nature are sometimes characterized as "speed" activities. As activity continues, cellular metabolism proceeds more toward oxidative processes and activities that are characterized as "endurance." All three energy systems and sources are utilized in varying degrees at all times, depending upon the intensity and length of time of the activity. It should be emphasized, however, that all systems of energy delivery support the reactions that phosphorylate ADP at all times. Nutritional practices should be modified to support the energy delivery system predominantly used in a particular activity in order to enhance performance.

2.1.2   ATP and CP

Many review sources and texts are available that outline currently accepted concepts in human energy metabolism and bioenergetics.[3–11] All include discussions of how substrates for utilization derived from food macronutrients (fats, carbohydrates, proteins) can ultimately be used to provide the phosphate groups and hydrogen ions necessary to phosphorylate adenosine nucleotides to regenerate the ATP molecule. ATP is the common chemical intermediate molecule in the cell that participates directly in receiving and supplying chemical energy to the reactions of the cellular machinery that can be converted into cell work. All energy systems must first transfer one or more phosphate groups to phosphate depleted forms of the ATP molecule before the cell can use the energy. The transfer of energy is a major limiting factor in physical activity.

The ATP molecule possesses an adenine and ribose portion to which three phosphate groups are linked. The phosphate groups are attached by high energy bonds that liberate a large amount of energy when they are broken. Enzymes, ATPases, catalyze the processes of bond formation and breakage. The formation and breakdown of the ATP molecule provide the energy that allows living cells to function.

The reactions of ATP usually involve hydrolysis, thereby emphasizing the importance of water to cellular metabolism. The exchange of the phosphate groups between the ATP molecule and phosphate donors to ADP and AMP allows activity to be sustained for long periods of time. As the ATP molecule releases its phosphate groups, energy in the form of kilocalories is released and then captured to perform biological work. In terms of physical activity, the support of the work of mechanical contraction in skeletal muscle is of greatest interest. The phosphate groups liberated from ATP to perform work must be continuously replaced to allow ongoing energy transfer. The processes leading to the phosphate attachment to ADP to resynthesize ATP is the most important consideration in understanding human energy metabolism, as ATP is the only substance that can be used for skeletal muscle contraction; ADP levels very much drive the process. The ATP stores alone are available for powerful, short-term activity. Supported by enzymes called ATPases, these reactions are rapid and immediate, and the cells uses them continuously.

Also available, in concentrations exceeding ATP by approximate factors of 3–5, is creatine phosphate (CP). Possessing one phosphate group, CP is capable of donating its phosphate immediately to support the phosphorylation of ADP, the nucleotide of ATP that has two phosphate groups attached. CP can be characterized as an intracellular energy shuttle that is catalyzed by the enzyme creatine kinase. Only CP can donate phosphates to ADP; however, once exercise commences this cannot proceed to a high degree until the exercise recovery period. Hence, other systems must provide energy. ATP and CP participate in coupled reactions, those that use the liberation of free energy in one reaction to drive a second reaction. The substances are frequently termed the phosphagens, a label that refers to their phosphate groups.

2.1.3   High Energy Phosphagen Utilization

The phosphagens ATP and CP enter into coupled energy transfer reactions by exchanging phosphate groups. At rest, the body is primarily in aerobic metabolism because most of the cellular need for oxygen is met by matched delivery by the cardiovascular system for appropriate blood flow. During this time, ATP is continuously resynthesized primarily by CP, particularly at the initiation of any sudden movement, but it is not overly stressed. When an activity begins, however, metabolic balance cannot be maintained and the CP stores of phosphate are immediately mobilized. The higher the intensity, the more rapidly stores will become depleted. In high-intensity work, it is difficult to deliver oxygen quickly to cells and the depleted phosphate groups must wait for the relatively slow mechanisms of the cardiovascular system to function to receive more adenosine nucleotides. Under these circumstances, approximately 80% of the ATP required for a 30-second activity may come from ATP derived anaerobically by quickly relying on glycolysis.[12]

During activity of any type, the immediate source of ATP is that which is already stored and the ADP, which may be coupled for acquisition of the phosphate group with CP. The phosphate groups may be removed from ATP in sequence with ADP, adenosine 5'-monophosphate (AMP), and adenosine remaining in varying ratios or proportions; however, exercise rarely uses phosphate groups to the complete depletion to adenosine. Energy can only be provided for brief periods of intense activity such as golf or tennis swings, sprints, or jumps because cellular stores of ATP are limited. However, the phosphate groups needed to resynthesize the adenosine forms are easily supplied in the exercise recovery period. Although CP is the immediate source of the phosphates and energy used to transform ADP to ATP, this coupled reaction cannot replete the system effectively until activity is diminished or terminated. During activity, other sources of phosphate besides CP must be used. While highly intense activity such as sprinting can deplete phosphate groups within seconds, a lower intensity activity will allow for primary use this system for several minutes. The fact remains, however, that the reformation of CP after it has been used in highly intense exercise can occur only during recovery and requires ATP. Once the system is "depleted," it cannot be fully restored until exercise intensity has been significantly diminished or terminated.

Myokinase — or adenylate kinase — an enzyme present in the cell, supports the immediate source of energy of the phosphagens. This enzyme is capable of facilitating a reaction in which two ADPs, which have a total of four phosphate groups, can be reconfigured to produce one ATP and one AMP. Although the total of phosphate groups at the end of the reaction is still four, the cell now has access to an ATP molecule that is capable of donating its phosphate group in an energy-requiring reaction.

Oxygen is not involved in the aforementioned reactions; therefore, some have termed the processes nonaerobic. The more common designation is anaerobic. The phosphagens are found in the cytosol of the cell, but their concentrations do not allow them to support activities that must be sustained. Other types of activities that use the immediate energy delivery system are power activities such as weightlifting, shot-put, and discus.

All humans have approximately the same ratio of CP to ATP, 5 to 1, which is related to muscle mass. The ATP is located at specific sites in muscle and tends to increase proportionately when the amount of muscle mass is increased. It appears that there is a ratio of ATP to muscle mass so that as muscle mass increases, so does the amount of ATP. Enhancement of ATP stores over and above this established ratio is controversial and the topic of much debate and investigation.

2.1.4   Nutritional Considerations of the Phosphagen Energy Delivery System

There is much interest in creatine supplementation to enhance performance.[13] Creatine in the form of creatine monohydrate is popular as a nutritional supplement. It is promoted as a substance that will enhance muscle development in activities that require strength and power. It is also thought that supplementation will delay fatigue and allow one to exercise longer, thereby improving performance due to exposure to an increased workload. Although several studies have been published, evidence for the ergogenic claims is still elusive.

Creatine is derived primarily from animal sources and can be synthesized from the amino acids arginine, glycine, and methionine. Muscle stores of total creatine (Cr) and CP are derived from ingested dietary sources synthesized in the liver that enter the bloodstream. An upper limit of Cr and CP seems to exist over and above which it does not seem to be possible to affect an increase.[14] Since it is known that fast twitch muscle has higher stores of creatine, the fiber-type composition of the individual will effect experimental results. It is also known that some interconversion of type of the sub-groups of fast twitch fiber can occur with exercise, thus studies that stimulate this response will be confounded by fiber-type transformation effecting results.

Although results of studies are inconclusive, there are several known effects.[13] Subjects who are studied who do not have near maximum levels of creatine stores will have measurable effects. Thus those who are mildly "deficient" may benefit from creatine supplements and those whose levels are near maximal seem to derive no benefit. Additionally, some individuals may be "nonresponders" to supplementation.[14] Some of the reported increases in muscle mass may be due to water retention and not protein synthesis.[15] Reports of dehydration leading to the need for medical intervention and possibly death exist and need further evaluation. Supplementation, if it works, will only enhance power activities of very short duration and high intensity; endurance and submaximal exercise performance may not be improved.

It has been shown that supplementation can increase intramuscular stores of CP, but the amounts that need to be ingested are high and initially in the order of 20 g per day. After loading, levels may be maintained by 2–5 g per day.[16] Whether the increased stores of CP will lead to improved performance is uncertain. It has been shown that supplementation may improve CP levels in the elderly,[17] but the cautions about dehydration are more acute in this population that is at risk.

Most studies show that repeated bouts of high-intensity, short duration exercise along with creatine supplementation increases average power outputs. However, reports of increases in peak power output are equivocal. Additionally, no evidence for a mechanism has been presented that can explain the already observed changes in power output.

Fatigue has be correlated with decreased CP in muscle.[18] At the same time, studies have shown a delay in fatigue when creatine supplements are used with repeated bouts of high-intensity, short duration work.[14,16,18,19]

Muscle biopsy studies have shown that supplements can modestly increase muscle CP and total creatine, however ATP stores appear unaffected.[20] It is widely accepted that there is little that can be done to effectively enhance and improve ATP regeneration by exercise training;[21] therefore, the search for a supplement, particularly one that allows CP to be more effective, to improve the phosphagen system of energy delivery is acute. However, the effects enhancing of the phosphagen system by creatine supplementation are equivocal. Nutritional or exercise training practices that allow higher amounts of ATP to be stored in muscle over and above established ratios of ATP to muscle mass do not appear to exist. Therefore, if muscle mass is increased, ATP and CP will also increase. There seems to be an upper limit for stores of the phosphagens in muscle, and there are no known nutritional practices that modify the upper limit of storage.

Reliable and noninvasive methods for estimating the amount of ATP and CP that can be derived from the phosphagen system have not yet been developed. Work continues in developing a good match between direct and indirect measurements of these substances so that many of the questions about methods of enhancing access to the system of immediate energy delivery may be answered.

Early theories of functioning of the phosphagen system suggested that CP was the exclusive substrate for ATP resynthesis in intense activity.[22,23] Figure 2.1 illustrates the relationships among the three systems for highly intense, short duration work. Prior to the start of exercise, energy is delivered primarily via aerobic sources that use fat as a substrate. As exercise begins, this homeostatic state is disrupted and unbalanced enough that energy delivery is compromised. This is the point at which Figure 2.1 begins, as it depicts the high delivery from the ATP-CP system, which quickly diminishes. Note that energy delivery from this system, ATP-CP, does not terminate but continues to contribute, albeit in a greatly diminished capacity, throughout exercise. As time continues, the glycolytic system generally "buys time" and alone is capable of supporting activity for a short period of time. However, note that aerobic energy delivery steadily increases its contribution until it dominates.

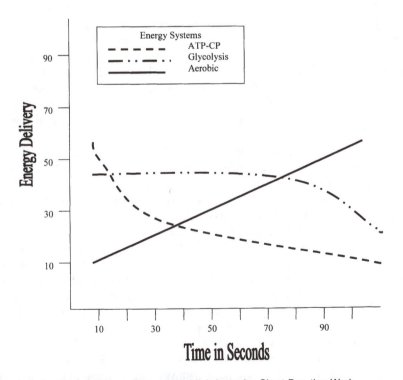

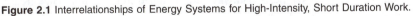

Figure 2.1 Interrelationships of Energy Systems for High-Intensity, Short Duration Work.

It is widely accepted that glycolysis is the next immediate system for energy transfer. However, experimental evidence shows that depletion of CP is not necessary for the mobilization of glycolysis and that CP degradation and anaerobic glycolysis are simultaneously activated.[24–26]

2.1.5 Glycolysis and Glycogenolysis

Exercise may be too intense and last too long for the phosphagen system to supply the ATP needed. At this point anaerobic processes that use glucose or glycogen, which degrades to glucose, are mobilized for ATP production. They generate both energy and, while anaerobic, lactate, which is the ionized form of lactic acid. Lactate is continuously formed in the cell and is easily transported to the blood stream due to its high permeability through cell membranes. Baseline amounts of lactate are established for normal individuals at rest such that the lack thereof is a clear sign of neuromuscular disease. If intensity is not high as activity ensues, lactate in the system is rapidly cleared by tissues of the body, including muscle, which keep blood levels minimal. The lactate can be used to resynthesize ATP. With high intensity and duration, lactate accumulation may be high enough to terminate activity by interfering with muscular contraction. It has long been accepted that this system predominates in activities that last from one to three minutes.

The first stages of glucose degradation are always anaerobic, without oxygen, thus the designation anaerobic glycolysis. Anaerobic glycolysis progresses to the formation of energy-rich pyruvate in the cytosol (cytoplasm) of the cell with no need for oxygen. If oxygen delivery is not or cannot be increased sufficiently, the process remains primarily anaerobic and pyruvate, the ionic form of pyruvic acid and precursor to lactate, is transformed to lactate when it acquires hydrogen ions. If the conversion of pyruvate to lactate occurs, anaerobic glycolysis results in very little energy transfer to produce a high net gain of ATP because the majority of the potential energy is left in the lactate. However, since this process is so rapid, the small amounts of ATP produced in the order of 2–3 moles of ATP per mole of glucose can supply a considerable amount of hydrogen ions for the rephosphorylation of ADP to ATP due to the speed of the reaction. Lactate is known to quickly cross the cell membrane into the blood where it can be cleared or taken out of the blood to resynthesize ATP elsewhere than in active muscle. Other cells in the body, particularly myocardium in the heart, use much of this lactate to form ATP for localized use. However, the rate of clearance can be exceeded by the rate of production, resulting in elevated blood lactate levels. Under these circumstances, exercise cannot continue for long periods because muscular contraction, which is highly pH-dependent will soon be hindered. High lactate levels are also associated with muscular fatigue, which will shorten the duration of exercise bouts.

During anaerobic glycolysis, nicotinamide adenine dinucleotide (NAD), which is derived from a B vitamin (niacin), plays an important role in transferring hydrogen ions. NAD is a co-enzyme, meaning it non-specifically reacts to capture two hydrogen ions at different steps in glycolysis. The captured hydrogen ions can be transferred to pyruvate to form lactate as just described. The hydrogen ions can also be transferred to the mitochondria, the organelle that provides ATPs through aerobic processes. When oxygen delivery improves, glycolysis can proceed aerobically. This is termed aerobic glycolysis. Lactate production is inhibited when cellular oxygen levels rise.

Should activity continue to the point of greater activation of the aerobic system, many more ATPs can be formed by utilization of the phosphorylating system found at the inner mitochondrial membrane. The number of ATPs generated is much higher and produces much more energy transfer so that duration of activity is sustained. Aerobic glycolysis, wherein glucose proceeds to aerobic metabolism, begins with pyruvate being converted to acetyl co-enzyme A instead of lactate. This can occur only when oxygen delivery to the cell increases sufficiently to inhibit pyruvate conversion to lactate. The end result is that aerobic glycolysis will yield 36–39 moles of ATP per mole of glucose, depending upon which ATP resynthesis pathways are included in the count. This greatly exceeds the yield from anaerobic glycolysis alone.

In activities where one remains in anaerobic glycolysis, glycogen may not be completely degraded aerobically to form water, a non-reversible end product of aerobic metabolism. The precursors of glycogen thus formed may then reassemble the glycogen molecule at the end of the activity. This eliminates the need to add high levels of carbohydrate to the diet immediately after activities of this type; elevated carbohydrate ingestion is more appropriately recommended for endurance activities.[27,28] Types of activities primarily utilizing anaerobic glycolysis include body-building, weightlifting, and resistance exercise. A more important concern in activities of this type is that increased glycogen storage induced by carbohydrate loading, if done immediately before a bout of intense exercise, may make the muscle compartment compressed due to the compensatory storage of water with the glycogen. Because water is not compressible, an injury such as a connective tissue tear of the epimysium that surrounds muscle may result.

Glycogen stored in muscle that can provide glucose or glucose brought directly into the cell exclusively fuel the glycolytic system. The subsequent degradation of glucose for energy transfer is rapid. It is known that carbohydrate stores in muscle in the form of glycogen can be enhanced by dietary practices that favor a high carbohydrate diet (carbohydrate loading), which will in turn increase the duration of a performance.[28] However, contrary to pronouncements made in the popular literature, not all activities benefit from this practice. Although all exercisers should consume slightly more carbohydrates than non-exercisers, the greatest benefit is derived when the activity is categorized as aerobic.

2.1.6 Nutritional Considerations of the Glycolytic Energy Delivery System

Glucose, fatty acids and amino acids derived from carbohydrates, fats, and proteins can all be converted to the two-carbon compound acetyl co-enzyme A. Acetyl co-enzyme A, a common intermediate into aerobic metabolism, proceeds through a series of reactions in the citric acid cycle. At this stage, carbon dioxide is produced that exits through the lungs, hydrogen ions and electrons are removed, and a small amount of ATP is produced by the conversion of guanosine triphosphate (GTP). Next, the reaction proceeds to the electron transport system (ETS), sometimes identified as cellular respiration, in which the majority of ATP resynthesis occurs. The electron carriers in the ETS are cytochromes that incorporate iron into their structures. Thus, iron deficiencies affect energy delivery fundamentally by hindering aerobic metabolism.

Carbon dioxide and water are formed during the end stage of aerobic metabolism. At this point, the glucose, fatty acids, and amino acids have become completely degraded and cannot be reconstituted through reversible reactions. Only new substrates can be used. Noteworthy is the fact that glucose is the only anaerobic substrate. Fats and proteins must, to a great degree, be degraded only in aerobic processes.

2.1.7 Aerobic Metabolism

When oxygen delivery is increased through the enhanced functioning of the cardiovascular system, substrates from glycolysis proceed to the mitochondria for subsequent oxidative phosphorylation, which results in much more ATP production. The pyruvate formed during anaerobic glycolysis is ultimately degraded to water and carbon dioxide, both nonfatiguing reaction byproducts. This produces approximately 18 times more ATP than that accrued through anaerobic glycolysis. Additionally, the enhanced aerobic metabolism will, through the process of oxidation, more efficiently clear the lactate previously produced. Thus lactate already accumulated and lactate that is produced will be diminished. At the end of aerobic glycolysis, the glycogen or glucose degraded to water and carbon dioxide cannot be changed back into glucose within the cell. Few precursor molecules will remain, and glycogen will not be reformed except through intake of carbohydrate, glucose, in the diet. If the exercise duration proceeds to predominance of the aerobic system, ATP is formed in great quantities at the inner mitochondrial membrane.

2.1.8 Nutritional Considerations of the Aerobic Energy Delivery System

This aerobic system does not rely heavily on carbohydrate. However, while the carbohydrate contribution to energy production may diminish, aerobic metabolism cannot continue without a carbohydrate contribution. Thus low carbohydrate states will hinder energy production. During aerobic metabolism, mitochondria can now process other substrates effectively, particularly fat (fatty acids). The hydrogens of fat are used for ATP production because fat contains great amounts of hydrogen, thus great amounts of ATP are produced (Figure 2.2) during long duration activity. Aerobic metabolism must first, however, be overloaded and then stressed over long periods of time to produce enhanced levels of enzymes necessary to use this pathway to a high degree at the cellular level. Protein (amino acids) can also be used for ATP production. This occurs to a greater extent in the aerobic exerciser than in the anaerobic exerciser.

CONTRIBUTION OF FAT AND CARBOHYDRATE SUBSTRATES
TO ENERGY DELIVERY AND LONG DURATION EXERCISES

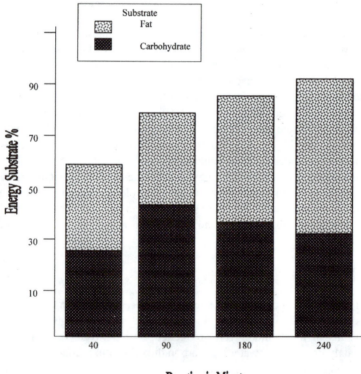

Figure 2.2 Contribution of Fat and Carbohydrate Substrates to Energy Delivery in Long Duration Exercise.

The interactions that occur between anaerobic and aerobic pathways that generate ATP are highly regulated and complex. Short duration, high-intensity activities rely more heavily on anaero-abic energy delivery, while long duration, low-intensity activities use aerobic sources. Conditioning or developing nutritional practices that support the metabolic pathway not stressed in an activity is counterproductive.

During low-intensity exercise, fats are known to be the primary fuel source. Conversely, carbohydrate use is primary for high-intensity exercise. However, neither is used exclusively. For example, at low intensities, approximately 70% of the ATPs may be derived from fat while 20%

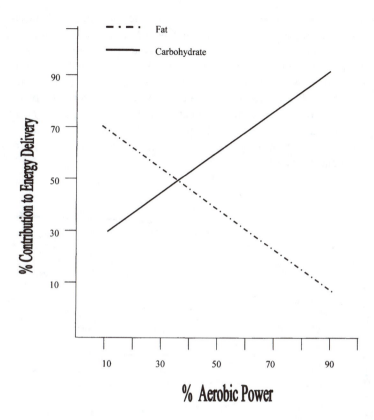

Figure 2.3 Fat and Carbohydrate Crossover During Increased Exercise Intensity.

may be derived from carbohydrate. As exercise intensity increases, fat utilization decreases and carbohydrate use increases. The point at which carbohydrate use becomes predominant as it increases is called the crossover point (Figure 2.3).[29] This shift occurs because more fast-twitch muscle fibers are recruited for higher-intensity tasks. Fast-twitch fibers have a more diminished ability to use fat as a substrate than the slow-twitch fibers recruited at lower intensities.

High-intensity exercise stimulates the production of epinephrine, which is known to increase glycogen use. The byproduct of glycogen breakdown, lactate, inhibits the metabolism of fat, thus further supporting the use of carbohydrate as a fuel source.

The endurance exerciser who participates in activities such as rhythmic aerobics, running, and other prolonged exercises needs to increase carbohydrate intake. Carbohydrate or glycogen loading may be considered in these activities on a limited basis, with the best practice being the conversion of the diet permanently to higher carbohydrate intake. A specificity of diet with respect to carbohydrate intake is suggested, based upon the metabolic pathway stressed in the activity; the need for carbohydrate is greater for the endurance exerciser than for the strength exerciser. This is an important concept for exercisers to understand if they are to use nutrition effectively to enhance activity performance.

2.1.9 Interactions of the Energy Delivery Systems

Aerobic metabolism requires that oxygen be delivered in greater quantities than were previously necessary during exercise, thus requiring a complex series of reactions to match cardiac output and capillary blood flow to the needs of the cell. With respect to speed of cellular metabolism, the aerobic pathway is slow to initiate and predominate during activity and is probably not used to a great degree until at least five minutes of continuous activity have elapsed. Although general principles of energy transitions have been known for some time, they are still not completely understood. One commonly misunderstood principle is that energy production is not a question of the three "systems" taking turns serially or being able to "skip" systems. Rather it is that all systems function at all times and while one predominates, the others participate in greater or lesser degrees. The interaction of the three systems of energy delivery in the first two minutes of exercise is complex and not completely understood (Figure 2.1). In long duration activity, the general patterns are clearer (Figure 2.4). Thus it is important for exercisers to understand which energy system or systems predominate in their activity and to follow specific dietary practices to enhance performance.

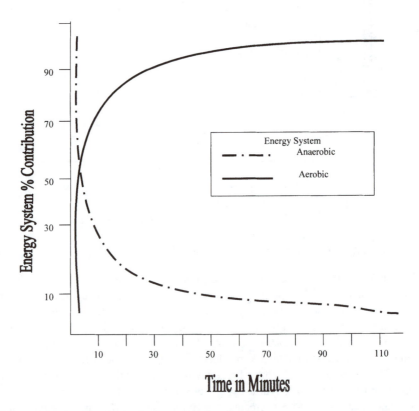

Figure 2.4 Energy System Contribution for Long Duration Activity.

2.2 SUBSTRATES FOR UTILIZATION: FAT, CARBOHYDRATE, PROTEIN

The three dietary sources of energy substrates are fat, carbohydrate, and protein. At rest and during normal daily activities, fats are the primary energy source, providing 80–90% of the energy, with carbohydrates and protein providing 5–18% and 2–5%, respectively.[9] During exercise, the proportion of each contribution will change as previously illustrated.

Highly intense, anaerobic activities that stress the phosphagen system and begin to immediately mobilize the glycolytic system may not directly use any of the three substrates when the activity begins. Post activity, the phosphagen system can be quickly restored, but this is impossible during the exercise bout. Anaerobic glycolysis does degrade some muscle glycogen, which is used to generate additional ATP to sustain the intense, anaerobic activities. Post exercise the muscle glycogen must be restored, much of it from glycogen precursors remaining in the cell.

When aerobic glycolysis becomes the principle pathway of energy production, the situation changes. Muscle glycogen is the initial source of glucose for aerobic energy; however, the duration of the activity may outlast the supplies stored within the muscle cell, and other substrates, fats and protein, must be used.

Whenever glycogen is degraded to water through aerobic glycolysis, it must be replaced through carbohydrates in the diet. All ingested carbohydrates degrade in the digestive system predominantly to glucose with lesser contributions from galactose and fructose. The majority of galactose and fructose are converted to glucose in the cells lining the small intestine, and most of the remainder is converted in the liver. Glucose is absorbed into the blood and transported to the body tissues for use or storage in the liver and muscles as glycogen.[30] Glucose must be brought into the cell and then strung together as glycogen; glycogen is composed of chains of individual glucose molecules that are linked together. The process of storage or replacement of glycogen is not immediate nor is it rapid and can take up to two days to complete.[31]

Excessive depletion of glycogen through exercise or diet may lead to insufficient carbohydrate available to provide glucose to regenerate muscle glycogen stores completely. If glucose supplies are low, muscle glycogen cannot be restored.[32] Glucose available in the blood will be spared for use by the brain, and muscle will be left deficient in carbohydrate stores. If glucose levels fall below the levels necessary for proper brain function, other sources of glucose will be used. Protein can be degraded to its amino acids in muscle and then be converted to pyruvate in the liver.[9] Two pyruvate molecules can be combined to form one glucose molecule that can then enter the blood and thus enter muscle. The primary source of protein for this process is muscle tissue, thus glucose may be provided for energy at the expense of muscle protein and muscle tissue. This reaction may occur when the body is in starvation, when the individual has low energy intake, or when the individual is under stress.

Storage fats, triglycerides, composed of glycerol and three fatty acids, can also be used to provide glucose. The glycerol can be converted to glucose while the fatty acids cannot. The fatty acids must be degraded aerobically or they become ketones.[30] Ketones in the blood are toxic in large quantities; therefore, depending upon fat for the generation of glucose is not desirable. The alternative use of protein and fat rather than carbohydrate for glucose or glycogen restoration has negative implications. It becomes clear that a person needs to ingest an adequate amount of carbohydrate to successfully participate in any activity.

During low-intensity activities, fats are the preferred substrate for utilization. But as intensity increases, carbohydrate utilization predominates (Figure 2.5). Fat is stored within the muscle cells and fat storage cells (adipocytes) as triglycerides. Fats also circulate in the blood as fatty acids. Triglycerides in adipocytes are easily liberated to the circulation for muscle use. The glycerol portion of a triglyceride can enter the glycolysis pathway in anaerobic metabolism and eventually become pyruvate to be used in aerobic glycolysis. The fatty acid portion of a triglyceride can undergo β-oxidation, which converts fatty acids to a compound that can be used in aerobic glycolysis to produce energy. Fatty acid use in aerobic metabolism results in far greater ATP production than that of carbohydrates. However, even when fats are the predominant energy source, carbohydrates must still be available. Carbohydrates are necessary to continuously prime the breakdown of fatty acids. Therefore, fats are never an exclusive energy source. Even when there is an overabundance of fat, if there are very low levels of carbohyrate, aerobic degradation of fat will stop. Other inhibitors of fat utilization are high insulin levels, such as those found after a large intake of simple sugars, and high lactate levels.[33]

Proteins can be converted to pyruvate and can be used for energy production during aerobic activities. Researchers disagree on how much energy protein can create; reported values have ranged from 5% to 15% of the total energy during aerobic activity. Greater amounts of protein may be used the longer one exercises.[34] It is generally agreed that the amount of ATP provided by protein is relatively small compared with fat and carbohydrate.

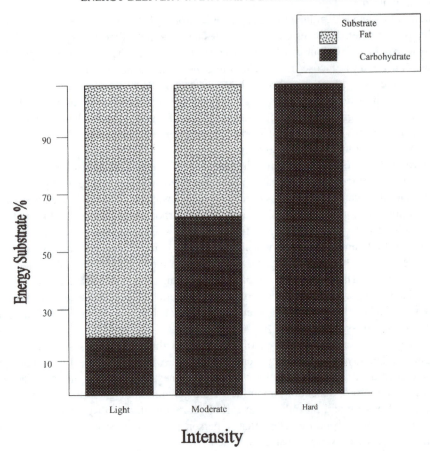

CONTRIBUTION OF FAT AND CARBOHYDRATE SUBSTRATE TO
ENERGY DELIVERY IN DIFFERING EXERCISE INTENSITIES

Figure 2.5 Contribution of Fat and Carbohydrate Sustrates to Energy Delivery in Differing Exercise Intensities.

It has been established that fat, carbohydrate, and protein can be utilized for energy production during physical activity. It is possible, and not uncommon, that energy intake of substrates outweighs the demand, particularly through dietary excess. Protein is utilized for cellular structure, enzymes (the molecules that govern the breakdown and buildup of other chemicals), hormones (chemical messengers), blood-borne carriers, and energy. Excess protein is not stored at any site in the body but may be converted to fat and stored in the adipocytes.

Carbohydrates are utilized for cellular structure, hormones, and energy. Excess carbohydrate is stored in muscle and liver as glycogen. A combination of a high carbohydrate diet and regular, activity-induced, depletion can increase these limited stores. When the glycogen storage capacity is exceeded, it is possible to convert carbohydrate to fat for storage in the adipocytes.

Fats are used for cellular structure, hormones, blood borne carriers, insulation, organ protection, and energy. Fats are the highest energy source available and the most easily stored. Fats are not usually converted to either protein or carbohydrate for storage. Fat storage occurs within muscle cells, for use during aerobic activity, and within adipocytes. Excess fat can also be found circulating in the blood and lining the walls of blood vessels. High levels of fat within the circulatory system are highly correlated with cardiovascular disease. It is clear that an excess of any one energy source may result in an increase in fat storage.

Interactions of the energy delivery system occur at all times, and it is often difficult to assess which system is being utilized for an activity. For example, walking, a simple activity, may place different demands upon the ability to deliver oxygen, and the energy intake and expenditure may not be the same under all conditions. As the speed of walking is increased and the time to cover a particular distance is shortened, the activity generates more power.[35] This results in an increased need for oxygen and energy production. One may have begun walking at a long duration and low enough intensity to predict fat as the major substrate for energy delivery, but if the activity generates high power, the shift will occur to short duration and high intensity to the extent that carbohydrate is the preferred substrate. It is crucial that the interelationships among frequency, intensity, and duration be considered.

All activity can be characterized by its frequency, intensity, and duration; understanding these relationships is fundamental to understanding the specificity of diet related to a particular activity. The influence of intensity of exercise on the substrate used to produce energy is great (Figure 2.5). Low-intensity activities will rely more upon fat for the generation of energy, while carbohydrate is utilized as power and intensity increases. There is also a relationship between duration of activity and substrate utilization (Figure 2.2). When exercise is prolonged, fat utilization predominates (Figure 2.6). It becomes clear that if the desire is to diminish fat stores in the body, low intensity and long duration activities should be chosen. The interactions between duration and intensity dictate which energy substrates will be utilized (Figure 2.7).

CONTRIBUTIONS OF FAT AND CARBOHYDRATE TO ENERGY
DELIVERY FOR LONG DURATION EXERCISE

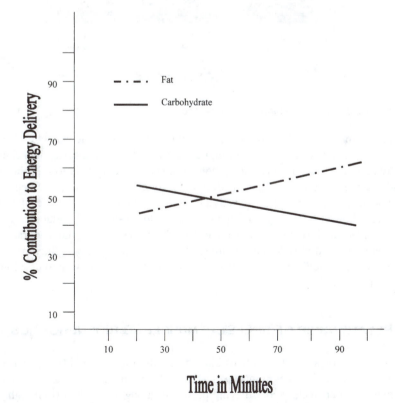

Figure 2.6 Contributions of Fat and Carbohydrate to Energy Delivery for Long Duration Exercise.

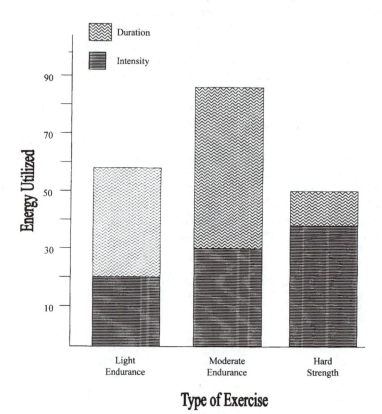

CONTRIBUTIONS OF DURATION
AND INTENSITY TO EXERCISE

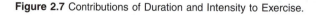

Type of Exercise

Figure 2.7 Contributions of Duration and Intensity to Exercise.

If hypertrophy of muscle is desired, activities should be chosen that generate more power. Observations made of cellular effects of the differences at the cell level that exist when conditioning for muscular strength or muscular endurance preclude, however, being able to mix the two types of activities and get maximum cellular benefit from both. Evidence has been presented that shows that at the cellular level, the two types of activities may not produce desired results. Although endurance training followed by strength training may not diminish either endurance or strength benefits at the cellular level, the converse may not be true. It has been shown that endurance training in previously strength-trained muscle may diminish the size of muscle fibers, thereby suggesting that aerobic conditioning should be undertaken cautiously in athletes who wish to develop strength and hypertrophy in muscle.[36]

2.3 RELATIONSHIP OF SKELETAL MUSCLE TO BIOENERGETICS

There is a direct relationship between nutritional practices aimed at modifying energy production and the specific characteristics of human skeletal muscle. Normal, nondiseased, human muscle is a mosaic of fiber types characterized as having properties along a spectrum from highly aerobic to highly anaerobic.[37] Due to the difficulty of characterizing subsets of fiber types that may number up to nine identifiable groups, simpler groupings are usually chosen for reporting that describe three major groups of fibers identified histochemically as types I, IIa, and IIb. Physiological, anatomical, and biochemical properties can be described and quantified. The fibers identified and studied by one method do not necessarily correlate with other systems of classification; i.e., not all fibers identified histochemically as type I will show the same aerobic characteristics when identified physiologically.[37]

Type I [slow-twitch (ST), slow-twitch-oxidative (SO), red, dark] fibers are those that have high aerobic energy production. These fibers are stressed in endurance activities such as running and cycling. All of the biochemical characteristics that support aerobic metabolism are high in these fibers. There are elevated amounts of carbohydrate (glycogen, glucose) and fat (neutral lipids, triglycerides), the substrates for aerobic energy production. Aerobic conditioning enhances the ability of type I fibers to use energy substrates by increasing the amount and activity of the enzymes in the pathways for substrate utilization. It has been reported that individuals participating for long periods of time in endurance activities such as marathons have higher than expected percentages of type I fibers.[38] Whether these greater percentages of type I fibers are genetically inherited or are converted with prolonged aerobic training remains an open question. The type I fiber, however, is not able to hypertrophy to a great degree, even if it is overloaded, perhaps due to the need to get oxygen to the center of the fiber.[36] The increase in cross-sectional area may reach a limit for efficient transport and diffusion of oxygen from the capillary to the center of the fiber. Thus, individuals who participate in and continually train using endurance activities stress the type I fiber and will find that the muscle hypertrophy is limited while body fat stores tend to diminish. There is also a need to keep glycogen stores high through dietary ingestion of carbohydrate. Although it has long been accepted that muscle glycogen stores are the most important factor in successful endurance performance, the adaptations to fat metabolism have been investigated with conflicting results.[38,39]

Type II fibers (fast-twitch, white, light) have two major subgroups, fast-twitch-oxidative-glycolytic (IIa, FTa, FOG) and fast-twitch-glycolytic (IIb, FTb, FG). Overall,. these fibers have high capabilities for producing energy anaerobically. However, the IIa also has a great ability for aerobic energy production, and therefore, is sometimes called "super fiber" in terms of performance. The IIa fiber, though fast-twitch, can provide aerobic metabolism and can hypertrophy the greatest of the type II subgroups. Type II fibers are stressed in resistance and power activities such as weightlifting and bodybuilding. All of the biochemical properties that support anaerobic metabolism are high in these fibers. Consequently, high amounts of glycogen are particularly found in the IIa fiber.[40] Conditioning enhances the ability of this fiber type to use energy substrates by increasing the amount and activity of enzymes that allow their use. It has not, however, been shown that individuals who participate in resistance activities over long periods of time have greater percentages of these fibers than those in the general population who do not train or condition to a high degree.[41] Transitions between the percentages of IIa and the IIb fiber types have been shown with exercise, along with significant and dramatic changes in size, thereby either enhancing the aerobic (IIa) or the anaerobic (IIb) capacity of the muscle as a whole.[42] The type II fiber will significantly hypertrophy with use and is responsible for the great increase in muscle mass seen in strength conditioning and bodybuilding. There is also an effect of the speed of movement used to stress the fiber, as slower movements show more rapid increases in power,[43] thereby increasing tension and hypertrophy to a greater degree than fast movements. It has been suggested that muscle fibers can split and increase their numbers (hyperplasia), but this has not been conclusively proved in humans and there is evidence to both prove and disprove this theory.[44] Individuals who stress the use of these fibers will find that their muscles will enlarge with conditioning and that carbohydrate stores must be adequate to support activity. There is also evidence that the amount of fat in the diet may directly affect testosterone production, which is known in turn to affect increases in muscle mass. Adequate fat in the diet may facilitate testosterone production, while low-fat diets are associated with clinically significant decreases in production.[45]

The composition of skeletal muscle with respect to fiber type affects the interpretation of dietary enhancement of performance. At low intensities, slow-twitch fibers that are more aerobic are recruited. At high intensities, recruitment quickly proceeds to fast-twitch, anaerobic fibers. Thus the interactions among exercise, skeletal muscle fiber-type percentages, and dietary manipulation are complex.

2.4 APPLICATIONS OF BIOENERGETIC PRINCIPLES

Measuring energy expenditure can be done by direct calorimetry, where the subject is placed into an enclosed container and heat production is measured directly. This is not usually done, as the rooms or enclosures necessary to collect these data for exercise are expensive and are not usually available to most researchers. The more practical method is that of indirect calorimetry in which the products of biological oxidation, carbon dioxide and oxygen, are collected and measured for certain periods of time. Since one liter of oxygen equates to use of 4.8 kcal (20.2 kJ), energy expenditure can be assessed.

Daily needs for energy (kcals) require assessment of basal metabolism, the minimal rate of energy expenditure necessary for life.[46] An accurate measurement requires standardizing rest conditions (8 hours of rest) and assuring that the subject is both post absorptive (12–18 hours) and quiet during measurement.[47] Practically, 3–4 hour post absorption differs little from the more rigorous data collection for normal individuals for whom weight loss or weight gain programs are not being recommended. Results show differences in males and females. Although males on average are heavier and taller than females, they tend to have almost one-third the body fat. Male lean body mass therefore is higher. Since this difference is made up of more muscle mass, which is more metabolically active that adipose tissue, males have higher resting oxygen consumptions. It is generally accepted that an average resting oxygen consumption $\dot{V}O_2$) is 3.5 ml/kg·min^{-1} (1 MET or metabolic equivalent). It is important to note that in reality, males have higher resting oxygen consumptions than females. As both genders age, the differences become more pronounced. It is more desirable to measure resting oxygen consumptions than to use the MET estimate when accurately assessing energy needs for weight loss or weight gain recommendations. In estimation there is a loss of precision, which might render dietary recommendations unsuccessful.

Although it is extremely important to understand the metabolic energy sources of activity for training and conditioning so that time is not wasted focusing on the wrong energy delivery system, it is also important to understand the overall energy needs of the body. Regardless of how precise one tries to calculate energy expenditure, energy need, and energy intake, it remains that in many individuals the energy equation, which states that energy in is equal to energy out, is simply not true. The body in many cases remains the proverbial scientific "black box," and all is not yet understood well enough to control all the variables. When steady state is perturbed, lean body mass can be modified upward by overfeeding, obesity, and in females, pregnancy and puberty. Lean body mass can be modified downward by such effects as androgens, underfeeding, anorexia, malnutrition, zero gravity, bed rest, aging and, in males, puberty. Exercise in and of itself is a very minor affector of total body fat.[48]

2.5 SUMMARY

Individuals who exercise need to understand how energy is transferred within the body and should choose modes of conditioning, training, and dietary practice that complement one another.[2,3,9,11,28,29,31,45] The high-energy phosphagens are utilized during immediate activity with transition to glycolysis and aerobic metabolism if exercise becomes more prolonged. Although the phosphagen system is not necessarily modified by nutritional practices,[13] glycolysis is enhanced by high carbohydrate intake, which promotes storage of muscle glycogen.[28,31,32] The aerobic system is enhanced by conditioning and training and can utilize fats, carbohydrates, and protein for ATP production.[47] Nutritional practices can be chosen to enhance performance in all three systems.[2,11]

Attention should be paid to the differences between muscular strength and muscular endurance activities, as they may not enhance each other.[36] The characteristics of the different types of muscle fibers should be understood with the intent of enhancing the capabilities of specific fiber types used in activity by conditioning and dietary regimens so that time and effort are used more effectively.

Assessing daily energy expenditure is difficult but can help in understanding nutritional needs of exercisers. Nutritional practices should be incorporated that support activity choices. Regardless of the choices, health should be a major concern.[48,49] It is now known that lower levels of activity than previously thought are sufficient to diminish the risk of disease.[49] A better understanding of metabolism and the nutritional practices that support the activity choices made will help to improve the quality of life for individuals who exercise.

ACKNOWLEDGMENT

Thanks are due to Sandra L. Cottle of California State University, Fresno for her assistance in the design and completion of all the figures in this chapter.

REFERENCES

1. Gollnick, P. D., Free fatty acid turnover and the availability of substrates as a limiting factor in prolonged exercise, in *The Marathon: Physiological Medical, Epidemiological, and Psychological studies,* Milvey, P., Ed., The New York Academy of Sciences, New York, 1977, 64.
2. Jackson, C. G. R. and Simonson, S., The relationships between human energy transfer and nutrition, in *Nutrition for the Recreational Athlete,* Jackson, C. G. R., Ed., CRC Press LLC, Boca Raton, FL, 1995, 19-36.
3. Brooks, G. A., Mammalian fuel utilization during sustained exercise, *Comp. Biochem. Physiol.,* Part B, 89,1998.
4. Brooks, G. A., Fahey, T. D., and White, T. P., *Exercise Physiology, Human Bioenergetics and Its Applications,* 2nd ed., Mayfield Publishing Company, Mountain View, CA, 1996, chap. 2.
5. Foss, M. L. and Keteyian, S. J., *Fox's Physiological Basis for Exercise and Sport,* 6th ed., McGraw-Hill, San Francisco, CA, 1998, chap. 2.
6. Greenhaff, P. L. and Timmons, J. A. Interaction between aerobic and anaerobic metabolism during intense muscle contraction, in *Exercise and Sport Science Reviews,* Holloszy, J. O., Ed., Williams and Wilkins, Baltimore, MD, 1998, 1-30.
7. Hargreaves, M., Ed., *Exercise Metabolism,* Human Kinetics, Champaign, IL, 1995.
8. Lamb, D. R. and Gisolfi, C. V., Eds., *Perspectives in Exercise Science and Sports Medicine: Volume 5, Energy Metabolism in Exercise and Sport,* Cooper Publishing Group, Carmel, IN, 1992.
9. McArdle, W. D., Katch, F. I., and Katch, V. L., *Exercise Physiology: Energy, Nutrition, and Human Performance,* 4th ed., Williams and Wilkins, Philadelphia, PA, sections 2 and 3.
10. Powers, S. K. and Howley, E. T., *Exercise Physiology, Theory and Application to Fitness and Performance,* 3rd ed., Brown and Benchmark, Dubuque, IA, chap. 3 and 4.
11. Wolinsky, I., Ed., *Nutrition in Exercise and Sport,* 3rd ed., CRC Press LLC, Boca Raton, FL, 1997.
12. Spriet, L. L., Anaerobic metabolism during high-intensity exercise, in *Exercise Metabolism,* Hargreaves, M., Ed., Human Kinetics, Champaign, IL, 1995, 1-36.
13. Zoeller, R. F. and Angeliopoulos, T. J., Creatine supplementation and exercise performance, in *ACSM Certified News,* Vol. 8, No. 2, 1, 1998.
14. Greenhaff, P. L., Casey, A., Short, A. H., Harris, R., Soderlund, K., and Hultman, E., Influence of oral creatine supplementation on muscle torque during repeated bouts of maximal voluntary exercise in man, *Clin. Sci.,* 84, 565, 1993.

15. Hultman, E., Soderlund, K., Timmons, J. A., Cereblad, G., and Greenhaff, P. L., Muscle creatine loading in man, *J. Appl. Physiol.,* 81, 232, 1996.
16. Harris, R., Soderlund, K., and Hultman, E., Elevation of creatine in resting and exercised muscles of normal subjects by creatine supplementation, *Clin. Sci.,* 83, 367, 1992.
17. Moller, P., Bergstrom, J., and Furst, P., Effect of aging on energy rich phosphagens in human skeletal muscle, *Clin. Sci.,* 58, 553, 1980.
18. Volek, J. S., Kraemer, W. J., Bush, J. A., Boetes, M., Incledon, T., Clark, K. L., and Lynch, J. M., Creatine supplementation enhances muscular performance during high intensity resistance exercise, *J. Am. Diet. Assoc.,* 97(7), 765, 1997.
19. Birch, R., Noble, D., and Greenhaff, P. L., The influence of dietary creatine supplementation on performance during repeated bouts of maximal isokinetic cycling in man, *Eur. J. Appl. Physiol.,* 69, 268, 1994.
20. Harris, R. C., Soderlund, K., and Hultman, E., Elevation of creatine in resting and exercised muscle of normal subjects by creatine supplementation, *Clin. Sci.,* 83, 367, 1992.
21. Nevill, M. S., Boobis, L. H., Brooks, S., and Williams, C., Effect of training on muscle metabolism during treadmill sprinting, *J. Appl. Physiol.,* 67, 2376, 1989.
22. Margaria, R., Cerretelli, P., and Mangili, E., Balance and kinetics of anaerobic energy release during strenuous exercise in man, *J. Appl. Physiol.,* 19, 623, 1964.
23. Margaria, R., Oliva, D., Di Prampero, P. E. and Cerretelli, P., Energy utilization in intermittent exercise of supramaximal intensity, *Eur. J. Appl. Physiol.,* 26, 752, 1969.
24. Boobis, L. H., Williams, C., and Wooton, S. A., Human muscle metabolism during brief maximal exercise, *J. Physiol. Lond.,* 338, 21P, 1982, Abstract.
25. Jones, N. L., McCartney, N., Graham, T., Spriet, L. L., Kowalchuk, J. M., Heigenhayuser, G. J. F., and Sutton, J. R., Muscle performance and metabolism in maximal isokinetic cycling at slow and fast speeds, *J. Appl. Physiol.,* 59, 132, 1985.
26. Saltin, B., Gollnick, P. D., Eriksson, B.-O., and Piehl, K. Metabolic and circulatory adjustments at onset of maximal work, in *Onset of Exercise,* Gilbert, A., and Guille, P., Eds., University of Toulouse Press, Toulouse, 1971, 63-76.
27. Hermansen, L., and Vaage, O., Lactate disappearance and glycogen synthesis in human muscle after maximal exercise, *Am. J. Physiol.,* 233, E422, 1977.
28. Bergstrom, J., Hermansen, L., Hultman, E., and Saltin, B., Diet, muscle glycogen and physical performance, *Acta Physiol. Scand.,* 71, 140, 1967.
29. Brooks, G. A. and Mercier, J., Balance of carbohydrate and lipid utilization during exercise: The "crossover" concept, *J. Appl. Physiol,* 76, 2253, 1994.
30. Guyton, A. C., *Textbook of Medical Physiology,* 8th ed., W. B. Saunders Co., Philadelphia, 1991, chaps. 67, 68.
31. Piehl, K., Time course for refilling of glycogen stores in human muscle fibers following exercise-induced glycogen depletion, *Acta Physiol. Scand.,* 90, 297, 1974.
32. Hultman, E., and Bergstrom, J., Muscle glycogen synthesis in relation to diet studied in normal subjects, *Acta Med. Scand.,* 182, 109, 1967.
33. Sharkey, B. J., *Coaches Guide to Sport Physiology,* Human Kinetics Publishers Inc., Champaign, IL., 1986, chap. 5.
34. Steinberg, D., Metabolism, in *Best and Taylor's Physiological Basis of Medical Practice,* West, J. B., Ed., Williams and Wilkins, Philadelphia, PA, 1990, 728.
35. Powers, S. K. and Howley, E. T., *Exercise Physiology: Theory and Application of Fitness and Performance* , 2nd ed., Brown and Benchmark, Dubuque, IA, 1994, chap. 4.
36. Jackson, C. G. R., Dickinson, A. L., and Ringel, S. P., Skeletal muscle fiber area alterations in two opposing modes of resistance-exercise training in the same individual, *Eur. J. Appl Physiol.,* 61, 37, 1990.
37. Romanul, F. C. A., Streter, F. A. , Salmons, S. , and Gergely, J., The effects of a changed pattern of activity on histochemical characteristics of muscle fibres, in *Exploratory Concepts in Muscular Dystrophy II,* Milhorat, E. A. T., Ed., Excerpta Medica, Amsterdam, 1974.
38. Costill, D., Daniels, J., Evans, W., Fink, W., Krahenbuhl, G., and Saltin, B., Skeletal muscle enzymes and fiber composition in male and female track athletes, *J. Appl. Physiol.,* 40, 149, 1976.
39. Hagenfeldt, L., Turnover of individual free fatty acids in man, *Fed. Proc.,* 34, 2236, 1975.

40. Jackson, C. G. R., Dickinson, A. W., Ringel S. P. and Morales, J., Histochemical profile of muscular cellular alterations following two modes of training in the same individual, In Press.

41. Jackson, C. G. R. and Dickinson, A. L., Adaptations of skeletal muscle to strength or endurance training, in *Advances in Sports Medicine and Fitness*, 1, Grana, W. A., Lombardo, J. A., Sharkey, B. J., and Stone, J. A., Eds., Year Book Medical Publishers Inc., Chicago, 1988, 45.

42. Dubowitz, V., *Muscle Biopsy, A Practical Approach,* 2nd. ed., Bailliere Tindall, Philadelphia, PA, 1988.

43. Coyle, E. F., Costill, D. L., and Lesmes, G. R., Leg extension power and muscle fiber composition, *Med. Sci. Sports.,* 11, 12, 1979.

44. Gollnick, P. D., Timson, B. F., Moore, R. L., and Riedy, M., Muscular enlargement and number of fibers in skeletal muscles of rats, *J. Appl. Physiol.,* 50, 936, 1981.

45. Ratzin, R. A., Effect of aerobic conditioning on resting serum testosterone levels and muscle fiber types in vegetarian and nonvegetarian sedentary males, Dissertation, University of Northern Colorado, Greeley, CO, 1990.

46. Durnin, J.V.G.A. and Passmore, R., Eds., *Energy Work, and Leisure*, Heinemann, London, 1967.

47. Bassett, D. R. and Nagle, F. J., Energy metabolism in exercise and training, in *Nutrition in Exercise and Sport,* 2nd ed., Wolinsky, I. and Hickson, J. F., Eds., CRC Press LLC, Boca Raton, FL, 1993.

48. Forbes, G. B., Body composition as affected by physical activity and nutrition, *Fed. Proc.*, 44, 343, 1985.

49. *1996 Surgeon General's Report on Physical Activity and Health*, Superintendent of Documents, P. O. Box 371954, Pittsburgh, PA, 15250-7954.

The Energy-Yielding Nutrients

CHAPTER **3**

Digestion and Absorption
of Energy-Yielding Nutrients

Alan J. Ryan

CONTENTS

3.1 INTRODUCTION

Athletes may need to consume, digest and absorb up to two to three times more calories each day compared with their sedentary counterparts. Ideally, an athlete's diet should contain sufficient calories to sustain the relatively high energy expenditures associated with vigorous exercise training. If sufficient calories are not consumed, the athlete's health or exercise performance may suffer. Thus, to meet the caloric demands of daily exercise, the athlete's gastrointestinal tract must be able to digest and absorb relatively large amounts of the three major energy-yielding nutrients: carbohydrates, proteins, and fats.

This chapter provides information on the dietary intakes of athletes as well as a general overview of the basic mechanisms involved in the digestion and absorption of carbohydrates, proteins, and fats. A clear understanding of these mechanisms is essential before specific dietary recommendations can be given to athletes. Unfortunately, very few studies describe the effects of exercise on digestion and absorption of fats and protein. There is, however, considerable information on gastric emptying and intestinal absorption of dilute carbohydrate solutions during exercise, and these topics are reviewed. Finally, gastrointestinal adaptations to dietary change are considered in view of the dietary practices of athletes.

3.2 DIETARY INTAKES OF ATHLETES: ENERGY, CARBOHYDRATE, PROTEIN, AND FAT

The energy demands of exercise can be tremendous, requiring large caloric intakes of carbohydrate, protein, and fat. The dietary intakes of Tour de France cyclists are of interest because they illustrate the nutritional requirements of humans who push the boundaries of exercise performance. Saris et al.[1] report food intake and energy expenditures of five male cyclists who completed the Tour de France, a 22-day race covering 4,000 km and 30 mountain passages. The elite cyclists weighed 69 kg with 11.5% body fat and a $\dot{V}O_{2\,max}$ of 79 ml/Kg/min. Cyclists consumed a daily average of 5,900 kcal, with carbohydrate, protein, and fat proportions equal to 62, 15, and 23% respectively of energy intake. Mean daily energy expenditure for the race was estimated to be 6,070 kcal, one of the highest energy values ever reported for a period exceeding one week. As shown, the daily energy intakes closely matched energy expenditures, and the high energy intakes resulted in high absolute values for carbohydrate (12 g/kg body wt/day), protein (3 g/kg body wt/day) and fat (2 g/kg body wt/day) intake. Due to their rigorous schedule, cyclists consumed much of their food during the race in-between meals, using a nibbling pattern in which small amounts of food were eaten continually throughout the day. A similar and more recent report describing energy expenditures and dietary intakes of Tour of Spain cyclists is available.[2]

The two main factors determining the energy needs of athletes are body size and the energy requirements of physical activity (type, intensity, frequency and duration of exercise).[3] Other important factors include age, sex, body composition, and basal metabolic rate. The energy intakes of most adult athletes range from 2,500 to 6,000 kcal per day, although there are rather large variations in energy intakes reported for specific athletic populations.[3–7] Although some of this variation may be related to methodological techniques used to gather data, much variation can be attributed to size, sex, and type of athlete. Thus, recent dietary reports and recommendations are specific for sex and type of athlete, and they are frequently normalized for body weight.

Economos et al.[4] provide a comprehensive review of elite athletes and report daily caloric intakes of male and female athletes engaged in endurance or strength and power sports. Male athletes reported caloric intakes of 45 to 87 kcal/kg/day for aerobic sports and 23 to 57 kcal/kg/day for anaerobic sports. Female athletes, on the other hand, reported lower caloric intakes of 30 to 46 kcal/kg/day for aerobic sports and 25 to 26 kcal/kg/day for anaerobic sports. The energy intakes of many female athletes (runners, dancers, gymnasts) and some male athletes (wrestlers, boxers) are thought to be insufficient to meet the energy demands of exercise training.[4,6,7] These low energy consumers generally engage in activities where body weight, body composition, and body appearance assumes a major role in successful performance. Other unique factors affecting caloric intakes of athletes include dietary customs (geographic location),[5] vigorous training habits (suppressed appetite, limited time and access to food), eating disorders (anorexia and bulimia nervosa),[4] and use of dietary supplements.[8] Economos et al.[4] recommend energy intakes of greater than 50 kcal/kg/day for male athletes who train for more than 90 minutes per day and 45 to 50 kcal/kg/day for female athletes with similar training scheldules.

Dietary surveys reveal that most athletes consume carbohydrates in amounts equal to 40 to 60% of total calories.[3] In general, athletes who consume insufficient calories are also likely to consume insufficient amounts of carbohydrates. A current recommendation for athletes is to consume carbohydrates equal to about 60 to 70% of total calories or 4.5 to 6.0 g/kg/day.[9] Carbohydrate intakes of up to 9 to 10 g/kg/day are recommended for rapid recovery from strenuous exercise that significantly depletes endogenous glycogen stores.[10] Hawley et al.[6] note that athletes who have large caloric intakes (5000 kcal/70 kg/day) may achieve adequate carbohydrate intake (more than 550 g per day) even though this nutrient intake comprises only 45% of total calories.

The proportion of protein in athletes' diets ranges from 10 to 36% of total calories consumed.[3] Protein intakes exceeding 1.0 to 2.0 g/kg/day are commonly observed for male and female endurance athletes and for athletes engaged in strength and power sports.[3-7] Although the protein requirements of athletes are actively debated, one recomendation is that dietary protein provide about 12 to 15% of total calories or 1.2 to 1.7 g/kg/day.[9] Athletes most at risk for inadequate protein intake are those who show inadequate energy intakes, especially female athletes who maintain low body weights for competition or who demonstrate an eating disorder.[4]

The contribution of fat in athletes' diets averages about 36% of calories consumed, though values may vary from about 20% to more than 50%.[3] Local dietary customs within different countries or regions are thought to explain some of the variation in fat content of athlete's diets.[3,5,7] However, most of the athletes surveyed report diets containing more than 30% of calories as fat. Because fat is calorie dense and food rich in complex carbohydrates can be bulky, many athletes may consume food rich in fat (animal and dairy products, fried foods, and confectioneries) in an effort to increase total caloric intake. Williams[9] notes that the high fat content of athletes' diets makes it likely that few succeed at achieving the recommended balance of saturated (less than 10% of total calories), monounsaturated (15%), and polyunsaturated (6%) fats. In recognizing fat as an important energy source, Economos et al.[4] recommend diets that contain 30% fat for athletes with high energy needs, and less than 25% fat for athletes with low energy needs (less than 2200 kcal per day).

The most important aspect of an athlete's diet is that it follows basic guidelines for being healthy and balanced.[3,4] The diet should contain sufficient calories to match the athlete's relatively large daily energy expenditures. Athletes who do not consume sufficient calories also probably do not consume enough carbohydrates and proteins. Diets low in either calories, protein, or carbohydrate do not promote good health or optimal exercise performance. As discussed later in this chapter, the human gastrointestinal tract may show structural and functional adaptations after it is exposed to high daily intakes of calories and carbohydrates. These adaptations may enhance intestinal absorptive capacity and may provide benefits for athletes who have high energy needs.

3.3 DIGESTION AND ABSORPTION

3.3.1 Carbohydrates

Carbohydrates are the main source of energy in human diets, comprising approximately 40–60% of energy intake. The major dietary sources of carbohydrates are starches and sucrose, with lesser amounts derived from lactose, glucose, and fructose. Before intestinal absorption can occur, carbohydrates must first be hydrolyzed to their constituient monosaccharides.[11,12] This digestive process begins in the mouth and is nearly complete in the jejunum. The secreted enzymes, salivary and pancreatic amylase, hydrolyze starches in luminal fluid while further hydrolysis of oligosaccharides and disaccharides is accomplished by enzymes located in the enterocyte brush border.

In the mouth, food is chewed and mixed with salivary secretions that contain amylase. This enzyme initiates the hydrolysis of amylose and amylopectin, the two primary components of plant starch granules. Amylose is a straight-chain polymer of glucose and a minor component (approximately 25%) of most starches, whereas amylopectin is a branched-chain polymer of glucose and a major component (about 75%) of most starches. Amylase activity (optimum pH = 6.9) splits starch to maltose, maltotriose, and alpha-limit dextrins (5–10 glucose units) with only small amounts of glucose. Chewing in the mouth and mixing processes in the stomach act to disrupt and hydrate starch granules, promoting starch hydrolysis, and the low gastric pH destroys salivary amylase activity. Thus, most starch hydrolysis is thought to occur within the duodenum and jejunum due to the action of pancreatic amylase. The pancreas produces and secretes amylase in excess.

The products of starch hydrolysis as well as the disaccharides sucrose and lactose are hydrolyzed by enzymes located in the enterocyte brush border. These membrane-bound enzymes are exposed to the intestinal luminal contents and are situated close to transport sites for released monosaccharides. This process of surface digestion takes place primarily in the upper and midjejunum, but activity extends from duodenum to ileum and thereby provides a safety margin. The products of starch digestion are further hydrolyzed to glucose by the glucoamylase and sucrase-isomaltase complexes. Sucrose is cleaved to glucose and fructose by the sucrase-isomaltase complex, whereas the milk sugar, lactose, is hydrolyzed to glucose and galactose by the enzyme lactase. With the exception of lactase activity in adult intestine, the activities of these hydrolytic enzymes are high and not rate-limiting for absorption.

All nutrients must transverse a thin layer of fluid, an unstirred water layer, before reaching the surface of the enterocyte for hydrolysis or transport.[13] The unstirred layer (30–40 μm) may provide a diffusion barrier to passage of nutrients, especially those not soluble in an aqueous medium, such as fats. The thickness of the unstirred layer largely depends upon mixing within the lumen (intestinal motility) and contractile activity of the villi. The effects of exercise on the unstirred layer are unknown.[14] Undigested fibre (non-starch polysaccharides) may increase the unstirred layer and thereby slow the rate of carbohydrate absorption.[12]

Transport of monosaccharides through the intestinal epithelium can occur by two routes: 1) passive solute and water movement between enterocytes by solvent drag (paracellular route), and 2) active transport or facilitated diffusion or passive diffusion of sugars through the brush border and basolateral enterocyte membranes (transcellular route). Although the paracellular route contributes to sugar transport,[15] the significance of this transport pathway is controversial.[16]

Carrier-mediated transport systems located in the enterocyte membranes transport most of the sugar through the entrocyte. These transporters are distributed throughout the small intestine, but they are highest in number and activity in the upper jejunum and duodenum. Sugar transporter activity correlates well with luminal substrate concentration: The jejunum is exposed to high nutrient loads and displays high transporter capacity, whereas the ileum, exposed to lower nutrient loads, displays lower capacity but higher transporter affinity.[17]

A model of intestinal hexose transport is as follows.[11] The Na^+-dependent glucose transporter (SGLT1) and Na^+-independent facultative fructose transporter (GLUT5) are located on the brush border membrane. Glucose and Na^+ absorption are driven by a transcellular Na^+ gradient established by a Na^+, K^+ ATPase, located on the basolateral membrane. Fructose transport occurs by a process of facilitated diffusion and is not coupled to Na^+ transport. A facultative hexose transporter (GLUT2) transports glucose or fructose out of the enterocyte through the basolateral membrane.

In addtion to hexose transport, this model indicates that glucose and Na$^+$ transport stimulates water absorption. Oral rehydration solutions contain both Na$^+$ and glucose because glucose-stimulated Na$^+$ absorption generates an osmotic gradient and therefore promotes absorption of water.[14] Fructose transport is not coupled to Na$^+$ transport, but fructose absorption does generate an osmotic gradient, which results in water absorption due to solvent drag. As described by Crane,[18] the enterocyte brush border functions as a digestive and absorptive unit. For example, glucose and fructose derived from sucrose hydrolysis may be transported more rapidly than glucose or fructose alone.

3.3.1.1 Factors Affecting Carbohydrate Digestion and Absorption

Reserachers are very interested in potential factors that influence the digestibility, absorption, and physiological properties of different carbohydrates, and new carbohydrate classification schemes are proposed to recognize this new information.[19,20] In particular, the forms in which carbohydrates are found in foods (raw, cooked, state of hydration), the ratio of starch components (amylose/amylopectin ratio), and the properties of food matrices (type and amount of dietary fibre) are thought to significantly affect gastric emptying, digestion and absorption, and physiological responses of ingested carbohydrates.[12,21,22]

Food factors that alter the rate of starch digestibility can alter the blood glucose response to foods. This information may be important for blood glucose control in diabetic patients and for athletes interested in carbohydrate supplementation before, during, and following exercise. Several of these factors, which are reviewed in detail by Walton and Rhodes[23] and Jenkins et al.,[22] are summarized below: 1) Amylose/amylopectin ratio[24] — foods that contain starches with high amylopectin content (barley, rice) are more susceptible to amylase activity and produce greater blood glucose responses compared with foods rich in amylose content (beans, peas, lentils). 2) Food preparation — cooking (boiling) foods ruptures granules and hydrates starches, whereas certain rendering processes (grinding, milling) reduce particle size and increase food surface area. Hydrated starches with high surface areas are susceptible to amylase hydrolysis and give more rapid glycemic responses. 3) Dietary fibre — the presence of soluble fibre in foods may increase volume and viscosity of chyme, delay gastric emptying, reduce small intestinal motility and transit, and reduce the glycemic response to starchy foods.[25–27] Thus, soluble fibre in foods is thought to delay delivery of starch to the intestines, reduce intestinal mixing and propulsion of chyme, and thereby reduce the rate and extent of starch hydrolysis by amylase.

3.3.2 Proteins

The gastrointestinal tract digests and absorbs protein efficiently. Each day, the small intestine is presented with large quantities of protein from exogenous and endogenous sources; dietary sources may provide approximately 100 g of protein per day, whereas 25 to 200 g per day are derived from secreted enzymes and sloughed mucosal cells. From the total protein presented to the small bowel, only 2 to 5% fails to be absorbed.[28]

Protein digestion begins in the stomach and is nearly complete in the jejunum. Digestion is accomplished by proteolytic enzymes secreted by the stomach and pancreas, and by peptidases located in both the enterocyte brush border and cytoplasm. Pepsin in gastric juice initiates digestion by cleaving proteins into large polypeptides. Further protein hydrolysis occurs in the upper small intestine by action of the pancreatic enzymes, trypsin, chymotrypsin, aminopeptidase, and carboxypeptidase. The pancreatic enzymes acting together with brush border peptidases produce a mixture of small peptides (2–6 amino acid residues) and amino acids. The final digestion products may be produced primarily in the upper small intestine, but absorption processes may extend into the ileum. Adibi and Mercer[29] report that significant amounts of peptides and some amino acids can be recovered from jejunal and ileal fluid as late as four hours after consumption of a meal containing 50 g of protein.

Amino acids and peptides are absorbed through various transporter systems located in enterocytes of the small intestine. The enterocyte brush border is thought to contain separate transporter systems with some specificity for acidic, basic, and neutral amino acids, for imino acids (such as proline), and for peptides.[30] Like glucose, most amino acid absorption appears to driven by a Na^+-dependent, active transport mechanism.[31] Peptide transporters, in contrast, may utilize an active transport mechanism that is driven by an electrochemical proton (H^+) gradient.[32] The role of the paracellular pathway for peptide and amino acid absorption in not known.[33]

Several features of peptide transport[35,35] are important to recognize. First, rates for amino acid uptake are frequently greater from di- and tripeptide solutions compared with equimolar solutions of free amino acids. This observation indicates that peptide absorption can result from two hydrolytic processes. Peptides can be hydrolyzed by brush border peptidases and then absorbed as free amino acids, or peptides can be absorbed and then hydrolyzed by cytoplasmic peptidases. Second, because the mechanisms used for mucosal uptake of peptides and amino acids are different and independent, the absorptive processes do not compete. Thus, the absorptive capacity of the small intestine is greater for mixtures of peptides and amino acids than for mixtures of amino acids alone. The separate mechanisms used for amino acid and peptide absorption may help explain why the small intestine efficiently absorbs the large amounts of protein typically presented from both dietary and endogenous sources.

3.3.2.1 Inclusion of Amino Acids in Sports Drinks?

Carbohydrate-electrolyte solutions containing amino acids (glycine or alanine) are used in oral rehydration solutions designed for treatment of diarrheal disease or severe dehydration.[36] These solutions are designed to maximize fluid absorption and provide an energy source. Inclusion of amino acids in these solutions is thought to be beneficial because amino acids are absorbed from the small intestine by multiple Na^+-dependent transport systems. These systems function independent of, but possibly additive to, the sodium-coupled glucose transport system. Should amino acids be included in sports drinks? Schedl et al.[14] discuss information relevant to including amino acids in sports drinks and cite several practical concerns, such as palatability and stability of amino acids in solution and potential toxicity with high doses of some amino acids.

3.3.3 Fats

The major types of fat in the Western diet are triglycerides (about 95%), phospholipids, and cholesterol. Digestion and absorption of fat are efficient processes, and they are mostly completed within the proximal small intestine. Each day, the gastrointestinal tract of an average healthy adult digests and absorbs more than 98% of the 60 to 100 g of ingested fat, as well as the 15 to 40 g of endogenous lipid (biliary secretions, sloughed mucosal cells) added to the intestinal lumen. Fats are insoluble in water, and this basic property affects their digestion, absorption, and transport in the blood.

The initial step in fat digestion is to disperse large, insoluble fat globules into smaller fat droplets and small emulsion particles.[37] The formation of droplets or emulsions with high surface areas provides better access for hydrolytic enzymes at the lipid-water interface. This process begins in the mouth where chewing food disperses fat and exposes lingual lipase to small fat droplets. Further digestion occurs in the stomach where vigorous mixing not only produces shear forces sufficient for emulsification but also exposes fat to lingual lipase and to emulsifying agents such as protein digestive products, polysaccharides, and phospholipids. Lingual lipase shows activity in the acidic gastric medium and in duodenal contents, acting on short and medium chain triglycerides to produce diacylglycerol and fatty acids; these products also act as emulsifying agents.

The final digestive step of the stomach is the propulsion of chyme through the small pyloric canal, producing strong shear forces and additional emulsification. Gastric delivery of fat digestive products in acid chyme stimulates duodenal endocrine cells to release the hormones cholesystokinin and secretin.[38] These and other gastrointestinal peptides play important roles in regulating gastrointestinal responses to food.[39] Cholesystokinin delays gastric emptying, stimulates pancreatic enzyme secretion, and promotes bile release from the gall bladder. Secretin acts to neutralize meal induced duodenal acidification by stimulating pancreatic bicarbonate secretion, delaying emptying, and inhibiting gastric acid secretion.

Most fat digestion occurs within the proximal small intestine under the action of pancreatic lipase and its co-factor, colipase.[37] The amount of pancreatric lipase activity in duodenal contents is extremely high and is more than is needed. Pancreatic lipase cleaves triglycerides to 2-monoacylglycerides and fatty acids. Bile salts above their critical micellar concentration inhibit pancreatic lipase activity, but activity is restored when colipase anchors lipase to the hydrophilic surface interface of bile salt micelles. Other pancreatic enzymes include cholesterol esterase, which hydrolyzes cholesterol esters to cholesterol and fatty acids, and pancreatic phospholipase, which cleaves lecithin to lysolecithin and fatty acids. Approximately 90% (7–22 g per day) of lecithin is derived from biliary secretions, while the remaining fraction comes from the diet. The products of pancreatic lipase, cholesterol esterase, and phospholipase activity are potent emulsifiers when incorporated into a shell of bile salts to form a mixed micelle. Within the duodenum and upper jejunum, the emulsification process is facilitated by the shearing/compression forces associated with peristaltic contractions.

The mixed micelle contains the products of fat digestion and serves as the vehicle for diffusion of lipids to the absorptive enterocytes. Adequate micellar formation is critical for lipid absorption and depends on numerous factors, including adequate bile salt concentrations and normal pH changes of chyme during passage through the duodenum. Once formed, the bile salt micelles are not absorbed as intact stuctures; rather, their lipid products must first dissociate and then pass through a series of diffusional barriers before reaching the enterocyte membrane. These barriers include the unstirred water layer, mucin gels, and the glycocalyx.

Lipids released from micelles may passively diffuse down their concentration gradients to the enterocyte membrane. Precisely how lipids leave the micelle, pass through the aqueous diffusion barriers and transverse the enterocyte membrane is not known. Several physicochemical models are used to explain this process.[37,40] Passage across the unstirred water layer is the rate limiting factor for absorption of long-chain fatty acids, cholesterol, lysolecithin, and monoglycerides. Short- and medium-chain fatty acids (less than 12 carbon atoms) are sufficiently water soluble to diffuse through the unstirred water layers without the assistance of the micelle.

To reach the systemic circulation, absorbed lipid must be transported in a water-soluble form. Short- and medium-chain fatty acids are bound to albumin and transported to the liver by the portal vein. The bulk of absorbed lipid, however, is processed within the enterocyte to form particles called chylomicrons. These particles are composed of resynthesized triglycerides (about 84%) and cholesterol esters (about 5%) in the core and phospholipids (about 8%), cholesterol (about 2%) and apolipoproteins in the outer coat. Chylomicrons enter the lymphatics and are transported to the systemic circulation via the thoracic duct.

The intestine may produce chylomicrons for up to nine or more hours following ingestion of a fatty meal. Cohn et al.[41] report that healthy subjects given a fat-rich meal (1 g fat/kg body wt) may show one, two, or more peaks in plasma triglycerides within a 12-hour period. In subjects showing a biphasic response, plasma triglycerides typically peak at three and nine hours and mirror the two peaks in plasma intestinal apolipoprotein (ApoB 48), a finding suggesting that plasma triglycerides are of intestinal origin and not from liver. Cohn et al.[41] suggest that the intestine may process fat in a pulsatile fashion, perhaps due to variations in intestinal motility and transit, fluctuations in phospholipid availability, differences between proximal and distal intestine to absorb fat and/or due to time required for synthesis of chylomicron apolipoprotein in the enterocytes.

3.3.4 Medium-Chain Triglycerides as an Energy Source for Athletes

Medium-chain triglycerides (MCTs), unlike long-chain triglycerides, are digested, absorbed and transported rapidly, and therefore may be considered a potential supplemental energy source for exercising endurance athletes. Briefly, MCTs are derived from coconut oil and contain fatty acids with chain lengths less than 12 carbon atoms.[42] Compared with long-chain triglycerides, MCTs are much more water soluble and are rapidly hydrolyzed by lingual lipase within the mouth, stomach, and duodenum. Medium-chain fatty acids pass rapidly through the unstirred water layer and enterocyte membranes and are transported bound to albumin via the portal circulation. Unlike long-chain fatty acids, medium-chain fatty acids require neither micelles nor chylomicrons for absorption. Unfortunately, compared to equimolar amounts of long-chain triglycerides, MCTs may acclerate intestinal transit and alter motility. And they are more likely to produce gastrointestinal symptoms such as cramps and diarrhea.[43,44]

Several studies have evaluated whether small amounts of MCT can be added to carbohydrate solutions to provide the benefit of two useable energy substrates for exercising athletes. Beckers et al.,[45] using single bolus (8 ml/kg body wt) ingestions of test drinks in resting subjects, report that gastric emptying is similar and not impaired by addition of MCT (0.8 to 2.4 g/100 ml) to maltodextrin (12 to 16%) solutions compared with emptying of an equicaloric maltodextrin solution. Further, this study shows that adding MCTs to carbohydrate solutions enhances delivery of energy (kcal) to the intestines compared with an equicaloric carbohydrate solution. These investigators[45] outline several other reasons for using MCTs as an energy source during prolonged, moderate intensity exercise.

First, in trained athletes cycling at 70% $\dot{V}O_{2\,max}$ for 80 minutes, Rehrer et al.[46] show that ingestion of a 17% glucose or 17% maltodextrin solution may double the amount of carbohydrate emptied from the stomach, but it will only slightly increase carbohydrate oxidation rates compared with values obtained during ingestion of a 4.5% glucose solution. Second, in trained athletes cycling at 65% $\dot{V}O_{2\,max}$ for 120 minutes, Wagenmakers et al.[47] show that ingestion of 12% or 16% maltodextrin solutions at rates providing more than 1 g carbohydrate per minute may provide little benefit because peak oxidation rates for exogenous carbohydrate rise to values of approximately 1 g per minute only during the final 30 minutes of exercise. These investigators suggest that ingesting carbohydrates at rates exceeding approximately1 g per minute may result in accumulation of exogenous carbohydrates in the gastrointestinal tract and/or in some other body pool. Because peak oxidation rates of ingested carbohydrates appear to be limited to approximately 1 g per minute during prolonged moderate intensity exercise and because consumption of excessive amounts of carbohydrates may produce gastrointestinal distress during exercise, the addition of MCTs to carbohydrate solutions offers the possibility of a readily absorbed, alternative energy source.

Using radioisotope tracers, Jenkendrup et al.[48] estimated rates of MCT oxidation in trained athletes cycling for 180 minutes at 57% $\dot{V}O_{2\,max}$. Cyclists ingested test drinks (1.375 l total) as an initial bolus (4 ml/kg body wt) at the start of exercise followed by serial feedings (2 ml/kg) every 20 minutes. Drinks consisted of MCT alone (29 g total) or MCT in two maltodextrin (11% or 15%) solutions. In these cyclists, MCTs were oxidized at rates equal to about 3 to 7% of total energy expenditure. MCT oxidation rates were greatest during the last 60 minutes of exercise and were higher when MCTs were ingested with carbohydrates. Van Zyl et al.[49] evaluated exercise performance in trained athletes who cycled for 120 minutes at 60% $\dot{V}O_{2\,max}$ while consuming two liters of either 10% glucose, 10% glucose containing 4.3% MCT, or 4.3% MCT. A 40-km timed performance ride was completed immediately after the 120-minute rides. Compared with the 10% glucose control trials, ingestion of the 10% glucose solution containing MCTs (about 86 g total) improved the 40-km time trial performance by about 2 minutes, whereas ingestion of the MCTs alone slowed the performance rides by about 5 minutes. Although these studies suggest that MCTs can be used as an additional energy source for exercising athletes, investigators warn that large quantities of MCTs (30–90 g in two to three hours) can produce gastrointestinal distress and hyperosmolar diarrhea in some individuals.

3.3.5 Regulation of Gastrointestinal Function

Gastrointestinal function is largely regulated by feedback control mechanisms, which act to match rates of nutrient delivery with rates of nutrient digestion and absorption. If nutrient delivery rates are too fast and exceed the functional capacity of the small intestine, malabsorption and diarrhea may occur. If delivery rates are too slow, the consumption of additional food is delayed.

Nutrient delivery is achieved by the propulsive activities of the stomach and small intestine, which in turn are largely controlled by neural and hormonal feedback signals originating from sensory nerves[50] and endocrine cells[39] located within the small intestinal mucosa. These specialized mucosal cells monitor the chemical and physical characteristics of chyme moving through the small intestinal lumen and generate feedback signals reflecting the quantity and quality of chyme components. The feedback signals are then integrated to stimulate pancreatic and biliary secretions, delay gastric emptying, reduce small bowel propulsion, and enhance intestinal mixing.

Feedback control ensures that the stomach adequately grinds and mixes food into an acidic chyme and then delivers the chyme into the duodenum at rates compatable with rates of intestinal digestion and absorption.[51] Feedback control also ensures that intestinal mixing produces a homogenous chyme that is amply exposed to the digestive and absorptive mucosal surface, while control of intestinal propulsion or transit through the small bowel permits sufficient time for absorption.[52] Three inhibitory feedback loops are recognized to control gastric and intestinal function. They are referred to as the duodenal, jejunal, and ileal brakes.

The duodenal brake is the first inhibitory feedback loop controlling the rate of gastric emptying. This control loop functions to match the rate of gastric emptying with the rate of duodenal digestion, absorption, and clearance.[53] Gastric emptying of liquid meals occurs in two phases: 1) an initial, rapid phase that is primarily dependent on volume or intragastric pressure, and 2) a relatively constant phase that is primarily dependent on duodenal feedback control.[54,55] In this control loop, the products of food digestion (fats, carbohydrates, and protein) as well as acidity and high osmolality are thought to stimulate sensory nerves or endocrine cells in the duodenal mucosa. Inhibitory signals generated by these duodenal receptors are then integrated and serve to slow gastric emptying by reducing gastric tone, enhancing pyloric tone, and switching from a propulsive to a mixing pattern. Cholesystokinin is one of several hormonal mediators of the duodenal brake.[56–58]

The jejunal brake is another inhibitory feedback loop controlling gastric delivery rates. Miller et al.[59] report that gastric emptying is inhibited to a similar extent when the jejunum is perfused with large (600 calorie) semi-elemental meals containing either protein (casein hydrolysates), carbohydrate (maltose), or lipid (oleate). In contrast, gastric emptying is inhibited by maltose, but not by protein or lipid, when smaller (300 calorie) meals are perfused.

Animal studies conducted by Lin et al.[60–62] suggest that nutrient contact area is an important determinant of feedback control. In these studies, perfusion of the small intestine with either oleate or glucose inhibits gastric emptying in a manner proportional to both nutrient concentration and the length of intestine exposed to unabsorbed nutrients. The full inhibitory effects of oleate or glucose are observed when the entire intestine is exposed to high nutrient concentrations. Exposure of the small intestine to fat will also inhibit intestinal transit in a dose- and length-dependent manner. Fat in the ileum more potently inhibits intestinal transit compared with fat in the jejunum.[63]

The ileal brake describes a potent feedback loop that alters gastric emptying and intestinal motility and transit. The ileal brake may be activated to compensate for defects resulting in the malabsorption of fats and carbohydrates. Studies show that ileal infusions of fat will delay gastric emptying,[64] reduce jejunal motility,[65,66] slow small intestinal transit,[64,65] and increase ileal chyme volume.[65] Spiller et al.[66] report that ileal infusions of corn starch hydrolysates (15 g) produce nausea and abdominal pain, possibly due to increased water secretion and intestinal distension. In a study of carbohydrate malabsorption, Layer et al.[67] used amylase inhibitors to delay digestion of ingested rice starch (50 g). Amylase inhibition increased the delivery of carbohydrate (mostly glucose polymers) to the jejunum and ileum, resulting in reduced intestinal water absorption and a doubling of gastric emptying time. Potential mediators of the ileal brake include neural or endocrine release of neurotensin, enteroglucagon and peptide YY.[65,66]

3.3.4.1 *Gastrointestinal Regulation During Exercise*

Can exercise adversely affect regulation of gastrointestinal function? The answer is probably yes in some cases of strenuous exercise. This question cannot be fully answered because the published literature is primarily descriptive in nature, and little is known about gastrointestinal regulation during exercise.[68] What is known is that many endurance athletes, especially runners, report symptoms such as vomiting, bloating, abdominal cramps, and diarrhea during strenuous training and competitive exercise.[69–71] Although the etiologies of these disturbances remain unknown, postulated causes include maldigestion and malabsorption, which in turn are possibly related to gastrointestinal ischemia, alterations in small intestinal motility and transit, and/or to improper food and fluid intake (foods rich in fibre and hypertonic drinks) during strenuous exercise.[72,73]

3.4 GASTRIC EMPTYING DURING EXERCISE

Factors influencing gastric emptying during rest and exercise have been reviewed extensively.[72,74,75] The following discussion will present a very brief review of this topic and will focus on emptying of carbohydrate solutions. Most evidence indicates that gastric emptying of dilute (up to 8%) carbohydrate solutions is not a limiting factor for replenishment of either fluids or energy during exercise and recovery. However, published guidelines[76] also suggest that there is no single sport drink that fulfills all requirements for fluid and carbohydrate supplementation during all exercise situations (pre-event, type and duration of event, and recovery). Little is known about the emptying of solid foods during exercise.

3.4.1 Liquids

The major factors influencing the emptying of liquids are solution composition and gastric volume. Solutions that are hypertonic or contain high acidity or high energy content are emptied more slowly than isotonic or neutral or calorie-free solutions.[53] Although fats (9 kcal/g) are calorie-dense and inhibit gastric emptying more than equivalent gram amounts of protein (4 kcal/g) or carbohydrate (4 kcal/g), these three substrates may leave the stomach at similar rates when isocaloric, isovolumic mixtures are ingested.[54] This finding suggests that energy delivery to the duodenum may be regulated at a constant rate. However, Hunt et al.[55] show that gastric delivery of calories is not constant, but it can be increased by increasing either the volume or the energy density of an ingested meal.

In a seminal study of gastric emptying, Costill and Saltin[77] report that single bolus feedings of solutions containing 2.5, 5.0, and 10.0% glucose slow gastric emptying compared with saline feedings. The effects of varying ingested volumes were also reported. When subjects ingested incremental volumes (200 to 800 ml) of the 2.5% glucose solution, emptying rates were found to increase by 3.7 ml/min for each 100 ml increase in gastric volume, up to a gastric volume of 600 ml. The 600 and 800 ml feedings produced similar maximal emptying rates of ~25 ml/min. The investigators suggested that the stomach should remain partially filled to maintain a high rate of gastric emptying during exercise.

More recent evidence supports this idea and emphasizes the importance of drinking patterns in controlling gastric emptying.[78] Compared with drinking a single bolus, repeated drinking will maintain high gastric volumes and will produce higher emptying rates of both fluids and nutrients. A repeated drinking pattern can produce high emptying rates from a variety of solutions containing small amounts of glucose, fructose, sucrose, and/or maltodextrins. The proportions of fluid and carbohydrate emptied from any particular drink depend largely on carbohydrate content. When a repeated drinking pattern is used, solutions containing more than 12% carbohydrate may impair emptying of fluids but enhance delivery of carbohydrates.[79]

Numerous studies show that repeated ingestion of small volumes (~150 to 350 ml every 20 minutes) of dilute carbohydrate (up to 8%) solutions can maintain relatively large gastric volumes and can provide high delivery rates of both fluids (15–20 ml/min) and carbohydrates (0.5 to 1.0 g/min) to the small intestine.[80–83] Notably, these fluid and carbohydrate delivery rates may closely match rates of sweating (0.5 to 1.5 l/h) and rates of blood glucose oxidation (0.5 to 1.0 g/min) in most competitive endurance athletes.[84,85] Noting that exogenous glucose oxidation rates rise to peak values of ~ 1g/min only after the first 90 minutes of exercise at 60–80% $\dot{V}O_{2\,max}$, Hawley et al[85] recommend a repeated drinking protocol using 2.5 to 5.0% carbohydrate solutions (providing 30g carbohydrate per hour) for the first 90 minutes of moderate exercise, followed by repeated consumption of 10 to 12% carbohydrate solutions (providing approximately 60 g carbohydrate per hour) after the first 90 minutes. Coyle and Montain[84] note that some competitive athletes may not drink repeatedly due to possible gastric discomfort and the loss of time associated with drinking large volumes.

Studies conducted over the past 25 years show that mild to moderate exercise has little effect on gastric emptying of either water or dilute carbohydrate solutions, whereas exercise exceeding 65–80% $\dot{V}O_{2\,max}$ may delay emptying of these liquids.[74,75,77] Compared with resting conditions, walking or moderate running is reported to enhance gastric emptying of a 400 ml bolus of water.[86] However, when a repeated drinking pattern is used, emptying of water or dilute carbohydrate solutions is similar during rest, moderate cycling, and moderate running.[82,87]

Though emptying is not altered by exercise below 65–80% $\dot{V}O_{2\,max}$, impairments in emptying may occur during such exercise when certain stressors are present. In particular, exercise combined with severe body fluid deficits (4–5% body wt) and/or hyperthermia (greater than 39°C) can impair gastric emptying when single feedings of either water or dilute carbohydrate solutions are given.[88,89] However, high emptying rates (about 18 ml/min) can be attained in hypohydrated (approximately 3% body wt), hyperthermic (38.6°C) subjects given multiple feedings of dilute carbohydrate solutions during moderate (65% $\dot{V}O_{2\,max}$) cycling in a cool environment.[90] These findings suggest that repeated drinking may overcome the inhibitory effects of exercise, fluid deficits, and hyperthermia on gastric emptying. Lastly, neither physical training[91] nor heat acclimation[88] are thought to improve gastric emptying during exercise.

3.4.2 Solid Foods

The proximal and distal regions of the stomach possess different roles for emptying solids and liquids.[51,92] Although both solid and liquid meals are emptied from the stomach at rates regulated by chemosensitive mechanisms of the small intestine, solid foods must first be converted into a liquefied chyme, whereas liquids can be emptied with little processing. The stomach's ability to discriminate liquids from solids is impaired by food components that produce a viscous gastric chyme, resulting in delayed emptying of both solids and liquids after ingestion of such foods.[25,92] When a meal is ingested, the proximal stomach (fundus and upper corpus) initially relaxes to accommodate the meal. Subsequent contractions of the fundus propells liquids into the duodenum and forces solid components into the distal stomach for mixing and grinding. The distal stomach (antrum and lower corpus) mixes and retains solid foods until particle sizes are reduced to less than 2 mm in diameter. Once formed, the liquefied chyme is propelled into the duodenum by antral contractions. Thus, solid foods generally empty from the stomach much more slowly than liquids.[93]

The effects of exercise on gastric emptying of solid foods are largely unknown. This information could benefit ultraendurance athletes (triathletes, cyclists, runners) who are known to ingest both solid and semi-solid foods during training or competition. Delayed emptying of solid foods seems likely to predispose competitive athletes to gastrointestinal distress. A practical recommendation is to limit intake of solid foods, especially foods high in fibre content, during the last three hours prior to exercise.[72]

3.5 INTESTINAL ABSORPTION DURING EXERCISE

The standard technique for studying small intestinal function in humans is a steady-state intraluminal perfusion technique using a multilumen tube positioned in the small intestine.[94] A major advantage of this technique is that it provides quantitative measurements of solute and water transport in the intestinal test segment under study. One disadvantage is that transport measurements describe only what occurs in the test segment, and these data may not accurately describe what occurs in more proximal or distal intestinal segments.[14]

3.5.1   Exercise Intensity

Using the perfusion technique, Fortran and Saltin[95] studied intestinal absorption in five subjects during 60 minutes of treadmill running at 64–78% $\dot{V}O_{2\,max}$. Four carbohydrate-electrolyte solutions were perfused (12 or 16 ml/min) into the jejunum or ileum, and only one or two subjects were perfused with a given solution. They report that exercise did not alter glucose, water, electrolyte, or water absorption and conclude that exercise does not affect active or passive intestinal transport. Gisolfi et al.[96] evaluated absorption from the duodenojejunum in six trained subjects during either rest, cycling for 60 minutes at 30, 50, or 70% $\dot{V}O_{2\,max}$, or cycling for 90 minutes at 70% $\dot{V}O_{2max}$. Either water or a 6% carbohydrate-electrolyte solution was perfused (15 ml/min) into the duodenojejunum (40 cm test segment) during rest, exercise, and recovery periods. Researchers found that exercise had no effect on water, carbohydrate, or electrolyte absorption in the duodenojejunum. Additional studies reported by these investigators support the contention that prolonged moderately intense exercise (85 minutes at 65% $\dot{V}O_{2\,max}$) does not affect absorption within the duodenojejunum.[90,97,98] Studies on intestinal absorption during rest and exercise have been carefully reviewed.[14,74,99]

3.5.2   Carbohydrate Absorption

Wagenmakers et al.[47] and Hawley et al.[100] estimate that ingested carbohydrates or intravenously infused glucose can be oxidized at rates as high as about 1 g/min during the latter stages (more than 90 minutes) of prolonged moderate intensity exercise. Can the intestines absorb carbohydrates at this rate? Using a triple-lumen tube with a 40-cm test segment, Duchman et al.[101] estimated maximum absorption rates while perfusing a 4.4% glucose-electrolyte solution into the duodenum of healthy subjects at rest. The test solution was perfused at three high rates: 21, 28.5, and 36 ml/min. These perfusion rates were generally well tolerated and did not produce diarrhea, though two of six subjects complained of mild abdominal cramps during the high (36 ml/min) rate. Despite large differences in perfusion rates, intestinal glucose absorption remained unchanged, with mean values ranging from 4.3 to 5.6 mmol/cm/h. Using these values and assuming a 100-cm length of duodenojejunum, glucose absorption rates from this solution were estimated to range from 1.3 to 1.7 g/min.

For comparison, other studies using 40-cm test segments, perfusion rates of 15 ml/min, and 2–8% carbohydrate-electrolyte solutions report carbohydrate absorption rates ranging from approximately 0.9 to 6.3 mmol/cm/h.[102–105] Gisolfi et al.[103] report that duodenojejunal perfusion of 2, 4, or 6% glucose solutions produce carbohydrate absorption rates equal to 1.5, 2.4, and 4.0 mmol/cm/h, whereas a hypertonic 8% glucose solution elicits a value of 3.2 mmol/cm/h. The high carbohydrate absorption rates of 5.2 or 6.3 mmol/cm/h were observed during duodenojejunal perfusions of solutions containing small amounts of electrolytes and either 1% glucose, 2% sucrose and 3% maltodextrins,[104] or 4% fructose and 4% sucrose.[105]

Using a novel technique designed to simultaneously measure gastric emptying and intestinal absorption,[97] Lambert et al.[98] report carbohydrate absorption rates of about 1 g/min in healthy subjects ingesting a 6% carbohydrate-electrolyte solution during 85 min of cycling at 64% $\dot{V}O_{2\,max}$.

Cyclists ingested the test solution (4% sucrose, 2% glucose, 18 meq Na$^+$, 3 meq K$^+$) as a bolus (380 ml) just before exercise, followed by serial feedings (190 ml) every 20 minutes (total = 23 ml/Kg body wt). This drinking pattern maintained gastric volumes at about 250 ml and elicited gastric emptying rates of 19 ml/min and 1.1 g carbohydrate/min.

Using the emptying rate as the intestinal perfusion rate, carbohydrate absorption rates from the duodenum (0–25 cm) and jejunum (25–50 and 50–75 cm) were found to be 6.0, 3.3, and 0.9 mmol/cm/h, respectively. Added together, these absorption rates show that 88 grams of carbohydrate were absorbed from the 75 cm test segment during 85 min of cycling exercise. These data are consistent with the idea that the stomach, acting under numerous feedback control loops, will deliver carbohydrates from a 6% carbohydrate-electrolyte solution to the intestine at rates that ensure adequate digestion and absorption.

Thus, the intestines of healthy subjects appear to be capable of absorbing carbohydrates at rates slightly exceeding 1 g/min when 6–8% carbohydrate solutions are perfused into the duodenum or repeatedly ingested during either rest or during prolonged moderate intensity exercise. Further, these high carbohydrate absorption rates may be attained from a variety of solutions containing glucose, fructose, sucrose, and maltodextrins. Whether intestinal absorption rates as high as 1 g carbohydrate per minute can be obtained from ingesting mixed meals or easily digestible foods is not known.

3.5.3 Water Absorption

Sport drinks should be designed to maximize absorption of both fluids and carbohydrates to offset fluid lost in sweat and to supplement endogenous carbohydrate stores. An important concern, especially for endurance athletes, is whether the amount or type of carbohydrate alters intestinal water absorption.

The two major factors governing water absorption in the small intestine are solute transport (Na$^+$ and carbohydrate) and osmolality. In general, solutions that are hypotonic promote more water absorption than isotonic solutions, whereas hypertonic solutions may promote water secretion. High rates of intestinal carbohydrate and Na$^+$ transport will increase water absorption.

Gisolfi et al.[103] report that isotonic solutions containing 2, 4, or 6% glucose, sucrose, maltodextrins, or corn syrup solids produce similar rates of water absorption from the duodenojejunum, whereas hypertonic solutions of 8% glucose or corn syrup solids, but not maltodextrins or sucrose, may reduce water absorption. These findings suggest that water absorption is independent of carbohydrate type for isotonic solutions containing up to 6% carbohydrate.

There is evidence that transport of Na$^+$ and carbohydrate may be more important than osmolality in determining intestinal water absorption from dilute carbohydrate solutions. Shi et al.[104] evaluated three 6% carbohydrate-electrolyte solutions and found that water absorption in the duodenojejunum correlated with Na$^+$ and carbohydrate absorption but not with osmolality. Water absorption was greatest for a hypertonic (403 mOsm/kg) solution containing 3.25% glucose and 2.75% fructose and lowest for a hypotonic (186 mOsm/kg) solution containing 1% glucose, 2% sucrose, and 3% maltodextrins.

Using duodenojejunal perfusions of nine 6–8% carbohydrate-electrolyte solutions, Shi et al.[105] report that solutions containing multiple transportable carbohydrates (fructose and glucose or sucrose) stimulate more water absorption than solutions with only one transportable carbohydrate (glucose or maltodextrins). Further, at any given osmolality of test solution (165–477 mOsmol/kg) perfusing the intestine, more water is absorbed from a solution that contains multiple transportable carbohydrate types than from a solution that contains only one carbohydrate type. Regression analysis revealed that total solute transport (Na$^+$ and carbohydrate) and osmolality accounted for 48% and 11% of the variance in water absorption rate. Thus, hypertonic solutions with multiple transportable carbohydrates may stimulate more water absorption than hypotonic solutions with only one transportable carbohydrate.

Can the small intestine absorb water from dilute carbohydrate-electrolyte solutions at rates sufficient to match rates of sweat production (0.5 to 1.5 l/h) commonly observed during exercise? Minimal estimates of water absorption rates can be derived from measurements made within the 40-cm duodenojejunum test segment. The duodenojejunum absorbs the major portion (about 70%) of fluid presented to the intestines, and perfusion rates used in most studies are reasonably matched with gastric emptying rates (15 ml/min). The following water absorption rates should be considered as minimal estimates because they do not account for water absorbed distal to the 40-cm or 75-cm duodenojejunum test segments.

Similar water absorption rates of approximately 13 ml/cm/h are reported for subjects perfused with a 6% carbohydrate-electrolyte solution during 60 minutes of cycling at 30, 50, or 70% $\dot{V}O_{2\,max}$.[96] The minimum rate of water absorption from this solution is estimated to be approximately 0.5 l/h. Likewise, in resting subjects, Shi et al.[104] report segmental water absorption rates equal to about 0.5, 0.5, and 0.6 l/h during perfusions of a hypotonic, isotonic, and hypertonic 6% carbohydrate-electrolyte solution. Gisolfi et al.[103] report that 2, 4, or 6% solutions containing glucose, sucrose, or corn syrup solids, or 8% solutions containing sucrose or maltodextrins (average of 7 carbon units) produce similar water absorption rates with values ranging from approximately 0.4 to 0.6 l/h.

Using simultaneous measures of gastric emptying and intestinal absorption in subjects cycling for 85 minutes at 60% $\dot{V}O_{2\,max}$, Lambert et al.[97] observed gastric emptying rates of 20 ml/min and water absorption rates equal to 0.8 l/h during repeated ingestion of a 6% carbohydrate-electrolyte solution. In a similar exercise study, Lambert et al.[98] report similar gastric emptying rates of about 19 ml/min and water absorption rates of about 0.9 l/min during repeated ingestion of either a water placebo or a 6% carbohydrate-electrolyte solution. Compared with a water placebo, the 6% carbohydrate-electrolyte solution produced greater solute (Na^+ and carbohydrate) flux and thus stimulated more water absorption in the jejunum. Water absorption rates from the duodenum (0–25 cm) and jejunum (25–50 cm and 50–75 cm) were 31, 4, and 3 ml/cm/h for water placebo and 15, 12, and 4 ml/cm/h for the 6% carbohydrate-electrolyte solution. In hypohydrated subjects cycling at 65% $\dot{V}O_{2\,max}$ for 85 minutes, Ryan et al.[90] found that repeated ingestion of a 6%, 8%, or 9% carbohydrate-electrolyte solution produced similar gastric emptying rates of about 18 ml/min; however, water absorption within the duodenojejunum differed markedly with values of approximately 0.7, 0.3, and 0.1 l/h, respectively.

Thus, most evidence indicates that water can be absorbed from healthy duodenojejunum at rates ranging from about 0.4 to 0.9 l/h when 2–8% carbohydrate-electrolyte solutions are perfused into the duodenum or repeatedly ingested during either rest or during prolonged moderate intensity exercise. In the studies cited, water absorption measurements were limited to the proximal small intestine (40-cm or 75-cm test segments) when solutions were presented to the intestine at rates of 0.9 l/h (perfusion studies) or about 1.2 l/h (repeated ingestion studies). Given the above considerations, values of 0.4 to 0.9 l/h compare favorably to sweat production rates (0.5 to 1.5 l/h) commonly observed during exercise. High water absorption rates may be obtained either from hypotonic or isotonic 2–8% carbohydrate-electrolyte solutions that contain single or multiple carbohydrate types, or from hypertonic 6–8% carbohydrate-electrolyte solutions that contain multiple transportable carbohydrates.

3.5.4 Fructose Malabsorption

The small intestine shows a limited capacity to absorb fructose. Fructose is absorbed at a slower rate than glucose and stimulates less water and sodium absorption.[106] Notably, glucose stimulates fructose uptake in a dose-dependent manner.[107] Natural products that contain fructose in excess of glucose include honey, apples, pears, and their fruit juices.[108] Fructose is also used commercially as a sweetener for confectionery and soft drinks (high-fructose corn syrup contains about 40–60% fructose).

Evidence shows that small amounts of fructose can cause malabsorption and gastrointestinal distress during both rest and exercise. In studies cited below, fructose malabsorption was determined by hydrogen (H_2) breath analysis: fructose that escapes absorption in small bowel serves as a substrate for colonic bacteria, generating H_2 as a product of fermentation. Ravich et al.[109] report that 50 g fructose given as a 10% solution produced intestinal malabsorption and cramps and diarrhea in six of 16 healthy resting subjects. In a study involving 10 resting subjects,[107] 10% solutions of 50, 25, and 10 g fructose produced malabsorption in eight, five, and one subjects, respectively. Addition of glucose to fructose solutions reduced malabsorption, whereas fructose given as sucrose did not produce malabsorption.

Fujisawa et al.[110] report that two 30-minute bouts of treadmill running (up to 70% $\dot{V}O_{2\,max}$) produced intestinal malabsorption in all 10 subjects who received 50 g fructose in 860 ml water. Subjects given glucose (50 g) or glucose + fructose (15 g + 35 g) solutions did not show malabsorption following the exercise stress. The investigators recommended limiting ingestion of pure fructose before or during exercise to quantities below 50 g. Thus, in some individuals, fructose malabsorption and gastrointestinal symptoms can occur with quantities as low as 10 to 50 g. However, fructose given as sucrose or in the presence of glucose appears to be better absorbed.

3.5.5 Intestinal Blood Flow

Strenuous exercise can reduce splanchnic blood flow to levels as low as 20% of resting values.[111] From a literature review, Brouns and Beckers[73] postulate that gut ischemia during prolonged, strenuous exercise, especially when conducted in a dehydrated state, may reduce intestinal absorption, promote secretion, and contribute to the development of abdominal cramps and diarrhea. So why do laboratory studies show that intestinal absorption is not altered by exercise? One reason is that these studies do not closely replicate factors that occur during training and competition. These factors may include exercise intensity and duration, degree of dehydration and hyperthermia, quantity and quality of food and fluid intake, and psychological stress. Another possible reason is that these studies examine intestinal absorption when the intestine is presented with relatively large volumes of carbohydrate solutions (15–20 ml/min of 6–8% carbohydrate solutions).

Ingestion of food increases intestinal blood flow by approximately 30 to 130% of fasting values.[112] Some evidence suggests that ingesting nutrients counters the reductions in intestinal blood flow observed during exercise. Qamar and Read[113] report that ingestion of a mixed meal (390 kcal) increases mesenteric artery blood flow by 56% in a group of 16 healthy subjects, whereas treadmill exercise (5 km/h, 20% grade, 15 minutes) reduces mesenteric flow by 43% of fasting control values. When the mixed meal was ingested during exercise, the meal-induced hyperemia was only slightly depressed at 42% above fasting values. Eriksen and Walker[114] report similar results for five subjects who first consumed a mixed meal (about 1500 kcal), rested for 30 minutes, and then cycled for 4 minutes at 150–200 W. These findings urge the question: Will ingestion of small liquid meals protect the gut during prolonged strenuous exercise?

3.6 GASTROINESTINAL ADAPTATIONS

Athletes frequently use dietary manipulations to maintain or improve their training or competitive efforts. As revealed by dietary surveys, body builders and strength athletes with the intent of repairing and constructing skeletal muscle will follow a high-protein diet and take protein supplements.[3] Endurance athletes often use the well-known carbohydrate loading regime to increase or maintain skeletal muscle and liver glycogen stores, and to improve exercise performance.[115] A recent proposal suggests that consumption of a high-fat diet for two to four weeks may be used to promote fat utilization and improve endurance exercise performance.[116,117] In addition, compared with sedentary people, athletes may consume up to two to three times more calories to meet the demands of their relatively large daily energy expenditures. While considerable attention is devoted to the physiological and performance enhancing effects of these dietary practices, little attention is given to the effects of these diets on the gastrointestinal tract.

This section will briefly review relevant human studies, present limited information on mechanisms of gastrointestinal adaptation, and highlight questions that may be of interest to exercise physiologists. Will the dietary practices of athletes, particularly their high daily carbohydrate and caloric intakes, produce structural and functional adaptations within the gastrointestinal tract? Can athletes use short-term dietary manipulations to enhance gastrointestinal function, improve gastric emptying and fluid and nutrient absorption during exercise, and thereby improve endurance exercise performance?

3.6.1 Human Studies

The gastrointestinal tract exhibits a tremendous capacity to adapt to changes in energy intake.[118] Some intestinal adaptations can be pronounced during extreme variations in energy intake. For example, in response to starvation, the intestines may show mucosal atrophy with reductions in digestive and absorptive surface area. On the other hand, adaptations that increase intestinal surface area, such as mucosal hypertrophy and increases in villi length and number, may occur within several weeks of hyperphagia. These adaptations are thought to provide a safety margin for nutrient absorption: Reductions in intestinal mass will save biosynthetic energy by eliminating unneeded mucosal absorptive capacity, whereas intestinal hypertrophy will ensure that mucosal absorptive capacity is maintained modestly above nutrient intake.[119,120]

Harris et al.[121] provide evidence that significant gastrointestinal adaptations are present in physically active males with high energy intakes. Orocecal transit time (hydrogen breath technique) of a mixed liquid meal (250 kcal/240 ml) was negatively correlated ($r = -0.69$) to daily energy intakes in 20 males with energy intakes ranging from 1,272 to 5,342 kcal/day. The food passage time from mouth to large intestine, measured during quiet rest, ranged from about 200 minutes to below 50 minutes for males with daily energy intakes of approximately 1300 and 4500 kcal/day, respectively. Orocecal transit of the liquid meal was related to total daily energy intake but not related to daily caloric intakes of protein, fat, or carbohydrate. Absorption of a nonmetabolizable sugar, xylose, was unrelated to daily energy intake. The investigators suggested that males with high energy intakes may display gastrointestinal adaptations that allow for rapid food transit without decrements in nutrient absorption.

Individuals with eating disorders often exhibit low caloric intakes, malnutrition, and impairments in gastrointestinal function. In particular, over 50% of patients with anorexia nervosa or bulimia nervosa demonstate delayed gastric emptying[122–124] and prolonged orocecal or whole-gut (radiopaque markers) transit[125] of solid and liquid meals. Patients report that consumption of meals often elicits symptoms such as nausea, vomiting, abdominal pain, and gastric fullness.[126] Gastric emptying of water or saline is typically normal and similar to control subjects.[123,124] Notable is that treatment of these patients with a nutritional program will improve gastric emptying of liquid and solid meals and will reduce gastrointestinal symptoms.[124,126] Although the gastrointestinal disturbances in these patients may result from both psychological and physiological mechanisms, the above findings do provide evidence for gastointestinal adaptation to acute changes in nutritional intake.

There is evidence that acute alterations in dietary intake of carbohydrates or fat will elicit gastrointestinal adaptations in healthy volunteers. Cunningham et al.[127] report that gastric emptying (by epigastric impedance) of a hypertonic glucose solution, but not a protein drink, can be enhanced by supplementation of a standard diet with 400 g glucose/day for three days. Total carbohydrate intake for the standard and supplemental diets was 287 and 687 g/day. In a later study,[128] using a more accepted measure of gastric emptying (scintigraphy), these investigators report that emptying of hypertonic glucose or fructose solutions (75 g/350 ml) can be enhanced by short-term (four to seven days) dietary supplementation with glucose (440 g/day). Dietary supplementation with glucose also resulted in greater increases in plasma glucose and insulin following ingestion of the hypertonic glucose drink. Cunningham et al.[129] also report that both gastric emptying and orocecal transit of a high-fat test meal are faster after 14 days on a high-fat diet (270 g/day) compared with

14 days on a low-fat diet (12 g/day). Gastric emptying and orocecal transit of the high-fat test meal was not altered by consumption of the high-fat diet for four days.

The investigators suggest that dietary history can be a contributing factor to inter- and intra-individual variations in studies of gastric emptying, orocecal transit, and oral glucose tolerance tests. They postulated that rapid (3–14 days) adaptations to changes in dietary intake could occur either by enhanced intestinal absorptive capacity, reduced intestinal chemoreceptor feedback to the stomach and intestines, desensitization of intestinal chemoreceptors, or by a combination of these mechanisms. The investigators have developed a rodent model that supports the proposal for desensitization of intestinal chemoreceptors.[130] In this model, four weeks of intermittent infusions of a lipid emulsion, but not infusions of the emulsion alone, resulted in delayed gastric emptying and small intestinal transit of a bean meal.

3.6.2 Mechanisms

Studies on the mechanisms of gastrointestinal adaptation show that the small intestine can rapidly adapt to changes in nutrient intake.[119] In general, these adaptations are nutrient-specific, they occur within several days of dietary change, and they are localized to the digestive and absorptive surface — the small intestinal epithelium. Intestinal adaptations may include both alterations in hydrolytic enzyme activities within the enterocyte brush border and changes in nutrient transporter number and activity within both the enterocyte brush border and basolateral membranes. Stimuli thought to be involved in regulating adaptive small-intestinal changes are large in number and diverse in scope, and they include the presence of luminal nutrients, pancreatic and biliary secretions, and gut hormones such as enteroglucagon, epidermal growth factor, and cholesystokinin.[131,132]

The time course for enterocyte adaptations (one to seven days) corresponds to time estimates for intestinal epithelial cell turnover in mammals and is compatable with regulation at the level of the intestinal crypt cells.[133] The largely undefined regulatory mechanisms are thought to act in some manner to closely match intestinal absorptive capacity to an average diet composition consumed over several days; that is, regulatory mechanisms do not switch adaptive changes on and off in response to each meal.[119] The following discussion briefly outlines selected research findings on specific adaptations to alterations in dietary carbohydrate, protein, and fat intake.

Acute changes in carbohydrate consumption can alter both digestive and absorptive functions of small intestinal epithelium. In human volunteers, as little as two to five days of supplemental feedings with sucrose or fructose, but not glucose, increases sucrase and maltase activities within the jejunal brush border membrane.[134] In rodents, increases in dietary carbohydrate intake, ranging from 0 to 68% of caloric intake, are associated with linear increases in glucose and fructose uptake across the jejunal bush border.[119,135,136] Increases in sugar absorption are rapid and observable within one to three days of dietary change. Glucose, galactose, fructose, and maltose appear to be equally effective inducers of glucose uptake, whereas fructose is the best inducer of fructose uptake.[137] These dietary-induced adaptations are associated with increases in the number and activity of hexose transporters within the brush border (SGLT1, GLUT5) and basolateral (GLUT2) membranes.

Dietary regulation of intestinal amino acid transporters is complex; however, there are two discernable patterns of regulation for nonessential and essential amino acids.[119] Nonessential amino acids show a regulatory pattern similar to that observed for sugars. In rodents, small-intestinal uptake of nonessential amino acids will increase in a linear fashion when dietary nitrogen intake increases from 0 to 68% of calories. In contrast, essential amino acid uptake by intestine decreases or remains unchanged when dietary nitrogen intake is low. When dietary intake is high, intestinal uptake increases only modestly. The amino acids also show a complex pattern regarding their ability to act as inducers. For example, dietary aspartate appears to be a good inducer of both acidic and basic amino acid transporters, whereas valine induces the neutral amino acid transporter, and arginine, a basic amino acid, induces the acidic amino acid transporter.[138]

Thompson et al.[139] measure intestinal transport function in rat jejunum following a two to three week diet rich in either saturated or polyunsaturate fats. Compared with the polyunsaturated diet or normal chow, the saturated fat diet resulted in enhanced jejunal uptake of fatty acids (palmitic, linoleic), cholesterol, and leucine, and reduced the uptake of glucose. The mechanisms by which dietary lipid manipulations result in altered intestinal transport remain largely unknown. Changes in dietary lipid intake can change the passive permeability properties of the enterocyte brush border membrane.[120] Alterations in membrane lipid composition and permeability properties may be important because small intestinal lipid absorption is thought to occur largely through a process of passive diffusion.

3.7 SUMMARY

An athlete's diet should follow accepted guidelines for eating healthily, and should contain sufficient calories to meet the demands of vigorous exercise training. The energy demands of daily exercise can be tremendous, requiring large caloric intakes of energy-yielding nutrients. Dietary surveys reveal that athletes who consume insufficient calories are also likely to consume insufficient amounts of proteins and carbohydrates. These low-energy consumers may therefore be at risk for problems with health and exercise performance.

The caloric demands of daily exercise requires an athlete's gastrointestinal tract to digest and absorb relatively large amounts of the major energy-yielding nutrients: carbohydrates, proteins, and fats. A review of the basic mechanisms of digestion and absorption shows that the human gastrointestinal tract efficiently digests and absorbs almost all of the carbohydrate, protein, and fat consumed each day. There is also some evidence that suggests that an athlete's gastrointestinal tract may show structural and functional adaptations in response to high daily intakes of calories and carbohydrates. These adaptations may enhance intestinal absorptive capacity and may provide benefits for athletes with high-energy needs.

Few studies describe the effects of exercise on digestion and absorption of either fats or proteins commonly found in solid or liquid foods. This lack of information hinders the development of specific dietary recommendations needed for formulation of the precompetition meal and for foods consumed during endurance and ultraendurance events.

On the other hand, there is considerable research that describes food properties that exert significant effects on gastric emptying, digestion and absorption, and physiological responses to foods containing carbohydrate. Food properties that alter the glycemic response to starchy foods may be of particular concern to athletes interested in carbohydrate supplementation before, during, and after exercise.

Several studies show that small amounts of medium-chain triglycerides can be added to carbohydrate solutions and thereby effectively used as an additional energy source for exercising athletes. A caveat is that large quantities of medium-chain triglycerides (30–90 g in two to three hours) are capable of producing gastrointestinal distress and hyperosmolar diarrhea in some individuals. The potential value of including amino acids in sports drinks is unknown. Glucose and the amino acids, alanine or glycine, are used in oral rehydration solutions designed for treatment of diarrheal disease or severe dehydration, and together they provide a theoretical advantage of maximizing water and energy absorption from the small intestine. Practical concerns include palatability and stability of amino acids in solution and potential toxicity with high doses of some amino acids.

A repeated drinking pattern can produce high gastric emptying rates from a variety of dilute solutions containing either glucose, fructose, sucrose and/or maltodextrins. Numerous studies show that repeated ingestion of small volumes (approximately 150 to 350 ml every 20 minutes) of dilute carbohydrate (up to 8%) solutions can provide high gastric delivery rates of both fluids (15–20 ml/min) and carbohydrates (0.5 to 1.0 g/min) to the small intestine. Notably, these delivery rates closely match rates of sweating (0.5 to 1.5 l/h) and rates of blood glucose oxidation (0.5 to 1.0

g/min) in most competitive endurance athletes. Gastric emptying of carbohydrate solutions does not appear to be altered by physical training or by heat acclimation, but emptying may be impaired by exercise exceeding 65–80% $\dot{V}O_{2\,max}$ and by slightly less intense exercise when severe body fluid deficits (4–5% body wt) and/or hyperthermia (greater than 39°C) are present.

Studies using the intestinal perfusion technique show that absorption of dilute carbohydrate solutions remains unaltered by exercise intenstities up to 70% $\dot{V}O_{2\,max}$ for 90 minutes. Perfusion studies also demonstrate that the healthy adult intestine can absorb carbohydrate at rates more than 1 g/min and water at rates greater than 0.4 to 0.9 l/h when 6–8% carbohydrate solutions are perfused into 40–75 cm segments of duodenojejunum. These intestinal absorption rates can be obtained from a variety of solutions containing glucose, fructose, sucrose and/or maltodextrins. Hypertonic solutions (more than 300 mOsmol/Kg) containing a single carbohydrate type may promote intestinal secretion whereas hypertonic solutions (less than 480 mOsmol/Kg) containing multiple carbohydrate types will promote water absorption. Nutrient malabsorption and intestinal ischemia are frequently cited as important etiological factors for the development of gastrointestinal disturbances during strenuous exercise. Considerable evidence shows that small amounts of fructose alone can cause malabsorption during both rest and exercise.

REFERENCES

1. Saris, W. H., van Erp-Baart, M. A., Brouns, F., Westerterp, K. R., and ten Hoor, F., Study on food intake and energy expenditure during sustained exercise: the Tour de France, *Int. J. Sports Med.*, 10 (suppl 1), S26, 1989.
2. Garcia-Roves, P. M., Terrados, N., Ferdundez, S. F., and Patterson, A. M., Macronutrient intake of top level cyclists during continuous competition—change in the feeding pattern, *Int. J. Sports Med.*, 19, 61, 1998.
3. Brotherhood, J. R., Nutrition and sports performance, *Sports Med.*, 1, 350, 1984.
4. Economos, C. D., Bortz, S. S., and Nelson, M. E., Nutritional practices of elite athletes. Pratical recommendations, *Sports Med.*, 16, 381, 1993.
5. Grandjean, A. C., Diets of elite athletes: has the discipline of sports nutrition made an impact?, *J. Nutr.*, 127, 874S, 1997.
6. Hawley, J. A., Dennis, S. C., Lindsay, F. H., and Noakes, T. D., Nutritional practices of athletes: are they sub-optimal?, *J. Sports Sci.*, 13, S75, 1995.
7. Van Erp-Baart, A. M., Saris, W. H., Binkhorst, R. A., Vos, J. A., and Elvers, J. W., Nationwide survey on nutritional habits in elite athletes. Part 1. Energy, carbohydrate, protein, and fat intake, *Int. J. Sports Med.*, 10 (suppl 1), S3, 1989.
8. Burke, L. M. and Read, R. S., Dietary supplements in sport, *Sports Med.*, 15, 43, 1993.
9. Williams, C., Macronutrients and performance, *J. Sports Sci.*, 13, S1, 1995.
10. Fallowfield, J. and Williams, C., Carbohydrate intake and recovery from prolonged exercise, *Inter. J. Sports Med.*, 3, 50, 1993.
11. Levin, R. J., Digestion and absorption of carbohydrates—from molecules and membranes to humans, *Am. J. Clin. Nutr.*, 59 (suppl), 690S, 1994.
12. Southgate, D. A., Digestion and metabolism of sugars, *Am. J. Clin. Nutr.*, 62 (suppl), 203S, 1995.
13. Levitt, M. D., Strocchi, A., and Levitt, D. G., Human jejunal unstirred layer: evidence for extremely efficient luminal stirring, *Am. J. Physiol.*, 262, G593, 1992.
14. Schedl, H. P., Maughan, R. J., and Gisolfi, C. V., Intestinal absorption during rest and exercise: implications for formulating an oral rehydration solution (ORS), *Med. Sci. Sports Exerc.*, 26, 267, 1994.
15. Pappenheimer, J. R., Paracellular intestinal absorption of glucose, creatine, and mannitol in normal animals: relation to body size, *Am. J. Physiol.*, 259, G290, 1990.
16. Ferraris, R. P., Yasharpour, S., Lloyd, K. C., Mirzayan, R., and Diamond, J.M., Luminal glucose concentrations in the gut under normal conditions, *Am. J. Physiol.*, 259, G822, 1990.
17. Spiller, R. C., Intestinal absorptive function, *Gut*, 35 (suppl. 1), S5, 1994.
18. Crane, R. L., Structural and functional organization of an epithelial cell brush border, in *Symposia of the International Society for Cell Biology*, Warren, K.B., Ed., New York, Acacemic Press, 1966, 71.

19. Asp, N., Nutritional classification and analysis of food carbohydrates, *Am. J. Clin. Nutr.*, 59 (suppl). 679S, 1994.

20. Cummings, H., Roberfroid, M. B., members of the Paris Carbohydrate Group, A., H., Barth, C., Ferro-Luzzi, A., Ghoos, Y., Gibney, M., Hermonsen, K., James, W. P., Korver, O., Lairaon, D., Pascal, G., and Voragen, A. G., A new look at dietary carbohydrate: chemistry, physiology, and health, *Eur. J. Clin. Nutr.*, 51, 417, 1997.

21. Annison, A. and Topping, D.L., Nutritional role of resistant starch: chemical structure vs. physiological function, *Ann. Rev. Nutr.*, 14, 297, 1994.

22. Jenkins, D. J., Josse, R. G., Jenkins, A. L., Wolever, T. M., and Vuksan, V., Implications of altering the rate of carbohydrate absorption from the gastrointestinal tract, *Clin. Invest. Med.*, 18, 296, 1995.

23. Walton, P. and Rhodes, E. C., Glycaemic index and optimal performance, *Sports Med.*, 23(3), 164-172, 1997.

24. Behall, K. M., Scholfield, D. J., and Canary, J., Effect of starch structure on glucose and insulin responses in adults, *Am. J. Clin. Nutr.*, 47, 428, 1988.

25. Benini, L., Castellani, G., Brighenti, F., Heaton, K. W., Brentegani, M. T., Casiraghi, M. C., Sembenini, C., Pellegrini, N., Fioretta, A., Minniti, G., Porrini, M., Testolin, G., and Vantini, I., Gastric emptying of a solid meal is acclerated by the removal of dietary fibre naturally present in food, *Gut*, 36, 825, 1995.

26. Cherbut, C., Varannes, S. B., Schnee, M., Rival, M., Galmiche, J., and Delort-Laval, J., Involvement of small intestinal motility in blood glucose response to dietary fibre in man, *Brit. J. Nutr.*, 71, 675, 1994.

27. Schonfeld, J., Evans, D., and Wingate, D. L., Effect of viscous fiber (guar) on postprandial motor activity in human small bowel, *Dig. Dis. Sci.*, 42, 1613, 1997.

28. Sleisenger, M. H. and Kim, Y. S., Protein digestion and absorption, *N. Eng. J. Med.*, 300, 659, 1979.

29. Adibi, S. A. and Mercer, D. W., Protein digestion in human intestine as reflected in luminal, mucosal, and plasma amino acid concentrations after meals, *J. Clin. Invest.*, 52, 1586, 1973.

30. Souba, W. W. and Pacitti, A. J., How amino acids get into cells: mechanisms, models, menus, and mediators, *J. P. E. N.*, 16, 569, 1992.

31. Hines, O.J., Bilchik, A.J., Ashley, S.W., Whang, E.E., Liu, C.D., Zinner, M.J. and McFadden, D.W., Amino acids mediate postprandial jejunal proabsorption, *J. Surg. Res.*, 58, 81, 1995.

32. Leibach, F. H. and Ganapathy, V., Peptide transporters in the intestine and the kidney, *Ann. Rev. Nutr.*, 16, 99, 1996.

33. Grimble, G. K., The significance of peptides in clinical nutrition, *Ann. Rev. Nutr.*, 14, 419, 1994.

34. Matthews, D. M., Intestinal absorption of peptides, *Physiol. Rev.*, 55, 537, 1975.

35. Matthews, D. M. and Adibi, S.A., Peptide absorption, *Gastroenterol.*, 71, 151, 1976.

36. Schedl, H. P., Scientific rationale for oral rehydration therapy, *Clin. Ther.*, 12 (Suppl. A), 14, 1990.

37. Carey, M. C., Small, D. M., and Bliss, C. M., Lipid digestion and absorption, *Ann. Rev. Physiol.*, 45, 651, 1983.

38. Hildebrand, P., Petrig, C., Burkhardt, B., Ketterer, S., Lengsfeld, H., Fleury, A., Hadvary, P., and Beglinger, C., Hydrolysis of dietary fat by pancreatic lipase stimulates cholecystokinin release, *Gastroenterol.*, 114, 123, 1998.

39. Green, D. W., Gomez, G., and Greely, G. H., Gastrointestinal peptides, *Gastroenterol. Clin. N. Am.*, 18, 695, 1989.

40. Thomson, A. B., Schoeller, C., Keelan, M., Smith, L., and Clandinin, M. T., Lipid absorption: passing through the unstirred layers, brush-border membrane, and beyond, *Can. J. Physiol. Pharmacol.*, 71, 531, 1993.

41. Cohn, J.S., McNamara, J.R., Krasinski, S.D., Russell, R.M., and Schaefer, E.J., Role of triglyceride-rich lipoproteins from the liver and intestine in the etiology of postprandial peaks in plasma triglyceride concentration, *Metabol.*, 38, 484, 1989.

42. Bach, A. C. and Babayan, V. K., Medium-chain triglycerides: an update, *Am. J. Clin. Nutr.*, 36, 950, 1982.

43. Ledeboer, M., Masclee, A. A., Jansen, J. B., and Lamers, C.B., Effect of equimolar amounts of long-chain triglycerides and medium-chain triglycerides on small-bowl transit time in humans, *JPEN*, 19, 5, 1995.

44. Verkijk, M., Gielkens, H. A., Lamers, C. B., and Masclee, A. A., Effects of medium-chain and long-chain triglycerides on antroduodenal motility and small bowel transit time in man, *Dig. Dis. Sci.*, 42, 1933, 1997.

45. Beckers, E. J., Jeukendrup, A. E., Brouns, F., Wagenmakers, A. J., and Saris, W. H., Gastric emptying of carbohydrate-medium chain triglyceride suspensions at rest, *Int. J. Sports Med.*, 13, 581, 1992.

46. Rehrer, N. J., Wagenmakers, A. J., Beckers, E. J., Halliday, D., Leiper, J. B., Brouns, F., Maughan, R. J., Westerterp, K., and Saris, W. H., Gastric emptying, absorption, and carbohydrate oxidation during prolonged exercise, *J. Appl. Physiol.*, 72, 468, 1992.

47. Wagenmakers, A. J., Brouns, F., Saris, W. H., and Halliday, D., Oxidation rates of orally ingested carbohydrates during prolonged exercise in men, *J. Appl. Physiol.*, 75, 2774, 1993.

48. Jeukendrup, A. E., Saris, W. H., Schrauwen, P., Brouns, F., and Wagenmakers, J. M., Metabolic availability of medium-chain triglycerides coingested with carbohydrates during prolonged exercise, *J. Appl. Physiol.*, 79, 756, 1995.

49. Van Zyl, G. G., Lambert, E. V., Hawley, J. A., Noakes, T. D., and Dennis, S. C., Effects of medium-chain triglyceride ingestion on fuel metabolism on cycling performance, *J. Appl. Physiol.*, 80, 2217, 1996.

50. Mei, N., Intestinal Chemosensitivity, *Physiol. Rev.*, 65, 211, 1985.

51. Minami, H. and McCallum, R. W., The physiology and pathophysiology of gastric emptying in humans, *Gastroenterol.*, 86, 1592, 1984.

52. Sarna, S. K. and Otterson, M. F., Small intestinal physiology and pathophysiology, *Gastroenterol. Clin. North Am.*, 18, 375, 1989.

53. Hunt, J. N., Mechanisms and disorders of gastric emptying, *Ann. Rev. Med.*, 34, 219, 1983.

54. Hunt, J. N. and Stubbs, D. F., The volume and energy content of meals as determinants of gastric emptying, *J. Physiol.*, 245, 209, 1975.

55. Hunt, J. N., Smith, J. L., and Jiang, C. L., Effect of meal volume and energy density on the gastric emptying of carbohydrates, *Gastroenterol.*, 89, 1326, 1985.

56. Jansen, J. B., Fried, M., Hopman, W. P., Lamers, C. B., and Meyer, J. H., Relation between gastric emptying of albumin-dextrose meals and cholesystokinin release in man, *Dig. Dis. Sci.*, 39, 571, 1994.

57. Liddle, R. A., Rushakoff, R. J., Morita, E. T., Beccaria, L., Carter, J. D., and Goldfine, I. D., Physiological role for cholesystokinin in reducing postprandial hyperglycemia in humans, *J. Clin. Invest.*, 81, 1675, 1988.

58. Schwizer, W., Asal, K., Kreiss, C., Mettraux, C., Borovicka, M. J., Remy, B., Guzelhan, C., Hartman, D., and Fried, M., Role of lipase in the regulation of upper gastrointestinal function in humans, *Am. J. Physiol.*, 273, G612, 1997.

59. Miller, L. J., Malagelada, J., Taylor, W. F., and Go, L. W., Intestinal control of human postprandial gastric function: the role of components of jejunoileal chyme in regulating gastric secretion and gastric emptying, *Gastroenterol.*, 80, 763, 1981.

60. Lin, H. C., Doty, J. E., Reedy, T. J., and Meyer, J. H., Inhibition of gastric emptying by glucose depends on length of intestine exposed to nutrient, *Am. J. Physiol.*, 256, G404, 1989.

61. Lin, H. C., Doty, J. E., Reedy, J., and Meyer, J. H., Inhibition of gastric emptying by sodium oleate depends on length of intestine exposed to nutrient, *Am. J. Physiol.*, 259, G1031, 1990.

62. Lin, H. C., Elashoff, J. D., Gu, Y., and Meyer, J. H., Nutrient feedback inhibition of gastric emptying plays a larger role than osmotically dependent duodenal resistance, *Am. J. Physiol.*, 265, G672, 1993.

63. Lin, H. C., Zhao, X., and Wang, L., Intestinal transit is more potently inhibited by fat in the distal (ileal brake) than in the proximal (jejunal brake) gut, *Dig. Dis. Sci.*, 42, 19, 1997.

64. Holgate, A. M. and Read, N. W., Effect of ileal infusion of intralipid on gastrointestinal transit, ileal flow rate, and carbohydrate absorption in humans after ingestion of a liquid meal, *Gastroenterol.*, 88, 1005, 1985.

65. Spiller, R. C., Trotman, I. F., Higgins, B. E., Ghatei, M. A., Grimble, G. K., Lee, Y. C., Bloom, S. R., Misiewicz, J. J., and Silk, D. B., The ileal brake—inhibition of jejunal motility after ileal fat perfusion in man, *Gut*, 25, 365, 1984.

66. Spiller, R. C., Trotman, I. F., Adrian, T. E., Bloom, S. R., Misiewicz, J. J., and Silk, D. B., Further characterization of the "ileal brake" reflex in man—effect of ileal infusion of partial digests of fat, protein, and starch on jejunal motility and release of neurotensin, enteroglucagon, and peptide YY, *Gut*, 29, 1042, 1988.

67. Layer, P., Zinsmeister, A. R., and DiMagno, E. P., Effects of decreasing intraluminal amylase activity on starch digestion and postprandial gastrointestinal function in humans, *Gastroenterol.*, 91, 41, 1986.

68. Moses, F. M., The effect of exercise on the gastrointestinal tract, *Sports Med.*, 9, 159, 1990.

69. Keeffe, E. B., Lowe, D. K., Goss, J. R., and Wayne, R., Gastrointestinal symptoms of marathon runners, *West J. Med.*, 141, 481, 1984.

70. Riddoch, C. and Trinick, T., Gastrointestinal disturbances in marathon runners, *Brit. J. Sports Med.*, 22, 71, 1988.

71. Worobetz, L. J. and Gerrard, D. F., Gastrointestinal symptoms during exercise in Enduro athletes: prevalence and speculations on the aetiology, *New Zeal. Med. J.*, 98, 644, 1985.

72. Brouns, F., Saris, W. H., and Rehrer, N. J., Abdominal complaints and gastrointestinal function during long-lasting exercise, *Int. J. Sports Med.*, 8, 175, 1987.

73. Brouns, F. and Beckers, E., Is the gut an athletic organ? Digestion, absorption and exercise, *Sports Med.*, 15, 242, 1993.

74. Gisolfi, C. V. and Ryan, A. J., Gastrointestinal physiology during exercise, in *Body Fluid Balance. Exercise and Sport*, Buskirk, E.R. and Puhl, S.M., Eds., New York, CRC Press LLC, 1996, 19.

75. Murray, R., The effects of consuming carbohydrate-electrolyte beverages on gastric emptying and fluid absorption during and following exercise, *Sports Med.*, 4, 322, 1987.

76. Gisolfi, C. V. and Duchman, S. M., Guidelines for optimal replacement beverages for different athletic events, *Med. Sci. Sports Exerc.*, 24, 679, 1992.

77. Costill, D. L. and Saltin, B., Factors limiting gastric emptying during rest and exercise, *J. Appl. Physiol.*, 37, 679, 1974.

78. Noakes, T. D., Rehrer, N. J., and Maughan, R. J., The importance of volume in regulating gastric emptying, *Med. Sci. Sports Exerc.*, 23, 307, 1991.

79. Mitchell, J. B., Costill, D. L., Houmard, J. A., Fink, W. J., Robergs, R. A., and Davis, J. A., Gastric emptying: influence of prolonged exercise and carbohydrate concentration, *Med. Sci. Sports Exerc.*, 21, 269, 1989.

80. Mitchell, J. B. and Voss, K. W., The influence of volume on gastric emptying and fluid balance during prolonged exercise, *Med. Sci. Sports Exerc.*, 23, 314, 1991.

81. Owen, M. D., Kregel, K. C., Wall, P. T., and Gisolfi, C. V., Effects of ingesting carbohydrate beverages during exercise in the heat, *Med. Sci. Sports Exerc.*, 18, 568, 1986.

82. Rehrer, N. J., Brouns, F., Beckers, E. J., Ten Hoor, F., and Saris, W. H., Gastric emptying with repeated drinking during running and bicycling, *Int. J. Sports Med.*, 11, 238, 1990.

83. Ryan, A. J., Bleiler, T. L., Carter, J. E., and Gisolfi, C. V., Gastric emptying during prolonged cycling in the heat, *Med. Sci. Sports. Exerc.*, 21, 51, 1989.

84. Coyle, E. F. and Montain, S. J., Carbohydrate and fluid ingestion during exercise: are there trade-offs?, *Med. Sci. Sports Exerc.*, 24, 671, 1992.

85. Hawley, J. A., Dennis, S. C., and Noakes, T. D., Carbohydrate, fluid and electrolyte requirements during prolonged exercise, in *Sports Nutrition. Minerals and Electrolytes*, Chapter 19, Kies, C. V. and Driskell, J. A., Eds., Boca Raton, FL, CRC Press LLC, 1995, 235.

86. Neufer, P. D., Young, A. J., and Sawka, M. N., Gastric emptying during walking and running: effects of varied exercise intensity, *Eur. J. Appl. Physiol.*, 58, 440, 1989.

87. Houmard, J. A., Egan, P. C., Johns, R. A., Neufer, P. D., Chenier, T. C., and Israel, R. G., Gastric emptying during 1 h of cycling and running at 75% $\dot{V}O_{2\,max}$, *Med. Sci. Sports Exerc.*, 23, 320, 1991.

88. Neufer, P. D., Young, A. J., and Sawka, M. N., Gastric emptying during exercise: effects of heat stress and hypohydration, *Eur. J. Appl. Physiol.*, 58, 433, 1989.

89. Rehrer, N. J., Beckers, E. J., Brouns, F., Hoor, F. T., and Saris, W. H., Effects of dehydration on gastric emptying and gastrointestinal distress while running, *Med. Sci. Sports Exerc.*, 22, 790, 1990.

90. Ryan, A. J., Lambert, G., Shi, X., Chang, R., Summers, R., and Gisolfi, C., Effect of hypohydration on gastric emptying and intestinal absorption during exercise, *J. Appl. Physiol.*, 84, 1581, 1998.

91. Rehrer, N. J., Beckers, E., Brouns, F., Ten Hoor, F., and Saris, W. H., Exercise and training effects on gastric emptying of carbohydrate beverages, *Med. Sci. Sports Exerc.*, 21(5), 540-549, 1989.

92. Read, N. W. and Houghton, L. A., Physiology of gastric emptying and pathophysiology of gastroparesis, *Gastroenter. Clin. North Am.*, 18, 359, 1989.

93. Lartigue, S., Bizais, Y., Varannes, S. B., Murat, A., Pouliquen, B., and Galmiche, J. P., Inter- and intrasubject variability of solid and liquid gastric parameters. A scintigraphic study in healthy subjects and diabetic patients, *Dig. Dis. Sci.*, 39, 109, 1994.

94. Modigliani, R., Rambaud, J. C., and Bernier, J. J., The method of intraluminal perfusion of the human small intestine. I. Principle and technique, *Digestion*, 9, 176, 1973.

95. Fordtran, J. S. and Saltin, B., Gastric emptying and intestinal absorption during prolonged severe exercise, *J. Appl. Physiol.*, 23, 331, 1967.

96. Gisolfi, C. V., Spranger, K. J., Summers, R. W., Schedl, H. P., and Bleiler, T. L., Effects of cycle exercise on intestinal absorption in humans, *J. Appl. Physiol.*, 71, 2518, 1991.

97. Lambert, G. P., Chang, R. T., Joensen, D., Shi, X., Summers, R. W., Schedl, H. P., and Gisolfi, C. V., Simultaneous determination of gastric emptying and intestinal absorption during cycling exercise in humans, *Int. J. Sports. Med.*, 17, 48, 1996.

98. Lambert, G. P., Chang, R. T., Xia, T., Summers, R. W., and Gisolfi, C. V., Absorption from different intestinal segments during exercise, *J. Appl. Physiol.*, 83, 204, 1997.

99. Gisolfi, C. V., Intestinal absorption of fluids during rest and exercise, in *Perspectives in Exercise Science and Sports Medicine. Fluid Homeostasis During Exercise.*, Gisolfi, C. V. and Lamb, D. R., Eds., Indianapolis, Benchmark Press, 1990, 129.

100. Hawely, J. A., Bosch, A. N., Weltan, S. M., Dennis, S. C., and Noakes, T. D., Effects of glucose ingestion or glucose infusion on fuel substrate kinetics during prolonged exercise, *Eur. J. Appl. Physiol. Occup. Physiol.*, 68, 381, 1994.

101. Duchman, S. M., Ryan, A. J., Schedl, H. P., Summers, R. W., Bleiler, T. L., and Gisolfi, C. V., Upper limit for intestinal absorption of a dilute glucose solution in men at rest, *Med. Sci. Sports Exerc.*, 29, 482, 1997.

102. Gisolfi, C. V., Summers, R. W., Schedl, H. P., Bleiler, T. L., and Oppliger, R. A., Human intestinal water absorption: direct vs. indirect measurements, *Am. J. Physiol.*, 258, G216, 1990.

103. Gisolfi, C. V., Summers, R. W., Schedl, H. P., and Bleiler, T. L., Intestinal water absorption from select carbohydrate solutions in humans, *J. Appl. Physiol.*, 7, 2142, 1992.

104. Shi, X., Summers, R. W., Schedl, H. P., Chang, R. T., Lambert, G. P., and Gisolfi, C. V., Effects of solution osmolality on absorption of select fluid replacement solutions in human duodenojejunum, *J. Appl. Physiol.*, 77, 1178, 1994.

105. Shi, X., Summers, R. W., Schedl, H. P., Flanagan, S. W., Chang, R., and Gisolfi, C. V., Effects of carbohydrate type and concentration and solution somolality on water absorption, *Med. Sci. Sports Exerc.*, 27(12), 1607-1615, 1995.

106. Shi, X., Schedl, H. P., Summers, R. M., Lambert, G. P., Chang, R., Xia, T., and Gisolfi, C. V., Fructose transport mechanisms in humans, *Gastroenterol.*, 113, 1171, 1997.

107. Rumessen, J. J. and Gudmand-Hoyer, E., Absorption capacity of fructose in healthy adults. Comparison with sucrose and its constituent monosaccharides, *Gut*, 27, 1161, 1986.

108. Rumessen, J. J., Fructose and related food carbohydrates. Sources, intake, absorption, and clinical implications., *Scand. J. Gastroenterol.*, 27, 819, 1992.

109. Ravich, W. J., Bayless, T. M., and Thomas, M., Fructose: incomplete intestinal absorption in humans, *Gastroenterol.*, 84, 26, 1983.

110. Fujisawa, T., Mulligan, K., Wada, L., Schumacher, L., Riby, J., and Kretchmer, N., The effect of exercise on fructose absorption, *Am. J. Clin. Nutr.*, 58(75), 75, 1993.

111. Rowell, L. B., Brengelmann, G. L., Blackmon, J. R., Twiss, R. D., and Kusumi, F., Splanchnic blood flow and metabolism in heat-stressed man, *J. Appl. Physiol.*, 24, 475, 1968.

112. Granger, D. N., Richardson, P. D., Kvietys, P. R., and Mortillaro, N. A., Intestinal blood flow, *Gastroenterol.*, 78, 837, 1980.

113. Qamar, M. I. and Read, A. E., Effects of exercise on mesenteric blood flow in man, *Gut*, 28, 583, 1987.

114. Eriksen, M. and Waaler, B. A., Priority of blood flow to splanchnic organs in humans during pre- and post-meal exercise, *Acta Physiol. Scand.*, 150, 363, 1994.

115. Sherman, W. M. and Costill, D. L., The marathon: dietary manipulation to optimize performance, *Am. J. Sports Med.*, 12, 44, 1984.

116. Lambert, E. V., Speechly, D. P., Dennis, S. C., and Noakes, T. D., Enhanced endurance in trained cyclists during moderate intensity exercise following 2 weeks adaptation to a high fat diet, *Eur. J. Appl. Physiol.*, 69, 287, 1994.

117. Lambert, E. V., Hawley, J. A., Goedecke, J., Noakes, T. D., and Dennis, S. C., Nutritional stategies for promoting fat utilization and delaying the onset of fatigue during prolonged exercise, *J. Sports Sci.*, 15, 315, 1997.

118. Williamson, R. C., Intestinal adaptation (first of two parts). Structural, functional and cytokinetic changes, *N. Eng. J. Med.*, 298, 1393, 1978.

119. Ferraris, R. P. and Diamond, J. M., Specific regulation of intestinal nutrient transporters by their dietary substrates, *Ann. Rev. Physiol.*, 51, 125, 1989.
120. Thomson, A. B., Keelan, M., and Wild, G. E., Nutrients and intestinal adaptation, *Clin. Invest. Med.*, 19, 331, 1996.
121. Harris, A., Lindeman, A. K., and Martin, B. J., Rapid orocecal transit in chronically active persons with high energy intake, *J. Appl. Physiol.*, 70, 1550, 1991.
122. Hutson, W. R. and Wald, A., Gastric emptying in patients with bulemia nervosa and anorexia nervosa, *Am. J. Gastroenterol.*, 85, 41, 1990.
123. McCallum, R. W., Grill, B. B., Lange, R., Planky, M., Glass, E. E., and Greenfield, D. G., Definition of a gastric emptying abnormality in patients with anorexia nervosa, *Dig. Dis. Sci.*, 30, 713, 1985.
124. Robinson, P. H., Clarke, M., and Barret, J., Determinants of delayed gastric emptying in anorexia nervosa and bulemia nervosa, *Gut*, 29, 458, 1988.
125. Kamal, N., Chami, T., Andersen, A., Rosell, F. A., Schuster, M. M., and Whitehead, W. E., Delayed gastroinestinal transit times in anoxexia nervosa and bulemia nervosa, *Gastroenterol.*, 101, 1320, 1991.
126. Rigaud, D., Bedig, G., Merrouche, M., Vulpillat, M., Bonfils, S., and Apfelbaum, M., Delayed gastric emptying in anorexia nervosa is improved by completion of a renutrition program, *Dig. Dis. Sci.*, 33, 919, 1988.
127. Cunningham, K. M., Horowitz, M., and Read, N. W., The effect of short-term dietary supplementation with glucose on gastric emptying in humans, *Brit. J. Nutr.*, 65, 15, 1991.
128. Horowitz, M., Wishart, J. M., Jones, K. L., and Hebbard, G. S., Gastric emptying in diabetes: an overview, *Diabet. Med.*, 13, S16, 1996.
129. Cunningham, K. M., Daly, J., Horowitz, M., and Read, N. W., Gastrointestinal adaptation to diets of differing fat composition in human volunteers, *Gut*, 32, 483, 1991.
130. Brown, N. J., Rumsey, R. D., and Read, N. W., Gastrointestinal adaptation to enhanced small intestinal lipid exposure, *Gut*, 35, 1409, 1994.
131. Jenkins, A. P. and Thompson, R. P., Mechanisms of small intestinal adaptation, *Dig. Dis.*, 12, 15, 1994.
132. Wolvekamp, M. C., Heineman, E., Taylor, R. G., and Fuller, P. J., Towards understanding the process of intestinal adaptation, *Dig. Dis.*, 14, 59, 1996.
133. Thomson, A. B., Keelan, M., Sigalet, D., Fedorak, R., Garg, M., and Clandinin, M. T., Patterns, mechanisms and signals for intestinal adaptation, *Dig. Dis.*, 8, 99, 1990.
134. Rosensweig, N. S., Herman, R. H., and Stifel, F. B., Dietary regulation of small intestinal enzyme activity in man, *Am. J. Clin. Nutr.*, 24, 65, 1971.
135. Cheeseman, C. I. and Harley, B., Adaptation of glucose transport across rat enterocyte basolateral membrane in response to altered dietary carbohydrate intake, *J. Physiol.*, 437, 563, 1991.
136. Diamond, J. M. and Karasov, W. H., Effect of dietary carbohydrate on monosaccharide uptake by mouse small intestine in vitro, *J. Physiol.*, 349, 419, 1984.
137. Solberg, D. H. and Diamond, J. M., Comparison of different dietary sugars as inducers of intestinal sugar transporters, *Am. J. Physiol.*, 252, G574, 1987.
138. Stein, E. D., Chang, S. D., and Diamond, J. M., Comparison of different dietary amino acids as inducers of intestinal amino acid transport, *Am. J. Physiol.*, 252, G626, 1987.
139. Thomson, A. B., Keelan, M., Clandinin, M. T., and Walker, K., Dietary fat selectively alters transport properties of rat jejunum, *J. Clin. Invest.*, 77, 279, 1986.

CHAPTER 4

Simple and Complex Carbohydrates in Exercise and Sport

J. Andrew Doyle and Charilaos Papadopoulos

CONTENTS

4.1 INTRODUCTION

Carbohydrates and fats provide the predominant substrates utilized for energy production during endurance exercise. The energy demands of competitive endurance training and competition generally exceed the rate at which fat can be oxidized, so carbohydrates are the predominant fuel source for these athletic activities. Carbohydrate is also the major source of energy for repetitive, high-intensity activities that utilize the anaerobic glycolytic energy system. It has been well-established that severely reduced carbohydrate stores, i.e. muscle glycogen, liver glycogen, and blood glucose, are closely associated with fatigue and impaired performance in prolonged endurance tasks.[4] Therefore, a considerable amount of research has focused upon methods to manipulate endogenous carbohydrate stores and to facilitate carbohydrate intake in an attempt to enhance carbohydrate oxidation and improve athletic performance in training and competition.

Research of carbohydrate manipulation has generally focused on one or more of the time periods when its alteration may have a significant impact on endurance exercise performance: 1) daily training, 2) the week before a prolonged event, 3) the hours (meal) before exercise, 4) during the exercise task, and 5) the post-exercise period (4–48 hours). The majority of this research has attempted to determine the optimal amount of carbohydrate to consume, the appropriate timing of the consumption, and within a fairly narrow focus, the appropriate type of carbohydrate. Studies of carbohydrate type have largely focused on the efficacy of different simple sugars (e.g., glucose and fructose) or polymers of glucose and the optimal concentration of those carbohydrates in a beverage. Comparably less attention has been given to carbohydrates in other forms, such as solid or semi-solid, or by their characterization as complex carbohydrates, and how their consumption may affect endurance exercise performance.

Rather than considering carbohydrates in the basic classification as simple or complex, a relatively recent approach in sports nutrition research has been to study carbohydrates by the physiological response they provoke, particularly the blood glucose and insulin response that results from their consumption. This categorization by glycemic response, known as the Glycemic Index,[30] may be a more appropriate way to look at carbohydrates, since not all simple carbohydrates provoke the same glycemic response and there is a wide range of responses among complex carbohydrates.

Training and competing athletes must make appropriate dietary decisions concerning carbohydrate intake: optimal amounts, timing, and types. They must consider the effect of carbohydrate intake on short-term training and competitive performance, but they must also keep in mind the potential effect of dietary choices on long-term health and fitness. This chapter examines the role of carbohydrates in exercise and sport and makes practical recommendations by which the athlete can choose a healthy fundamental diet and can further optimize carbohydrate intake to potentially enhance exercise performance.

4.2 SIMPLE AND COMPLEX CARBOHYDRATES

Carbohydrates can be characterized by their structure and by the number of sugar molecules as either monosaccharides, disaccharides, or polysaccharides. Monosaccharides, containing one sugar molecule, such as glucose and fructose, are simple sugars. Disaccharides, such as sucrose, contain two sugar molecules, are also characterized as simple carbohydrates. Simple carbohydrates and typical sources in the diet are listed in Table 4.1.

Table 4.1 Simple Carbohydrates

Carbohydrate	Comments
Monosaccharides:	
Glucose	Also known as dextrose; found in plant foods, fruits, honey
Fructose	Also known as fruit sugar; found in plant foods, fruits, honey
Galactose	Product of lactose digestion
Disaccharides:	
Sucrose	Also known as white or table sugar; composed of glucose and fructose; used as a sweetener
Lactose	Composed of galactose and glucose; found in milk and dairy products
Maltose	Composed of 2 glucose molecules; a product of starch digestion

Polysaccharides, with many glucose units chained together, are considered complex carbohydrates. Starches, dextrins, fiber, and processed concentrated sugars compose complex carbohydrates. Malto-dextrins are polysaccharides — glucose polymers — but contain no starch or fiber and are metabolized like simple sugars. Complex carbohydrates and typical dietary sources are listed in Table 4.2.

Table 4.2. Complex Carbohydrates

Carbohydrate	Comments
Polysaccharides:	
Amylopectin	Starch; found in plant foods and grains
Amylose	Starch; found in plant foods and grains
Carrageenan	Soluble fiber; found in the extract of seaweed and used as food thickener and stabilizer
Cellulose	Insoluble fiber; found in the bran layers of grains, seeds, edible skins and peels
Corn Syrup	Hydrolyzed starch; found in processed foods
Dextrins	Starch; found in processed foods
Glycogen	Animal starch; found in meat, liver
Hemicellulose	Insoluble fiber; found in the bran layers of grains, seeds, edible skins and peels
Inulin	Soluble fiber; found in Jerusalem artichokes
Invert Sugar	Hydrolyzed sucrose; found in processed foods
Lignin	Insoluble fiber; found in plant cell walls
Pectins	Soluble fiber; found in apples

4.2.1 Digestion and Absorption

A wide variety of factors, alone and in combination, can affect the digestion and absorption of carbohydrates, including the form of the carbohydrate, the type and content of fiber, the type of starch, the presence of other nutrients, the size of the food particles, and the methods of cooking and processing.[8] A brief overview is presented here.

Digestion and absorption of carbohydrates begins to a small degree in the mouth. Salivary amylases begin the process of digestion for complex carbohydrates by initiating the breakdown of starches and dextrins. Chewing, or mastication, is also an important part of the digestive process to reduce foods to smaller sized particles. Mechanical action of the stomach continues this process of size reduction, which influences both rate of gastric emptying of food into the small intestine, and the surface area of the food particles accessible to intestinal enzymes.

The majority of carbohydrate digestion and absorption occurs in the small intestine. After moving into the small intestine, the monosaccharides (glucose, fructose, and galactose) are absorbed directly into the capillaries within the intestinal villi. The disaccharides (sucrose, lactose, and maltose) are split into their constituent monosaccharides by disaccharidases and are then directly absorbed into the blood. The complex carbohydrates are acted upon by pancreatic amylase and brush border enzymes that reduce polysaccharides to monosaccharides, which are then absorbed as above. The monosaccharides that are absorbed into the intestinal circulation are transported to the liver via the hepatic portal vein. From this point forward, carbohydrate is utilized by the body either as glucose or is stored as glycogen.

Not all of the carbohydrate content of foods is digested and absorbed. The amount that is not absorbed may be because of the form of the food, the type of starch, and the amount of fiber present in the food. Undigested and unabsorbed carbohydrates go to the large intestine, where they may be digested by colonic bacteria or excreted in the feces. Large amounts of indigestible carbohydrates, or excessive amounts of simple sugars consumed rapidly, may result in excessive gas production or gastrointestinal disturbances, such as cramping and diarrhea. The fiber content of carbohydrate foods, which is largely indigestible by humans, plays an important role in maintaining appropriate gastric transit, may influence the eventual glycemic response to the foods consumed, and has important long-term health implications.

4.2.2 Glycemic Index

Under normal circumstances, the physiological result of carbohydrate consumption, digestion, and absorption is a postprandial increase in blood glucose, followed by an increase in glucose uptake by tissues in the body, which is facilitated by insulin secretion by the pancreas. The time course and magnitude of this glycemic response are highly variable with different foods and do not follow the basic structural characterization of carbohydrates as simple or complex. For example, the consumption of identical amounts of two simple sugars, glucose and fructose, results in very different blood glucose responses. Glucose ingestion provokes a rapid and large increase in blood glucose, which in turn rapidly returns to baseline levels. Fructose consumption, on the other hand, results in a much slower and lower glycemic response. This variability in postprandial glycemic response with different foods has important implications, particularly for people who must carefully control their blood glucose level, such as people with diabetes. Because the glycemic response to carbohydrate consumption is not easily predictable by their characterization as simple or complex, the concept of the Glycemic Index (GI) was created, tested on a variety of foods, and initially published by Jenkins, et al. in 1981.[30]

The Glycemic Index is a ranking based upon the postprandial blood glucose response of a particular food compared to a reference food. Specifically, the GI is a percentage of the area under the glucose response curve for a specific food compared to the area under the glucose response curve for the reference food:[29]

$$GI = \left(\frac{\text{Blood glucose area of test food}}{\text{Blood glucose area of reference food}} \right) \times 100$$

Glucose or white bread containing 50 g of carbohydrate is typically used as the reference food. Test foods contain an identical amount of carbohydrate, and the blood glucose response is determined for either two or three hours after consumption of the meal.[52] Extensive testing of foods has resulted in the publication of tables of glycemic indices for a wide variety of foods.[20] Glycemic Index has become an important reference tool for prescribing appropriate diets for clinical populations that have a need for close regulation of blood glucose, such as people with diabetes. The GI is based upon physiological measurement; therefore, a high degree of precision cannot be expected. However, reviews of numerous GI studies indicate a high degree of consistency of response with the same foods, within approximately 10–15 units of measurement for most foods.[52] The GI of glucose (GI = 100) and fructose (GI = 23) clearly demonstrates the vast difference in glycemic response that can occur with the consumption of these two structurally similar monosaccharides.

Athletes may also benefit from considering the GI of the carbohydrates they consume as well as whether they are categorized as simple or complex carbohydrates. There may be specific situations in which an athlete would want to consume high glycemic index foods and provoke a large blood glucose and insulin response (e.g., when attempting to synthesize muscle glycogen quickly).[7] Conversely, there may be occasions when an athlete may want to consume lower GI foods and avoid large increases in glucose and insulin. There is controversial evidence that the hyperglycemia and hyperinsulinemia associated with high GI foods consumed shortly before the onset of endurance exercise suppresses fat oxidation and may have a negative impact upon subsequent performance.[51] Therefore, the concept of the Glycemic Index will be revisited in the sections on carbohydrate manipulation that follow.

4.3 CRITICAL PERIODS FOR CARBOHYDRATE MANIPULATION

Substantial research has been published on the effect of carbohydrate intake on exercise performance. In general, carbohydrate manipulation has been shown to be most effective for prolonged endurance activities (more than two hours) where carbohydrate stores and oxidation may limit performance or is related to fatigue. A few studies have indicated a potential ergogenic effect of carbohydrate loading, pre-exercise meals, or intake during exercise on shorter duration, high intensity activity,[35] but the evidence is not sufficiently strong to definitively recommend carbohydrate use for improving performance in these types of activities.

An athlete must contemplate two major considerations when making dietary plans concerning carbohydrate intake. First, for maintenance of long-term health, most major health organizations recommend that carbohydrate make up the majority of energy intake. Second, athletes must consider the demands of their sport or activity and determine if it is appropriate to further manipulate carbohydrate intake to positively influence physical performance in training or competition.

Research of carbohydrate manipulation has typically used simple carbohydrates in beverages when consumption of other forms of carbohydrate (e.g., solid food) may be difficult or poorly tolerated. Use of complex/solid carbohydrate during exercise may not be necessary unless the exercise task is very prolonged, to the point that satiety and satisfaction is improved with solid food intake (e.g., ultramarathons). An examination of the critical dietary periods for carbohydrate intake follows, with reference where applicable, to recommendations about complex versus simple carbohydrate intake.

4.3.1   The Daily Training Diet

The first consideration for an athlete's daily training diet is to conform to recommendations for a long-term healthy dietary intake. Carbohydrates should make up the bulk of total energy intake, primarily in the form of grain products, vegetables, and fruits. This concept is represented visually by the Food Guide Pyramid (Figure 4.1). Individuals should further seek to limit total fat, saturated

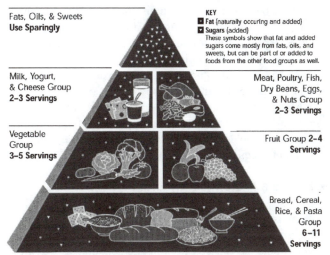

Figure 4.1   The Food Guide Pyramid: A Guide to Daily Food Choices

fat, and cholesterol in their diet. The Dietary Guidelines for Americans[36] further recommend that people choose a diet that is moderate in sugars. The implication with this recommendation is an emphasis on complex carbohydrates and some simple sugars as consumed in grains, vegetables, and fruits and a reduction in the intake of simple sugars that are typically consumed in soft drinks and snack foods. There is an emphasis on complex carbohydrates because several studies[41,42] have shown an increased risk of chronic disease, particularly Non-insulin-dependent Diabetes Mellitus (NIDDM), with a long-term dietary intake of foods with a high glycemic load, especially in conjunction with low fiber consumption. By emphasizing food choices from the base of the Food Guide Pyramid, athletes can easily consume a varied diet that is adequate in carbohydrate and also contains sufficient vitamins, minerals, and fiber.

To reduce the risk of chronic disease and promote long-term health, several health organizations make basic dietary recommendations that apply to athletes. For reduced risk of heart disease, the American Heart Association recommends the diet consist of 55–60% or more of energy intake from carbohydrates, with an emphasis on complex carbohydrates. It further recommends that fat comprise 30% or less of the diet, with 8–10% from saturated fats.[1] To reduce one's risk of various common forms of cancer, the American Cancer Society recommends the diet be mainly composed of foods from plant sources, with a minimum of five servings of fruits and/or vegetables each day, coupled with a limited intake of high-fat foods.[48] These dietary guidelines are well-suited for active and athletic populations, giving a dietary foundation for long-term health, as well as providing a varied diet that is predominately composed of carbohydrates for fueling exercise.

Athletes must further consider if the carbohydrate content of their diet is sufficient to support optimal performance in training and competition. The recommendation of The American Dietetic Association and The Canadian Dietetic Association[2] is that, in general, the diet should be 60–65% carbohydrate, and elevated to 65–70% if the individual is engaged in exhaustive training. It is important to note that total energy intake must be sufficient to obtain the necessary amount of carbohydrate. If total caloric intake is too low, even a diet that is more than 70% carbohydrate may yield an inadequate number of grams of carbohydrate. Therefore, carbohydrate consumption should be considered on an absolute basis (number of grams for each kilogram of body weight) to ensure adequate intake.

Carbohydrate content of the diet should be sufficient to maintain muscle glycogen stores during periods of intense training or muscle glycogen concentrations progressively decline.[10] Inadequate muscle glycogen levels may be associated with diminished training and competitive performance.[3] For athletes engaged in exhaustive training, it is apparent that the diet may need to contain up to 10 grams of carbohydrate per kilogram of body weight each day to adequately replace the muscle glycogen used during daily training.[45] People involved in activities or training of lesser intensity and duration do not need to consume this much carbohydrate, but they should maintain their carbohydrate intake at 7 grams per kilogram of body weight or more, depending upon their level of activity. It may be difficult to consume this large amount of carbohydrate as food, and athletes may want to consider using carbohydrate supplements, particularly in liquid form, to increase their intake. Liquid carbohydrate supplements have the added advantage of increasing fluid intake, helping the athlete maintain adequate hydration levels.

4.3.2   The Week Before a Prolonged Endurance Event

Manipulation of exercise and carbohydrate content of the diet over a week's time has been shown to result in supranormal levels of muscle glycogen, which in turn enhances carbohydrate oxidation and improves endurance capacity in prolonged endurance activities such as cycling and running.[3,44] This strategy is known as "carbohydrate loading," or "muscle glycogen supercompensation." Most studies of muscle glycogen supercompensation have shown an increase in "time to exhaustion" during exercise at a moderate-to-high intensity, but few have assessed the effect on more valid and reliable measures of endurance performance.

Early studies showed a near doubling of muscle glycogen following the strategy referred to as the "classical" carbohydrate-loading method[3] However, this method has some onerous exercise and dietary demands that may be unacceptable to the athlete preparing for an important competition. Muscle glycogen is depleted with prolonged, exhaustive exercise and is maintained in a suppressed state for the next three days with a virtually carbohydrate-free diet. Depleting exercise is performed again to further reduce glycogen stores, after which the athlete rests and consumes a carbohydrate-rich diet for the three days before the event. While resulting in the highest muscle glycogen stores, this method of carbohydrate loading may have other adverse physical and psychological effects that may not be advantageous for subsequent performance.

Because of the extreme exercise and dietary manipulations of the classical carbohydrate-loading method, many athletes may choose a more palatable method referred to as "modified" carbohydrate loading[44] (Figure 4.2). In this method, athletes taper their training, following a more realistic exercise preparation during the week before an important event. Early in the week when athletes exercise for longer duration, the diet is manipulated to include a higher percentage of fat and protein and less carbohydrate (approximately 50% of total calories). The final three days before the event, when the athlete exercises the least, the amount of carbohydrate in the diet increases to 70% or more, stimulating muscle glycogen storage. The amount of muscle glycogen synthesis following this modification is nearly as great as with the classical method, but the difficulties associated with exhaustive exercise and a period of very low carbohydrate diet are avoided.

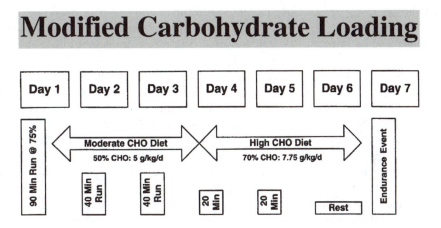

Figure 4.2   The Modified Carbohydrate Loading strategy. Adapted with permission from Sherman et al.

The earliest studies[3,44] did not describe in detail the composition of the diet used, but the carbohydrate content apparently consisted of a combination of complex and simple carbohydrates. Two more recent studies have investigated the efficacy of one type of carbohydrate over the other,[6,40] and both concluded there was no advantage of either a predominately simple or a predominately complex carbohydrate diet in the three-day high carbohydrate period of the loading phase. Both types of carbohydrate in the diet increased muscle glycogen similarly and had a similarly positive impact on subsequent endurance exercise. Carbohydrate loading is a short-term, relatively infrequent manipulation of diet and exercise, and the incorporation of simple sugars during this period should not pose any significant dietary health risk for the athlete. It is recommended, however, that long-term dietary composition be composed mostly of complex carbohydrates with a lower glycemic load because of the relationship of chronic low fiber, high glycemic diets to increased risk of NIDDM.[41,42]

4.3.3 The Meal Before Exercise

The meal consumed just prior to a training bout or competitive event may also be used to maximize carbohydrate stores in an attempt to improve performance. If these meals consist primarily of carbohydrate, they act to maximize muscle and liver glycogen stores before the onset of exercise. It has been conclusively demonstrated that fasting before prolonged endurance events results in diminished performance,[14] so it is important for the athlete to consume a meal in the hours before long training sessions or competitive efforts. The meal should provide adequate energy and carbohydrate to support the metabolic demands of the exercise, be consumed in adequate time before the onset of exercise to allow for gastric emptying, digestion, and absorption, and be palatable and acceptable to the athlete.

Carbohydrate meals of 1–2 g per kilogram body weight eaten one hour before exercise, and meals containing up to 4.5 g of carbohydrate per kilogram body weight consumed three to four hours before exercise have been shown to improve endurance performance.[43,46,53] There appears to be a positive additive effect when pre-exercise meals are consumed in conjunction with carbohydrate intake during exercise, leading to substantially better performance than when no carbohydrate is consumed or when carbohydrate is consumed only before or only during exercise.[53]

A current area of investigation is the potential effect foods of differing glycemic indices may have upon subsequent performance because of the potential for hyperglycemia and hyperinsulinemia at the onset of exercise.[51] Meals high in carbohydrate, particularly high glycemic foods, consumed in the hour or so before exercise result in high insulin and decreasing blood glucose at the time that exercise begins. It has been hypothesized that this glycemic response, coupled with the enhanced glucose uptake by exercising muscle, may result in a "rebound" hypoglycemia, inhibition of FFA oxidation, and may impair endurance exercise performance. This concern has stimulated a considerable amount of recent research and has led to recommendations to consume only low glycemic index foods prior to exercise.[23,51]

Studies generally show that consuming high GI foods within an hour of beginning exercise does result in hyperglycemia and hyperinsulinemia before exercise compared with low GI foods. At the onset of exercise, this results in a lowering of blood glucose, a decrease in FFA release and oxidation, and a greater reliance on carbohydrate oxidation during the exercise. However, there are two major reasons why this should not concern athletes. First, most studies show a decrease in blood glucose in the first 30 to 60 minutes of exercise, but blood glucose does not decrease to the low levels at which symptoms of hypoglycemia are experienced (neuroglucopenia), and very few studies have shown an impairment in subsequent performance.[49] If the exercise continues for sufficient duration, blood glucose and insulin generally return to normally expected levels, and most studies show that carbohydrate consumption one hour before exercise improves performance, regardless of the glycemic index.[18,21,22,25,28,35,47,49,50]

Second, from a practical perspective, most athletes would not choose to eat within an hour of beginning a long exercise bout. To allow time for adequate gastric emptying and to avoid gastrointestinal discomfort, most people tend to eat three to four hours before exercise. This additional time allows for the return of glucose and insulin toward baseline levels and diminishes any lingering effects of the GI of the meal consumed.[12]

In summary, it is important for an athlete to consume a meal before prolonged exercise. The meal should be timed so that it is largely cleared from the gastrointestinal tract before the onset of exercise to minimize the possibility of gastric upset, usually three to four hours. The meal should be largely composed of carbohydrate and should consist of food(s) the athlete is familiar with and used to eating. This strategy should be employed consistently in training; new foods or meal patterns should not be instituted before important competitive events. The glycemic index of the foods consumed is not as important as the familiarity with, tolerance of, and timing of the meal. For example, in the early morning hours before a marathon, it would be more practical for a runner to consume a familiar high carbohydrate breakfast food such as oatmeal (GI = 61), rather than attempting to meet an unwarranted recommendation to consume a low glycemic index meal by consuming a bowl full of lentils (GI = 30).

4.3.4 During Prolonged Endurance Exercise

Endogenous stores of carbohydrate will eventually become depleted during prolonged moderate to high-intensity exercise; therefore, carbohydrate must be consumed to maintain a high rate of carbohydrate oxidation. A large body of research provides evidence that consuming carbohydrate during exercise maintains blood glucose levels and carbohydrate oxidation and significantly improves both endurance capacity and performance.[9] Carbohydrate consumption during cycling exercise apparently does not reduce reliance on muscle glycogen but maintains blood glucose as a fuel source for oxidation late in exercise and clearly results in enhanced endurance capacity.[13] A study of runners utilizing an endurance performance protocol with published reliability[16] showed a significant improvement in time trial performance when a carbohydrate beverage was consumed.[15]

Improvements in endurance capacity or performance have been seen when 0.5 to 1.0 grams of carbohydrate are consumed per kilogram of body weight every hour during exercise. Most studies have focused on carbohydrate intake as simple sugars or maltodextrins in beverages, while few studies have investigated complex carbohydrate or solid food consumption during exercise. Glucose and glucose polymers (maltodextrins) have been shown to be effective, particularly compared to low GI carbohydrates such as fructose.[34]

Consuming carbohydrate in the form of a liquid beverage, or sports drink, is common during exercise. The consumption of other forms of carbohydrate (e.g., solid food) may be difficult or poorly tolerated during activities such as running. Other activities, such as cycling, may provide the opportunity for consumption of solid food with less discomfort. The few studies of solid food consumption during endurance exercise show improvements in performance[19,24] compared with a placebo, but there is no evidence that solid, or semi-solid carbohydrate consumption has any physiological or performance advantage over carbohydrate intake in liquid form.[32,38] There may be circumstances, such as during ultra endurance events, when the consumption of solid food may enhance the feelings of satiety.

Drinking carbohydrate beverages conveys an additional benefit of aiding fluid replacement and thermoregulation if exercise is performed in a thermally challenging environment. The beverage must be formulated to reach a balance between carbohydrate energy delivery and gastric emptying and absorption. Beverages of higher concentration deliver more energy, but they empty from the stomach more slowly.[33] It is apparent, however, that athletes may consume carbohydrate beverages in concentrations up to 10% without impairing thermoregulation.[37] Popular commercially available sports drinks typically contain 6-8% carbohydrate and can therefore be used effectively during endurance exercise. As with pre-exercise meals, athletes should incorporate this feeding strategy during their regular training, particularly during training sessions of long duration, to become accustomed to carbohydrate intake during exercise and to determine their individually appropriate volume of consumption. Sudden introduction of unfamiliar carbohydrate feeding during exercise may result in gastrointestinal distress, cramping, diarrhea, and/or vomiting, which would likely result in poorer, rather than improved performance.

4.3.5 Immediately After Exercise

Rapid replacement of carbohydrate stores, especially muscle and liver glycogen, may be important for many athletes. An athlete who competes in an occasional prolonged endurance event like the marathon may not need to resynthesize muscle glycogen rapidly, but one who participates in multiple, frequent activities that tax carbohydrates stores, such as weekend soccer tournaments, may require fast recovery. Rapid replacement of the body's carbohydrate stores can be achieved if carbohydrate is consumed quickly after depleting exercise. Delay for as little as two hours may result in significantly less muscle glycogen synthesis.[27] Therefore, an athlete seeking fast recovery should consume carbohydrates as soon as practicable after the depleting exercise.

Studies of muscle glycogen synthesis rates in the hours after exhaustive exercise have shown very rapid resynthesis when carbohydrates in amounts from 0.75 to 1.6 g per kilogram body weight are consumed every hour for four hours.[17,26] When carbohydrate is consumed in a large meal every two hours, several studies indicate the larger amount of carbohydrate intake does not increase the glycogen synthesis rate any further.[5,26] However, at least one study has shown higher rates of synthesis when smaller carbohydrate meals were consumed more frequently (every 15 minutes).[17] Although rapid muscle glycogen synthesis was seen with this feeding amount and strategy, athletes should be aware that the rapid consumption of large amounts of carbohydrates after exercise may cause gastrointestinal upset.

The form in which the carbohydrate is consumed after exercise may have some effect on the muscle glycogen replenishment rate. Although considered a simple sugar, fructose has a low glycemic response, and its consumption has been shown to result in a slower rate of muscle glycogen synthesis.[5] Carbohydrate consumed in equivalent amounts in liquid and solid form appears to result in similar replacement rates for muscle glycogen.[31,39] Studies of simple versus complex carbohydrates have shown no difference in the amount of muscle glycogen resynthesized in the first 24 hours after exhaustive exercise,[11] but that a diet in which the carbohydrate content was 70% complex carbohydrates resulted in greater muscle glycogen content 48 hours after exhaustive running. In a study emphasizing the Glycemic Index of foods, Burke, et al.[7] demonstrated that high GI foods resulted in significantly greater muscle glycogen synthesis in the 24 hours after exhaustive cycling compared to low GI foods. The increased insulin and blood glucose response seen after consumption of high GI foods may stimulate a greater short-term synthesis of muscle glycogen, but there does not appear to be any advantage to their consumption after the first 24 hours.

Athletes requiring rapid replacement of carbohydrate stores should eat or drink as soon as possible after depleting exercise. They should choose carbohydrates with a high Glycemic Index and preferably consume them in small, more frequent meals rather in large amounts at one time. After this initial replacement period, the normal predominately complex carbohydrate diet can be resumed.

4.4 PRACTICAL RECOMMENDATIONS

1. The basic diet should be consistent with the recommendations for chronic disease prevention and long-term health promotion. This diet is a high carbohydrate (greater than 55% of total calories), low fat diet (less than or equal to 30% of total calories), emphasizing a wide variety of foods from the base of the Food Guide Pyramid: bread, cereal, rice, pasta, fruits, and vegetables.
2. Evaluate the demands of the sporting or athletic activity, both for training and for competition. If the activity is of high intensity and is repeated frequently or it is of prolonged duration, additional manipulation of carbohydrate in the diet may be called for during appropriate time periods.
3. Carbohydrate intake should be determined as an absolute amount based upon the athlete's body weight; i.e., grams of carbohydrate per kilogram or pound of body weight (see recommended amounts in Table 4.3). A diet containing a high percentage of carbohydrate may be too low in actual grams of carbohydrate if the total energy intake is insufficient.
4. The majority of carbohydrate intake should be from a variety of foods from the base of the Food Guide Pyramid. However, if carbohydrate intake needs are extreme, as with intense, prolonged training, consider using carbohydrate supplements.
5. Consider manipulating carbohydrates during each of the critical time periods for training and competition. Practice these strategies during training; don't introduce any new foods or dietary practices before important competitive events.

Table 4.3 Practical Recommendations for Manipulation of Carbohydrate Intake

Time Period	Carbohydrate	Comments
Daily Training	7–10 g·kg^{-1}·day^{-1} (3.2–4.5 g per pound)	Amount depends upon duration and intensity of daily training; may need to supplement
Carbohydrate Loading	5 g·kg^{-1}·day^{-1} for three days then 8 + g·kg^{-1}·day^{-1} for three days (2.3 then 3.6 + g per pound)	For prolonged events (more than 2 hours); depleting exercise bout followed by tapered training for six days
Pre-exercise Meal	1–2 g·kg^{-1} one to two hours before, or up to 4–5 g·kg^{-1} three to four hours before (.45–.90 or 1.8–2.3 g per pound)	Consume familiar foods; time meal before exercise to insure complete digestion
During Exercise	.5–1.0 g·kg^{-1}·hour^{-1} (.23–.45 g per pound)	For prolonged events (more than 2 hours); sports drinks up to 10% concentration
After Exercise	.75–1.5 g·kg^{-1}·hour^{-1} (.34–.68 g per pound)	Evaluate need for rapid replacement of muscle glycogen; small, frequent feedings beginning as soon as possible for two to four hours

4.5 FUTURE DIRECTIONS FOR RESEARCH

1. Studies of carbohydrate manipulation have predominately used exercise protocols that measure time to exhaustion at a fixed exercise intensity, a measure of endurance capacity. Few studies have determined the effects of carbohydrate consumption on valid and reliable measures of endurance performance.[16] Additional research is needed to confirm the ergogenic advantage of carbohydrate consumption using exercise protocols that more closely mimic the demands of competitive athletic performance.

2. Further research is needed to clarify whether the Glycemic Index of pre-exercise meals is an important determinant of subsequent performance. Recommendations to avoid high GI foods before exercise are based upon what are perceived to be the adverse metabolic responses to these meals, while few studies have assessed their impact on endurance performance using valid and reliable protocols.

REFERENCES

1. American Heart Association, Dietary guidelines for healthy American adults: a statement for physicians and health professionals by the Nutrition Committee, *Circulation*, 7, 721A, 1988.

2. Benardot, D. and Plomden, M. S., Position of the American Dietetic Association and the Canadian Dietetic Association: Nutrition for physical fitness and athletic performance for adults, *J. Am. Dietetic Assoc.*, 93(6), 691, 1993.

3. Bergström, J., Hermansen, L., Hultman, E., and Saltin, B., Diet, muscle glycogen and physical performance, *Acta Physiologica Scandinavica*, 71, 140, 1967.

4. Bergström, J., and Hultman, E., A study of the glycogen metabolism during exercise in man, *Scand. J. Clin. Lab. Invest.*, 19, 218, 1967.

5. Blom, P. C. S., Costill, D. L., and Vøllestad, N. K., Exhaustive running: inappropriate as a stimulus of muscle glycogen supercompensation, *Med. and Sci. in Sports and Exercise*, 19(4), 398, 1987.

6. Brewer, J., Williams, C., and Patton, A., The influence of high carbohydrate diets on endurance running performance, *Eur. J. Appl. Physiol.*, 57, 698, 1988.

7. Burke, L. M., Collier, G. R., and Hargreaves, M., Muscle glycogen storage after prolonged exercise: effect of the glycemic index of carbohydrate feedings, *J. Appl. Physiol.*, 75(2), 1019, 1993.

8. Christian, J. L. and Greger, J. L., *Nutrition for Living*, The Benjamin/Cummings Publishing Company, Inc., Redwood City, CA, 1991.

9. Coggan, A. R. and Coyle, E. F., Carbohydrate ingestion during prolonged exercise: effects on metabolism and performance, in *Exercise and Sport Science Reviews*, John O. Holloszy, Ed., Williams & Wilkins, Baltimore, 1991, 1.

10. Costill, D. L., Bowers, R., Branam, G., and Sparks, K., Muscle glycogen utilization during prolonged exercise on successive days, *J. Appl. Physiol.*, 31(6), 834, 1971.

11. Costill, D. L., Sherman, W. M., Fink, W. J., Maresh, C., Witten, M., and Miller, J. M., The role of dietary carbohydrates in muscle glycogen resynthesis after strenuous running, *Am. J. Clin. Nutr.*, 34, 1831, 1981.

12. Coyle, E. F., Substrate utilization during exercise in active people, *Am. J. Clin. Nutr.*, 61(Supplement), 968S, 1995.

13. Coyle, E. F., Coggan, A. R., Hemmert, M. K., and Ivy, J. L., Muscle glycogen utilization during prolonged strenuous exercise when fed carbohydrate, *J. Appl. Physiol.*, 61(1), 165, 1986.

14. Dohm, L. G., Beeker, R. T., Israel, R. G., and Tapscott, E. B., Metabolic responses to exercise after fasting, *J. Appl. Physiol.*, 61(4), 1363, 1986.

15. Doyle, J. A. and Elliott, M. B., Distance running performance is improved with carbohydrate intake, *Med. Sci. in Sports and Exercise*, 28(5), S129, 1996.

16. Doyle, J. A. and Martinez, A. L., Reliability of a protocol for testing endurance performance in runners and cyclists, *Res. Quart. Exer. and Sport*, 69(3), 304, 1998.

17. Doyle, J. A., Sherman, W. M., and Strauss, R. L., Effects of eccentric and concentric exercise on muscle glycogen replenishment, *J. Appl. Physiol.*, 74(4), 1848, 1993.

18. Febbraio, M. A. and Stewart, K. L., CHO feeding before prolonged exercise: effect of glycemic index on muscle glycogenolysis and exercise performance, *J. Appl. Physiol.*, 81(2), 1115, 1996.

19. Fielding, R. A., Costill, D. L., Fink, W. J., King, D. S., Hargreaves, M., and Kovaleski, J. E., Effect of carbohydrate feeding frequencies and dosage on muscle glycogen use during exercise, *Med. Sci. in Sports and Exer.*, 17(4), 472, 1985.

20. Foster-Powell, K. and Miller, J. B., International tables of glycemic index, *Am. J. Clin. Nutri.*, 62, 871S, 1995.

21. Goodpaster, B. H., Costill, D. L., Fink, W. J., Trappe, T. A., Jozsi, A. C., Starling, R. D., and Trappe, S. W., The effects of pre-exercise starch ingestion on endurance performance, *Int. J. Sports Med.*, 17(5), 366, 1996.

22. Guezennec, C. Y., Satabin, P., Duforez, F., Koziet, J., and Antoine, J. M., The role of type and structure of complex carbohydrates response to physical exercise, *Int. J. Sports Med.*, 14(4), 224, 1993.

23. Guezennec, C.Y., Oxidation rates, complex carbohydrates and exercise, *Sports Medicine*, 19(6), 365, 1995.

24. Hargreaves, M., Costill, D. L., Coggan, A., Fink, W. J., and Nishibata, I., Effect of carbohydrate feedings on muscle glycogen utilization and exercise performance, *Med. Sci. in Sports and Exer.*, 16(3), 219, 1984.

25. Horowitz, J. F. and Coyle, E. F., Metabolic responses to pre-exercise meals containing various carbohydrates and fat, *Am. J. Clin. Nutri.*, 58, 235, 1993.

26. Ivy, J. L., Lee, M. C., Brozinick, J. T., and Reed, M. J., Muscle glycogen storage after different amounts of carbohydrate ingestion, *J. Appl. Physiol.*, 65(5), 2018, 1988.

27. Ivy, J. L., Katz, A. L., Cutler, C. L., Sherman, W. M., and Coyle, E. F., Muscle glycogen synthesis after exercise: effect of time of carbohydrate ingestion, *J. Appl. Physiol.*, 64(4), 1480, 1988.

28. Jarvis, J. K., Pearsall, D., Oliner, C., and Schoeller, D. A., The effect of food matrix on carbohydrate utilization during moderate exercise, *Med. Sci. in Sports and Exer.*, 24(3), 320, 1992.

29. Jenkins, D. J. A., Wolever, T. M. S., Jenkins, A. L., Josse, R. G., and Wong, G. S., The glycaemic response to carbohydrate foods, *Lancet*, 388, August 18, 1984.

30. Jenkins, D. J. A., Wolever, T. M. S., Taylor, R. H., Barker, H., Fielden, H., Baldwin, J. M., Bowling, A. C., Newman, H. C., Jenkins, A. L., and Goff, D. V., Glycemic index of foods: a physiological basis for carbohydrate exchange, *Am. J. Clin. Nutri.*, 34, March, 362, 1981.

31. Keizer, H. A., Kuipers, H., van Kranenburg, G., and Geurten, P., Influence of liquid and solid meals on muscle glycogen resynthesis, plasma fuel hormone response, and maximal physical working capacity, *Inter. J. Sports Med.*, 8, 99, 1987.

32. Mason, W. L., McConell, G., and Hargreaves, M., Carbohydrate ingestion during exercise: liquid vs solid feedings, *Med. Sci. in Sports and Exer.*, 25(8), 966, 1993.

33. Murray, R., The effects of consuming carbohydrate-electrolyte beverages on gastric emptying and fluid absorption during and following exercise, *Sports Medicine*, 4, 322, 1987.

34. Murray, R., Paul, G., L., Seifert, J. G., Eddy, D. E., and Halaby, G. A., The effects of glucose, fructose, and sucrose ingestion during exercise, *Med. Sci. Sports and Exer.*, 21(3), 275, 1989.

35. Neufer, D. P., Costill, D. L., Flynn, M. G., Kirkwan, J. P., Mitchell, J. B., and Houmard, J., Improvements in exercise performance: effects of carbohydrate feedings and diet, *J. Appl. Physiol.*, 62(3), 983, 1987.

36. Nutrition and your health: dietary guidelines for Americans, in *Home & Garden Bulletin*, 4, US Dietary Guideline Committee, US Department of Agriculture, US Department of Health and Human Services, Ed., 1995, 232.

37. Owen, M. D., Kregel, K. C., Wall, P. T., and Gisolfi, C. V., Effects of ingesting carbohydrate beverages during exercise in the heat, *Med. Sci. Sports and Exer.*, 18(5), 568, 1986.

38. Peters, H. F. P., van Schelven, W. F., Verslappen, P. A., de Doer, R. W., Bol, E., Erich, W. B.M., van der Togt, C. R., and de Vries, W. R., Exercise performance as a function of semi-solid and liquid carbohydrate feedings during prolonged exercise, *Inter. J. Sports Med.*, 16(2), 105, 1995.

39. Reed, M. J., Brozinick, J. T., Lee, M. C., and Ivy, J. L., Muscle glycogen storage post-exercise: effect of mode of carbohydrate administration, *J. Appl. Physiol.*, 66(2), 720, 1989.

40. Roberts, K. M., Noble, E. G., Hayden, D. B., and Taylor, A. W., Simple and complex carbohydrate rich diets and muscle glycogen content of marathon runners, *Eur. J. Appl. Physiol.*, 57, 70, 1988.

41. Salmerón, J., Ascherio, A., Rimm, E. B., Colditz, G. A., Spiegelman, D., Jenkins, D. J., Stampfer, M. J., Wing, A. L., and Willett, W. C., Dietary fiber, glycemic load, and risk of NIDDM in men, *Diabetes Care*, 20(4), April, 545, 1997.

42. Salmerón, J., Manson, J. E., Stampfer, M. J., Colditz, G. A., Wing, A. L., and Willett, W. C., Dietary fiber, glycemic load, and risk of non-insulin-dependent diabetes mellitus in women, JAMA, 277(6), 472, 1997.

43. Sherman, W. M., Brodowicz, G., Wright, D. A., Allen, W. K., Simonsen, J., and Dernbach, A., Effects of 4 h preexercise carbohydrate feedings on cycling performance, *Med. Sci. in Sports and Exer.*, 21(5), 598, 1989.

44. Sherman, W. M., Costill, D. L., Fink, W. J., and Miller, J. M., Effect of exercise-diet manipulation on muscle glycogen and its subsequent utilization during performance, *Inter. J. Sports Med.*, 2(2), 114, 1981.

45. Sherman, W. M., Doyle, J. A., Lamb, D. R., and Strauss, R. H., Dietary carbohydrate, muscle glycogen, and exercise performance during 7 d of training, *Am. J. Clin. Nutri.*, 57, 27, 1993.

46. Sherman, W. M., Peden, M. C., and Wright, D., Carbohydrate feedings 1 h before exercise improves cycling performance, *Am. J. Clin. Nutri.*, 54, 866, 1991.

47. Sparks, M. J., Selig, S. S., and Febbraio, M. A., Pre-exercise carbohydrate ingestion: effect of the glycemic index on endurance exercise performance, *Med. Sci. in Sports and Exer.*, 30(6), 844, 1998.

48. The American Cancer Society, Nutrition guidelines, CA - *A Journal for Clinicians*, 46(6), 325, 1996.

49. Thomas, D. E., Brotherhood, J. R., and Brand, J. C., Carbohydrate feeding before exercise: effect of glycemic index, *Inter. J. Sports Med.*, 12(2), 180, 1991.

50. Thomas, D. E., Brotherhood, J. R., and Miller, J. B., Plasma glucose levels after prolonged strenuous exercise correlate inversely with glycemic response to food consumed before exercise, *Inter. J. Sport Nutri.*, 4, 361, 1994.

51. Walton, P. and Rhodes, E. C., Glycaemic index and optimal performance, *Sports Medicine*, 23(3), 164, 1997.

52. Wolever, T. M. S., Jenkins, D. J. A., Jenkins, A. L., and Josse, R. G., The glycemic index: methodology and clinical implications, *Am. J. Clin. Nutri.*, 54, 846, 1991.

53. Wright, D. A., Sherman, W. M., and Dernbach, A. R., Carbohydrate feedings before, during, or in combination improve cycling endurance performance, *J. Appl. Physiol.*, 71(3), 1082, 1991.

CHAPTER 5

Dietary Fiber in Sports Nutrition

Daniel D. Gallaher

CONTENTS

5.1 INTRODUCTION

Dietary fiber is a heterogeneous mixture of plant carbohydrates that, when consumed, have several important physiological effects. Consumption of dietary fiber alters metabolism of carbohydrates, lipids, and proteins, although the magnitude of these changes varies dramatically with the quantity and type of fiber ingested. Numerous studies indicate that dietary fiber can impact the incidence and treatment of various chronic diseases, such as diabetes, colon cancer, and heart disease. The possibility that dietary fiber may improve athletic performance, however, is a relatively new concept in the study of dietary fiber. Nonetheless, several studies indicate that consumption of certain types of dietary fiber prior to exercise may increase athletic endurance. This chapter describes the different types of dietary fiber in our diets and their physical properties and physiological effects, and it reviews the studies in which the role of dietary fiber in athletic performance has been examined.

5.2 DIETARY FIBER — DEFINITION AND TYPES

Dietary fiber is generally agreed to derive from plant materials, which is evident from the definitions put forth over the years. One well-known and commonly accepted definition is plant material resistant to hydrolysis by the digestive enzymes of humans.[1] Because this definition relies on the resistance of a plant material to enzymatic degradation, this represents a physiological definition. Other definitions, however, focus on the common chemical characteristics of dietary fiber, e.g., the sum of nonstarch polysaccharides and lignin.[2] Some controversy has existed over the years as to whether lignin should be considered part of the definition of fiber. Lignin is a highly branched and cross-linked polymer based on oxygenated phenylpropane units and consequently is not a carbohydrate. However, because the lignin content of most foods is quite low, in practical terms, this distinction is rarely important.

There are several polymeric plant carbohydrates that represent the common types of dietary fiber. These include cellulose, the hemicelluloses, β-glucans, pectins, and gums (Figure 5.1). Cellulose is a linear polymer of glucose molecules joined by a $\beta(1\rightarrow4)$ linkage. In contrast, amylose, a highly digestible linear polymer of glucose, is composed of $\alpha(1\rightarrow4)$ linkages. Mammalian amylases are unable to hydrolyze a $\beta(1\rightarrow4)$ linkage. Hemicelluloses, which are not biosynthetically related to cellulose, are highly branched polymers consisting mainly of glucurono- and 4-O-methylglucuro-xylans.[3] β-Glucans are mixed linkage $(1\rightarrow3)$, $(1\rightarrow4)$ β-D-glucose polymers found primarily in cereals, particularly oats and barley.[4] Pectins are a group of polysaccharides composed primarily of D-galacturonic acid,[5] which is methoxylated to variable degrees. Finally, the gums represent a broad array of different branched structures. Guar gum, one of the best known and frequently used gums, is a galactomannan. Other gums, such as gum arabic and gum acacia, have quite different structures.

There are several substances, both natural and synthetic, that fit into one or more definitions of dietary fiber. These include such things as Maillard reaction products, formed during heating of proteins in the presence of reducing sugars, modified celluloses such as methyl cellulose, indigestible animal products such as chitosan, and oligosaccharides such as inulin and oligofructose. Each substance shares some characteristics with what can be thought of as traditional dietary fibers, yet has a significant difference in other ways. None of these substances has universally been accepted as dietary fiber, but nonetheless they are sometimes described as such.

5.3 DIETARY FIBER IN FOODS

Attempts to measure dietary fiber go back to the late 1800s, when methods were being developed to quantitate the indigestible components of feed forages. In an attempt to simulate the acid conditions of the stomach and the alkaline conditions of the small intestine, forages were exposed to concentrated acid, followed by strong base. This method was named crude fiber. However, it accurately measured only cellulose, certain hemicelluloses, and lignins. Although this was acceptable for forages, which contain little of the other types of fiber, crude fiber is unacceptable as a measure of dietary fiber in foods consumed by humans.

As the importance of dietary fiber in human nutrition became apparent, efforts were made to develop methods that measured all types of dietary fiber. Although several accurate methods now exist for fiber measurement, the procedure known as Total Dietary Fiber (TDF)[6,7] has become the

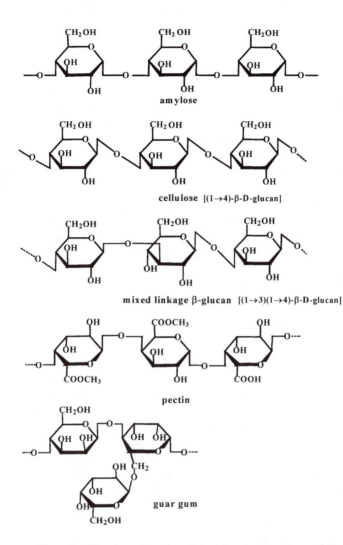

Figure 5.1 Structure of amylose (starch) and several types of dietary fiber.

most accepted method in the United States. TDF is a FDA-approved method, and values generated using this method may be used on food labels.

Different dietary fibers are frequently classified as either soluble or insoluble. This dichotomous classification arose from the observation that dietary fibers that lowered cholesterol levels could be solubilized in water (although technically they are in suspension), whereas cellulose and wheat bran, which are insoluble, can not. The TDF method, in its original form, did not give separate values for soluble and insoluble fiber in a food. However, a modification of the TDF method has subsequently been developed that does allow measurement of both the insoluble and soluble fiber content of a food.[8] Most values for the soluble fiber content of food have been generated using this modified TDF method.

Many foods commonly consumed in the United States and Western Europe have now been analyzed for dietary fiber content. Consequently, most food databases have relatively complete entries for dietary fiber. Using this information, daily dietary fiber consumption in the United States has been estimated at 10–15 g per day.[9] On average, most people in Western cultures consume about 75% of their fiber as insoluble types and 25% as soluble types.

5.4 IMPORTANT PHYSICOCHEMICAL CHARACTERISTICS OF DIETARY FIBER

5.4.1 Solubility

Given that dietary fiber is a mix of heterogeneous types of plant carbohydrates, it is not surprising that fibers differ in their physical and chemical characteristics. The physical characteristic that has received the most attention, as discussed above, is solubility in water. Cellulose and certain hemicelluloses represent insoluble forms of dietary fiber. β-Glucans, pectins, gums, and modified celluloses are to a great degree water soluble. However, the viscosity they impart on the solution differs dramatically among soluble fiber types. For example, guar gum is extremely viscous and is used as a thickener in foods because of this. Yet other gums range from being only somewhat viscous, such as gum arabic, to gums that have virtually no viscosity at all, such as gum acacia. The viscosity of a gum depends on both the chain length of the polymer and the degree of branching. Longer chain length and less chain branching both lead to greater viscosity. Hydrolysis of soluble fibers, either by chemical means or enzymatically, will greatly reduce the viscosity of these fibers in solution.

Pectins can exhibit a high viscosity in solution, but this is greatly influenced by the degree of methoxylation of the uronic acids it contains. The viscosity of pectins derives from the formation of cross-linked gels in solution. These gels are weak, however. Consequently, the extent of gel formation under physiological conditions is uncertain.

5.4.2 Susceptibility to Fermentation

Susceptibility to microbial fermentation is another important, but highly variable, characteristic of dietary fibers. Although this is not, strictly speaking, a physicochemical characteristic, the physical and chemical characteristics of a fiber determine its susceptibility to fermentation. For example, cellulose, a glucose polymer, is resistant to fermentation and consequently is only partially degraded within the colon. Yet, β-glucans, another glucose polymer, are highly susceptible to fermentation and are rapidly and completely degraded in the colon. This difference can be ascribed to the tight packing of the glucose chain in cellulose, making it inaccessible to bacterial cellulases. In general, the insoluble fibers, such as cellulose and many hemicelluloses, are resistant to fermentation. In contrast, most soluble types of fiber are rapidly fermentable. Examples include guar gum, pectins, and β-glucans. However, some soluble fibers, such as psyllium, are only slightly fermentable, and the highly soluble modified celluloses, such as methylcellulose, are not fermentable at all. Thus, the solubility of a dietary fiber does not equate with a susceptibility to fermentability.

5.4.3 Water-Holding Capacity

Most dietary fibers will absorb water. The quantity of water that can be absorbed is referred to as the water-holding capacity (WHC). Interest in the WHC of fibers developed early from studies indicating that the swelling power, which is related to the WHC, of certain fibers approximated the laxative effects of certain fibers.[10] Several methods have been developed to measure the WHC. For example, an early method involved soaking the fiber in water for 24 hours, followed by centrifugation. The difference between the dry fiber and the pellet obtained after centrifugation constitutes the WHC.[11] Another technique places the fiber in a dialysis bag and uses polyethylene glycol in the medium to create an osmotic suction approximating the absorption of water in the colon.[12] Subsequently, this method was modified to include *in vitro* fermentation of the fiber with a fecal inoculum prior to determination of the WHC by suction dialysis, a measure referred to as the potential WHC.[13] As might be expected, different methods for determining the WHC give quite different values, leading to difficulty in interpretation. More important, none the methods developed to date is highly predictive of the stool weight produced *in vivo* by consumption of the fibers. Thus, the physiological significance of WHC determined *in vitro* is uncertain.

5.5 PHYSIOLOGICAL EFFECTS OF DIETARY FIBER AND THEIR RELATIONSHIP TO PHYSICOCHEMICAL CHARACTERISTICS

Dietary fibers have several important physiological effects, which vary with the type and quantity of fiber consumed. Because dietary fiber, by definition, is not absorbed, all these effects have their primary effect within the gastrointestinal tract. However, due to the ability of some fibers to alter the rate and degree of absorption of nutrients and to be fermented within the colon, profound metabolic effects can occur beyond the intestine. In many cases, these physiological effects can be understood by relating the physicochemical characteristics of a fiber to events within the intestine. That is, a physical or chemical characteristic of a fiber will lead to an alteration in the intestinal milieu, which then leads secondarily to a metabolic alteration in a different organ. In this section, this relationship will be described for several of the well-known physiological effects of dietary fiber.

5.5.1 Fecal Bulking and Transit Time

The laxative effect of dietary fiber is certainly its best-known physiological effect. In modern times, this effect was recognized as early as 1840, when John Burne recommended that "coarse brown and bran bread is very efficacious, the bran acting as a salutory stimulus to the peristaltic action of the intestines."[14] This laxative effect is related to the fecal bulking produced by a fiber, but not in a simple way. Transit time, the time required for a consumed substance to be excreted, has a curvilinear relationship to fecal wet weight.[15] At fecal wet weights of 60 g per day or less, transit times commonly exceed 90 hours. As fecal wet weight increases, transit time decreases but reaches a plateau at 40–50 hours when fecal wet weight is between 150 and 200 g per day. Fecal wet weights in the United States are highly variable, but they are 120 g or less in many individuals.[16,17] Addition of fecal bulking agents, such as dietary fiber, would be expected to increase laxation significantly for these people.

All dietary fibers provide some fecal bulking. However, the degree to which they increase fecal wet weight varies with the type and form of fiber. Based on a summary of several studies, Cummings[18] reported that wheat (mainly as bran) gives the largest increase in fecal output, followed by fruits and vegetables, gums, and oats and corn. Purified pectin gave the smallest increment in fecal output (Figure 5.2). The form of wheat bran has an influence on fecal output, as course wheat

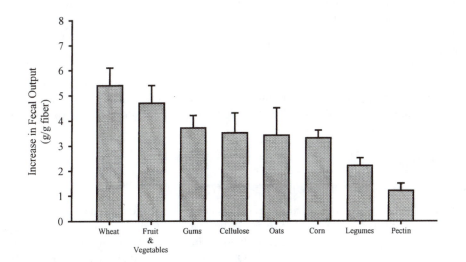

Figure 5.2

bran has a somewhat greater bulking effect than fine wheat bran.[18] The effect of particle size has not been examined extensively for other fiber sources.

The increase in stool weight brought about by dietary fiber occurs for several reasons. For fibers that are not completely degraded by colonic microflora, such as wheat bran and cellulose, the persistence of indigestible material in the colon contributes greatly to fecal bulking. In addition, these fibers have some water-holding capacity, which further contributes to the increase in bulk. Increasing bulk in the colon promotes laxation. However, many fibers, such as pectin, guar gum, and β-glucans, are completely fermented in the colon and consequently contribute no bulk or have no water-holding capacity. These fibers produce an increase in bulk by promoting the growth of colonic microflora. In individuals consuming Western diets, the microflora account for approximately half the weight of fecal solids.[19] Thus, changes in colonic microbial growth have the potential for significantly altering fecal bulking. Finally, increased fermentation in the colon leads to the production of a number of end products, including gases such as H_2, CH_4, and CO_2. These gases can become entrapped in the colonic contents and contribute to the fecal bulk. However, as can be seen by the far greater fecal bulking effect of wheat bran and cellulose compared to pectin, fibers that are incompletely fermented are superior bulking agents.

5.5.2 Effects on Intestinal Absorption

5.5.2.1 Carbohydrates

Numerous studies have established that certain dietary fibers flatten the postprandial blood glucose and insulin curves. This flattening is not due to malabsorption of glucose, but to a delayed rate of glucose absorption.[20,21] Fibers that most reproducibly demonstrate this effect are guar gum[21] and β-glucans.[22] Both fibers are characterized by a very high viscosity in water. Fibers such as wheat bran or cellulose, which are insoluble and therefore have no viscosity, produce either a modest or undetectable effect on the postprandial blood glucose or insulin curves.[23,24] A high correlation between the viscosity of pectin and its ability to flatten the glucose curve has been found in rats.[25] Such findings suggest that viscosity is the primary characteristic of fiber responsible for the delayed absorption of glucose.

An obvious explanation for the delayed absorption of glucose by viscous fibers is a slowed rate of glucose diffusion within the intestinal lumen to the mucosa, the site of absorption. Studies using isolated lengths of jejunum in rats found a delayed rate of glucose absorption in the presence of a perfusate containing guar gum compared with one containing no fiber,[26] thus supporting this concept. However, studies in which viscous fibers were infused directly into the intestine of human subjects to examine the decrease in glucose diffusion have yielded conflicting results.[27,28] Thus, the importance of slowed glucose diffusion as an explanation for the flattening of the postprandial glucose and insulin curves is uncertain. In contrast, several studies clearly demonstrate that viscous fibers slow stomach emptying.[28–31] Thus, viscous fibers appear to flatten the postprandial glucose curve primarily by slowing the rate of entry of a meal from the stomach into the small intestine.

5.5.2.2 Lipids

The effect of dietary fiber on absorption of cholesterol has been examined, either directly or indirectly, for several fiber types. Purified pectin has been found to reduce cholesterol absorption,[32] but a pectin-rich citrus fraction did not (N. Osterberg and D. Gallaher, unpublished), suggesting that the food matrix in which the fiber is held is important. Guar gum reduces cholesterol absorption, whereas psyllium does not[32] (N. Osterberg and D. Gallaher, unpublished). Hydroxypropyl methylcellulose, a modified and highly soluble form of cellulose, has been shown to reduce cholesterol absorption linearly as a function of the logarithm of the intestinal contents viscosity that it produces.[33] Overall, it appears that viscous fibers are effective in reducing cholesterol absorption, although the mechanism by which they do so has yet to be established.

Several studies have reported that dietary fibers or fiber-rich foods decrease pancreatic lipase activity in vitro, yet in most cases the lipase activity in vivo is increased.[34] This paradoxical situation points to the importance of studying the effects of dietary fiber in vivo whenever possible. Triacylglycerol absorption may be delayed or impaired in spite of normal or elevated levels of lipase, for several reasons, including interference with enzyme-substrate interactions, micelle formation, or diffusion of micelles to the intestinal mucosa. The finding that triacylglycerol excretion was increased in ileostomy fluid by 36% by pectin feeding[35] but was unaltered by wheat bran feeding[36] suggests that viscous fibers do indeed interfere with the process of triacylglycerol absorption. Consistent with this is the finding of a delayed disappearance of triolein from the small intestine in rats fed guar gum or glucomannan, two viscous fibers, compared to cellulose.[37] Although decreased lipid absorption by viscous dietary fibers has been demonstrated, the physiological significance of this phenomenon is uncertain.

5.5.2.3 Vitamins and Minerals

Fat-soluble vitamins are absorbed similarly to triacylglycerol, in that fat-soluble vitamins are dissolved in the lipid phase within the intestine, then become incorporated into mixed micelles for transport and ultimate absorption by the intestinal mucosa. Given the ability of certain dietary fibers to delay triacylglycerol absorption, described above, one might expect an altered absorption of fat-soluble vitamins as well. However, results of studies on the effect of fiber on fat-soluble vitamin absorption are inconsistent. Long-term studies of vitamin A absorption have found that wheat bran consumption either increased[38] or decreased[39] serum vitamin A concentrations. Limited information exists on the effects of long-term fiber consumption on the absorption of other fat-soluble vitamins. However, the available evidence does not suggest that fiber consumption is likely to induce a significant malabsorption.

Absorption of water-soluble vitamins is less understood than fat-soluble vitamins. However, it is known that, in most cases, water-soluble vitamin absorption involves an active uptake at the mucosa. The effect of fiber on their absorption has been examined only superficially for most. Wheat bran had no effect, and psyllium even appeared to increase riboflavin absorption after a pharmacological dose.[40] Pectin consumption had no negative influence on utilization of vitamin B_6[41] or urinary ascorbic acid concentration.[42] Folic acid absorption was unaffected by wheat bran.[43]

Several studies have been conducted examining the effect of various types and levels of dietary fiber on mineral absorption. The results of these studies are rather inconsistent. Although the possibility that consumption of fiber could impair mineral status has been raised many times over the years, it has been argued persuasively by Gordon et al.[44] that evidence to support this contention is lacking.

At present, there is no compelling evidence that consumption of any particular dietary fiber type significantly impairs absorption of vitamins or essential minerals.

5.5.3 Fermentation of Fiber in the Colon

Dietary fiber can be fermented and thereby degraded in the colon by the microflora present, yielding many products are produced, including gases (H_2, CO_2, CH_4) and short-chain fatty acids (SCFA) (primarily acetic, propionic, and butyric acids). The degree of fermentation varies considerably with fiber type. For example, lignin and the synthetic celluloses, such as methylcellulose, are essentially entirely resistant to fermentation. Cellulose is fermented to approximately 30 to 50%, hemicelluloses 50 to 80%, and pectins and gums essentially 100%. Because lignin and synthetic celluloses normally represent only a small fraction of the dietary fiber intake, increasing fiber intake would necessarily lead to an increase in fermentation in the colon.

Increased fermentative activity in the colon will lead to an increase in bacterial mass. Since bacteria account for 35 to 50% of the volume of the colon in humans,[19] this increased activity results in an expansion of the fecal mass, as discussed in Section 5.4. Because of the increased microbial metabolic activity, large increases in SCFA may occur. SCFA have a tropic effect on the colon, leading to hypertrophy of the colonic mucosa.[45] Increases in SCFA also lead to acidification of the colon contents, which has been linked epidemiologically with a reduced risk of colon cancer.[46]

Propionate, a SCFA that is absorbed into the portal circulation and metabolized in the liver, has been proposed to be responsible for the hypocholesterolemic effect of fermentable fibers, such as guar gum and oat bran.[47] Propionate has been found to decrease cholesterol synthesis rates in cultured hepatocytes.[48] However, in whole animals, dietary propionate did not alter cholesterol synthesis.[49] Presently, the available evidence does not support a role for cholesterol lowering by propionate.[50]

5.6 INTAKE PATTERNS OF DIETARY FIBER IN ATHLETES

Although many studies have examined the macronutrient intake of athletes, few have included a measure of dietary fiber as part of the analysis. Table 5.1 lists studies where dietary fiber has been included as part of the dietary assessment. In all cases, the nutrient intake was based on dietary

Table 5.1   Dietary Fiber Intake in Athletes

Subjects	Number	Sex	Method of determination of fiber intake	Dietary fiber intake (g/d)	Intake of comparison group (g/d)	Comparison group	Reference
Marathon runners	291	M	3-day food record	20.9 ± 0.7[a]	18.5	"National average"[c]	65
Marathon runners	56	F	3-day food record	17.1 ± 1.2	11.5	"National average"	65
Distance runners	14	M	7-day food record	31 ± 11*	21.4	Sedentary men	66
Distance runners	14	M	4-day food record	20.6 ± 2.1	N/A	None	67
Distance runners	10	F	4-day food record	14.7 ± 1.6	N/A	None	67
Ultradistance runners	150	M	1-day food record	25.7 ± 12.8*	21.0 ± 11.4	Sedentary men	68
Ultradistance runners	23	F	Two 24-hour food records	21.4 ± 10.2*	15.9 ± 7.4	Sedentary women	68
"Well-trained men"	20	M	7-day food record	24 ± 8[b]	21	Swedish National Food Balance Sheets[d]	69
Gymnasts, figure skaters, runners, 11- to 12-year-olds	43	F	4-day food record	17.1 ± 6.0	15.9 ± 4.8	No supervised sports training	70
Ice hockey, 12- to 13-year-olds	49	M	4-day food record	20.5 ± 6.4	19.2 ± 9.0	No supervised sports training	70

a	Values represent means ± SD; * indicates significantly different from the comparison group (p < 0.05).
b	Estimated from Figure 5.2 in the report.
c	Comparison to results for the USDA Nationwide Food Consumption Survey, Continuing Survey of Food Intakes by Individuals, 1985.
d	Estimated dietary fiber intakes for Sweden for 1988.[71]

records, ranging from one to seven days in length. In several studies, sedentary controls were recruited and analyzed concurrently with the analysis of the nutrient intake of the athletes; in other cases no comparison group was reported. Only in those studies where a control group was included was a statistical comparison of intake possible. Most studies utilized runners as subjects. However, one study used athletes defined as "well-trained"[69] and another used children in early puberty, where the boys were ice hockey players and the girls were gymnasts, skaters, or runners.[70]

As can be seen from Table 5.1, fiber intake ranged from approximately 15 to over 30 g per day in the athletes. In all cases, the intake of dietary fiber by the athletes was greater than that of the comparison group. In the two studies of adults where a sedentary control group was included,[66,68] this difference in intake was statistically significant.

One obvious explanation for the increased intake of dietary fiber is that athletes simply eat more, as their energy needs are higher than that of non-athletes. However, in a study by Nieman et al.,[65] marathon runners reported that they presently consumed more fruits, vegetables, and whole grains than they did before they began serious running. If this were true, one would expect to see an increase in the ratio of dietary fiber to (digestible) carbohydrate, as fruits, vegetables, and whole grains are fiber-rich foods. Interestingly, the nutrient intake data do not support this altered pattern. In the study by Peters and Goetzche,[68] the ratio of dietary fiber to carbohydrate, expressed as a percentage, was 8.5% for both male athletes and controls and 9.6% for female athletes versus 9.5% for female controls. Using the "national average" as the comparison group, the ratio in the study of Nieman et al.[65] was 6.4% in male athletes versus 7.0% in the male national average. For females, the ratio in the athletes was 7.0% and 6.4% in the national average. Only in the study of Sutherland et al.[66] was there a suggestion of a difference in the ratio — 9.2% in the athletes versus 8.0% in the sedentary controls. Thus, although athletes do appear to consume somewhat more dietary fiber than non-athletes, these results do not support a change in the dietary pattern of the athlete to one containing more fiber-rich foods.

5.7 INFLUENCE OF DIETARY FIBER ON ATHLETIC PERFORMANCE AND CARBOHYDRATE OXIDATION RATES

It is well established that carbohydrates are important sources of energy for contracting muscles and that fatigue can develop during intense and prolonged exercise after depletion of muscle and liver glycogen. It has become clear in recent years that ingestion of carbohydrate before and during endurance exercise can enhance performance.[51] However, there is some debate about the most appropriate type of carbohydrate to consume prior to exercise. Foods that lead to a rapid digestion and absorption of carbohydrate (high Glycemic Index) produce a drop in blood glucose concentrations at the onset of exercise.[52] This is due to the hyperinsulinemia that results from consumption of high glycemic index foods, which in turn stimulates glucose uptake by contracting muscles.[53,54] It has been argued that the hypoglycemia that occurs with the onset of exercise does not lead to muscle weakness or impair performance.[55] Nevertheless, several investigators have been interested in whether consumption of a carbohydrate that yields a slow release of carbohydrate, and thereby avoids hyperinsulinemia, might be beneficial for increasing endurance in prolonged exercise.

As discussed in Section 5.5.2.1, viscous dietary fibers slow the absorption of glucose, leading to a blunted postprandial blood glucose and insulin curve. Jarvis et al.[56] showed that, compared to liquid glucose, consumption of a refined cereal with added soluble fiber 30 minutes prior to exercise reduced the peak insulin response and slowed exogenous glucose oxidation in subjects walking a treadmill at 40% $\dot{V}O_{2\,max}$. Thus, consumption of a viscous dietary fiber that slows glucose absorption appears to be a means of attenuating the hyperinsulinemia that normally occurs with exercise onset. This slowed glucose absorption may be of benefit by increasing glucose availability later in exercise to meet the need for carbohydrate oxidation.[72]

Table 5.2 shows the results of several studies that have examined the effect of either a soluble fiber or a fiber-rich food with a low Glycemic Index on exercise endurance and the rate of carbohydrate oxidation. Low glycemic foods are those that yield a reduced rate of glucose absorption compared to glucose.[57] Foods may exhibit a low glycemic index for many reasons, including a reduced rate of gastric emptying,[58] a high amylose starch content,[59] or the presence of antinutrients.[60,61] Because low glycemic foods produce the same effect on glucose absorption as does a viscous dietary fiber, both can be viewed as similar in terms of a potential effect on athletic performance.

Table 5.2   Effect of Dietary Fiber on Exercise Endurance and Carbohydrate Oxidation Rate

Subjects	Number, Sex	Exercise Intensity (% $\dot{V}O_{2\,max}$)	Time of Ingestion Before Exercise (min)	Substance Consumed	Glycemic Index	Exercise Time (min)	Carbohydrate Oxidation Rate (g/min)	Reference
Trained cyclists	5 M	65–70	60	Water	N/Aa	99 ± 11b	1.85	72
				Glucose	100	108 ± 10	2.13	
				Potato	98	97 ± 11	2.04	
				Lentils	29	117 ± 11*	1.96	
Trained cyclists	6 M	65–70	60	Potato flakes	100	90 ± 11	NR	73
				Rice cereal	73	101 ± 12	NR	
				Lentil flakes	36	97 ± 13	NR	
				Bran cereal	30	90 ± 8	NR	
Adults of above-average aerobic power	6 M,6F	60	90	Fasted	NR	10.6 ± 0.2c	NR	74
				Corn cereal	NR	10.5 ± 0.2	NR	
				Oat cereal	NR	10.5 ± 0.2	NR	
				Wheat cereal	NR	10.7 ± 0.3	NR	
Recreationally active, college age	6 F	60	45	Water	NR	225 ± 8	1.89	75
				Whole oat flour	NR	251 ± 12	1.90	
				Rolled oats	NR	266 ± 13*	1.94	
Trained for endurance-based activities	5 M	65	2-3	Water	NR	2.7 ± 0.9d	0.85	76
				Glucose	NR	6.2 ± 2.6*	1.71	
				Maltodextrin	NR	7.5 ± 3.1*	1.79	
				Glucose + guar gum	NR	7.2 ± 2.6*	1.74	
				Maltodextrin + guar gum	NR	8.1 ± 2.8*	1.69	

a   Abbreviations are: N/A, not applicable; NR, not reported.

b   Values represent mean $\pm$ SEM. *, significantly different from water control group ($p < 0.05$).

c   Values represent time to complete a 6.4 km ride after 90 minutes of exercise at 60% of $\dot{V}O_{2\,max}$.

d   Values represent a timed ride to exhaustion at 75% $\dot{V}O_{2\,max}$ after completion of 90 minutes of exercise.

The results of the studies on the effect of fiber or low Glycemic Index (GI) foods are mixed. In one study of trained male cyclists, who consumed either water, glucose, potato (high GI), or lentils (low GI) an hour before exercise, time to exhaustion at 65–70% $\dot{V}O_{2\,max}$ was significantly longer when lentils were consumed compared to the other three substances.[72] The rate of carbohydrate oxidation did not differ among the groups. However, a subsequent trial of male cyclists, in which foods with a range of GI from 30 to 100 were consumed, using essentially the identical protocol, failed to find an increase in the time to exhaustion.[73] Another study examined the effect of consumption of oats, which are rich in β-glucans, a viscous fiber known to flatten the postprandial glucose and insulin curves.[62] College-aged, recreationally active females consumed water, whole oat flour, or rolled oats one hour before exercising to exhaustion at a $\dot{V}O_{2\,max}$ of 60%.[75] Although time to exhaustion was increased by both oat-containing meals, only the increase in the group consuming rolled oats reached statistical significance. The rate of carbohydrate oxidation did not differ among the groups. Two additional studies examined the effect of fiber or fiber-rich foods on exercise endurance using a slightly different protocol. In a group of male and female adults described as being of above average aerobic power, subjects were either given water or fed a corn-, oat-, or wheat-based cereal 90 minutes before exercising.[74] The subjects cycled for 90 minutes at 60% $\dot{V}O_2$ $\dot{V}O_{2\,max}$, then performed a timed 6.4 km ride. The time to complete this ride did not differ among the groups, suggesting that none of the cereal meals provided any benefit in terms of endurance. Finally, in the only study reported that used a purified fiber source, male subjects trained for endurance-based activities were given either water or drinks containing glucose, maltodextrin, glucose + guar gum, or maltodextrin + guar gum.[76] These were given two to three minutes before the initiation of 90 minutes of exercise at 65% $\dot{V}O_{2\,max}$. After a 10-minute rest, a timed ride to exhaustion at 75% $\dot{V}O_{2\,max}$ was conducted. All four carbohydrate-containing drinks substantially increased the length of the timed ride; however, there were no significant differences among these drinks. It is worth noting that the length of the timed ride was longer with both drinks containing guar gum than in the drinks with the same carbohydrate without guar gum, i.e., glucose + guar gum was longer than glucose alone, and maltodextrin + guar gum was longer than maltodextrin alone. A two-way analysis of variance may have determined whether guar gum had a statistically significant effect on time to exhaustion; however, this was apparently not done.

The evidence indicating that a slowed rate of glucose absorption, mediated by either viscous fiber or low Glycemic Index foods, increases athletic endurance is intriguing but not compelling. Particularly troublesome is the inconsistent effect of the low Glycemic Index foods on endurance in the two studies of trained cyclists that were conducted using essentially the same protocol.[72,73] Thus, there is not a strong basis for advocating consumption of viscous fibers or low GI foods prior to endurance exercise to enhance performance. However, viewed another way, there is also no evidence that it in any way impairs performance. A definitive answer to the utility of consuming such foods must await further research.

5.8 EFFECT OF DIETARY FIBER AND EXERCISE ON RISK FACTORS FOR DISEASE

Only one study has examined dietary fiber consumption and exercise on risk factors for disease in a systematic manner. In this study, the effect of wheat bran and exercise on plasma lipids and body weight and fat in moderately overweight men was determined.[63] The high fiber period included 0.5 g wheat bran per kg initial body weight, and during the low fiber period 0.2 g wheat bran per kg was consumed. The groups were to cross over after six weeks. The exercised group took part in a 12-week training program of walking and running 12 miles per week. A group that maintained their normal level of activity served as sedentary controls. Thus, both the exercised group and sedentary groups consumed both the high- and low-fiber diets. The fiber content of the diets had no influence on either total plasma cholesterol or triglycerides or upon the cholesterol concentration in any lipoprotein fraction. Fiber content also had no effect on body weight or percentage body fat. Body weight and percentage body fat decreased in the exercised group, whereas these parameters slightly increased in the sedentary group. However, these differences were not statistically significant. HDL cholesterol concentrations increased over the 12-week period in the exercised group, whereas there was no change in the sedentary group. There were no apparent interactions between fiber and exercise for any of the parameters measured. Thus, in this study, there was no potentiation of the effect of exercise on plasma lipids or body composition by a high insoluble fiber diet.

In a study of glycemic control by dietary fiber, insulin-dependent diabetic children were rotated through low-, medium-, or high-fiber diets, spending two days on each. The increase in fiber was as bran, wholemeal bread, and apple. In addition, all children were asked to exercise for an hour the first day and rest for an hour the second day of each two-day diet period. Blood glucose concentrations were measured at intervals after breakfast and mid-morning snack. Exercise had no significant effect on blood glucose concentrations. However, the medium- and high-fiber diets significantly reduced blood glucose concentrations at 60 minutes after breakfast and through an hour after the mid-morning snack. The reduction was approximately the same for both. Thus, some benefit in glucose control was gained by consumption of increased amounts of fiber, but the inclusion of exercise did not add further to this. However, as the role of exercise in improving blood glucose control in insulin-dependent diabetics is controversial,[64] there may not have been a strong basis for expecting an interaction between fiber and exercise.

From the very limited evidence available, an interaction between dietary fiber and exercise on risk factors for disease has not been shown. However, this is an area that clearly warrants further attention, given the potential benefit of both. Different types of dietary fiber, more intense exercise programs, and risk factors for other diseases all need to be explored.

5.9 CONCLUSION

Dietary fiber is composed of a mixture of plant materials that resist hydrolysis by mammalian digestive enzymes[1] and, thus, pass through the small intestine unabsorbed. Fibers differ greatly in their physical and chemical properties, which gives rise to different physiological effects. The best established of these effects include fecal bulking,[18] reduction in the postprandial blood glucose and insulin curves,[21,22] and a reduction in cholesterol absorption.[32,33]

Several studies have been reported in which athletic endurance was significantly prolonged when soluble dietary fiber or foods that slowed glucose absorption were consumed before exercise.[72,75] However, several other studies reported no increase in endurance.[73,74] There are no studies reporting negative consequences to consuming a dietary fiber-rich meal 45 to 60 minutes before exercise. Thus, a definitive answer to the question of the role of dietary fiber in athletic performance must await further study.

REFERENCES

1. Trowell, H., Definition of fiber, *Lancet*, i, 503, 1974.
2. Spiller, G. A., Definition of dietary fiber, *CRC Handbook of Dietary Fiber in Human Nutrition*, first edition, Spiller, G. A., CRC Press LLC, Boca Raton, 1986, 15.
3. Selvendran, R. R., The plant cell wall as a source of dietary fiber: chemistry and structure, *Am. J. Clin. Nutr.*, 39, 320, 1984.
4. Wood, P. J., Physicochemical characteristics and physiological properties of oat $(1\rightarrow3)$, $(1\rightarrow4)$-β-D-glucan, *Oat Bran*, Wood, P. J., American Association of Cereal Chemists, St. Paul, 1993, 83.
5. Kay, R. M., Dietary fiber, *J. Lipid Res.*, 23, 221, 1982.
6. Prosky, L., Asp, N.-G., Furda, I., DeVries, J., Schweizer, T. F., and Harland, B., Determination of total dietary fiber in foods, food products and total diets: interlaboratory study, *J. Assoc. Off. Anal. Chem.*, 67, 1044, 1984.
7. Prosky, L., Asp, N.-G., Furda, I., DeVries, J., Schweizer, T. F., and Harland, B., Determination of total dietary fiber in foods and food products: collaborative study, *J. Assoc. Off. Anal. Chem.*, 68, 677, 1985.
8. Prosky, L., Asp, N.-G., Schweizer, T. F., DeVries, J. W., and Furda, I., Determination of insoluble, soluble, and total dietary fiber in foods and food products: interlaboratory study, *J. Assoc. Off. Anal. Chem.*, 71, 1017, 1988.
9. Lanza, E., Jones, Y., Block, G., and Kessler, L., Dietary fiber intakes in the U.S. population, *Am. J. Clin. Nutr.*, 46, 790, 1987.

10. Tainter, M. L., and Buchanan, O. H., Quantitative comparisons of colloidal laxatives, *Annals N. Y. Acad. Sci.*, 58, 438, 1954.
11. McConnell, A. A., Eastwood, M. A., and Mitchell, W. D., Physical characteristics of vegetable foodstuffs that could influence bowel function, *J. Sci. Fd. Agric.* 25, 1457, 1974.
12. Stephen, A. M., and Cummings, J. H., Water holding capacity of dietary fibre in vitro and its relationship to fecal output in man, *Gut*, 20, 722, 1979.
13. McBurney, M. I., Horvath, P. J., Jeraci, J. L., and Van Soest, P. J., Effect of an *in vitro* fermentation using human fecal inoculum on the water holding capacity of dietary fibre, *Br. J. Nutr.*, 53, 17, 1985.
14. Burne, J., *A Treatise on the Causes and Consequence of Habitual Constipation*, Longman, Orme, Brown, Green & Longmans, London, 1840.
15. Spiller, G. A., Suggestions for a basis on which to determine a desirable intake of dietary fiber, *CRC Handbook of Dietary Fiber in Human Nutrition*, second edition, Spiller, G. A., CRC Press LLC, Boca Raton, 1993, 351.
16. Burkitt, D. P., Walker, A. R. P., and Painter, N. S., Effect of dietary fibre on stools and transit-times, and its role in the causation of disease, *Lancet*, ii, 1408, 1972.
17. Marlett, J. A., Balasubramanian, R., Johnson, E. J., and Draper, N. R., Determining compliance with a dietary fiber supplement, *J. Natl. Cancer Inst.*, 76, 1065, 1986.
18. Cummings, J. H., The effect of dietary fiber on fecal weight and composition, *CRC Handbook of Dietary Fiber in Human Nutrition*, second edition, Spiller, G. A., CRC Press LLC, Boca Raton, 1993, 263.
19. Stephen, A. M. and Cummings, J. H., The microbial contribution to human faecal mass, *J. Med. Microbial.*, 13,45, 1980.
20. Holt, S., Heading, R. C., Carter, D. C., Prescott, L. F., and Tothill, P, Effect of a gel fibre on gastric emptying and absorption of glucose and paracetamol, *Lancet*, i, 636, 1979.
21. Jenkins, D. J. A., Wolever, T. M. S., Leeds, A. R., Gassull, M. A., Dilawari, J. B., Goff, D. V., Metz, G. L., and Alberti, K. G. M. M., Dietary fibers, fiber analogues, and glucose tolerance: importance of viscosity, *Brit. J. Med.*, 1, 1392,1978.
22. Wood, P., Braaten, J., Scott, F., Riedel, D., and Poste, L., Comparisons of viscous properties of oat and guar gum and the effects of these and oat bran on glycemic index, *J. Agric. Food Chem.*, 38, 753, 1990.
23. Wahlqvist, M. L., Morris, M. J., Littlejohn, G. O., Bond, A., and Jackson, R. V. J., The effects of dietary fibre on glucose tolerance in healthy males, *Aust. N. Z. J. Med.* 9, 154, 1979.
24. Vachon, C., Jones, J. D., Wood, P. J., and Savoie, L., Concentration effect of soluble dietary fibers on postprandial glucose and insulin in the rat, *Can. J. Physiol. Pharmacol.*, 66,801, 1988.
25. Ebihara, K., Masuhara, R., Kiriyama, S., and Manabe, M., Correlation between viscosity and plasma glucose- and insulin-flattening activities of pectins from vegetables and fruits in rats, *Nutr. Rep. Intl.*, 23, 985, 1981.
26. Blackburn, N. A. and Johnson, I. T., The effect of guar gum on the viscosity of the gastrointestinal contents and on glucose uptake from the perfused jejunum in the rat, *Br. J. Nutr.*, 46, 239, 1981.
27. Blackburn, N. A., Redfern, J. S., Johnson, I. T., and Read, N. W., The mechanism of action of guar gum in improving glucose tolerance in man, *Clin. Sci.*, 66, 329, 1984.
28. Leclère, C. J., Chapm, M., Boillot, J., Guille, G., Lecannu, G., Molis, C., Bornet, F., Krempf, M., Delort-Laval, J., and Galmiche, J.-P., Role of viscous guar gums in lowering the glycemic response after a solid meal, *Am. J. Clin. Nutr.*, 59, 914, 1994.
29. Ray, T K., Mansell, K. M., Knight, L. C., Owen, L. S., and Boden, G., Long-term effects of dietary fiber on glucose tolerance and gastric emptying in noninsulin-dependent diabetic patients, *Am. J. Clin. Nutr.* 37, 376, 1983.
30. Leatherdale, B. A., Green, D. J., Harding, L. K., Griffin, D., and Bailey, C. J., Guar and gastric emptying in non-insulin dependent diabetes, *Acta Diabet. Lat.*, 19, 339, 1982.
31. Torsdottir, I., Alpsten, M., Andersson, H., and Einarsson, S., Dietary guar gum effects on postprandial blood glucose, insulin, and hydroxyproline in humans, *J. Nutr.*, 119, 1925, 1989.
32. Fernandez, M. L., Distinct mechanisms of plasma LDL lowering by dietary fiber in the guinea pig: specific effects of pectin, guar gum, and psyllium, *J. Lipid Res.*, 36, 2394, 1995.
33. Carr, T. P., Gallaher, D. D., Yang, C-H., and Hassel, C. A., Increased intestinal contents viscosity reduces cholesterol absorption efficiency in hamsters fed hydroxypropyl methylcellulose, *J. Nutr.*, 126, 1463, 1996.

34. Schneeman, B. O. and Gallaher, D., Effects of dietary fiber on digestive enzymes, *CRC Handbook of Dietary Fiber in Human Nutrition*, 2nd ed., Spiller, G. A., CRC Press LLC, Boca Raton, 1993, 111.

35. Sandberg, A.-S., Andersson, H., Hallgren, B., Hasselblad, K., Isaksson, B., and Hultén, L., The effects of citrus pectin on the absorption of nutrients in the small intestine, *Hum. Nutr. Clin. Nutr.,* 37C, 171, 1983.

36. Sandberg, A.-S., Andersson, H., Hallgren, B., Hasselblad, K., Isaksson, B., and Hultén, L., Experimental model for in vivo determination of dietary fibre and its effects on the absorption of nutrients in the small intestine, *Br. J. Nutr.*, 45, 283, 1981.

37. Ebihara, K. and Schneeman, B. O., Interaction of bile acids, phospholipids, cholesterol, and triglycerides with dietary fibers in the small intestine of rats, *J. Nutr.*, 119, 1100, 1989.

38. Rattan, J., Levin, N. E., Graff, N., Weizer, T., and Gilat, N., A high fiber diet does not cause mineral and nutrient deficiencies, *J. Clin. Gastroenterol.*, 3, 389, 1981.

39. Wahal, P. K., Singh, R., Kishore, B., Prakash, V., Maheshwari, B. B., Gujral, V. K., and Jain, B. B., Effect of high fibre intake on serum vitamin A levels, *J. Assoc. Physicians India*, 34, 269, 1986.

40. Roe, D. A., Kalkwarf, H., and Stevens, J., Effect of fiber supplements on the apparent absorption of pharmacological doses of riboflavin, *J. Am. Dietetic Assoc.*, 88, 210, 1988.

41. Miller, L.T., Schultz, T. D., and Leklem, J. E., Influence of citrus pectin on the bioavailability of vitamin B_6 in man, *Fed. Am. Soc. Exp. Biol.,* 39, 797, 1980.

42. Keltz, F. R., Kies, C., and Fox, H. M., Urinary ascorbic acid excretion in the human as affected by dietary fiber and zinc, *Am. J. Clin. Nutr.*, 31, 1167, 1978.

43. Kegy, P. M., Shane, B., and Oace, S. M., Folate bioavailability in humans: effects of wheat bran and beans, *Am. J. Clin. Nutr.*, 47, 80, 1988.

44. Gordon, D. T., Stoops, D., and Ratliff, V., Dietary fiber and mineral nutrition, *Dietary Fiber in Health and Disease*, Kritchevsky, D. and Bonfield, C., Eds., Eagan Press, St. Paul, 1995, 267.

45. Sakata, T., Stimulatory effect of short-chain fatty acids on epithelial cell proliferation in the rat intestine: a possible explanation for trophic effects of fermentable fibre, gut microbes, and luminal trophic factors, *Br. J. Nutr.*, 58, 95, 1987.

46. Malhotra, S. L., Faecal urobilinogen levels and pH of stools in population groups with different incidence of cancer of the colon, and their possible role in aetiology, *J. R. Soc. Med.*, 75, 709, 1982.

47. Chen, W.-J., Anderson, J. W., and Jennings, D., Propionate may mediate the hypocholesterolemic effects of certain soluble plant fibers in cholesterol-fed rats, *Soc. Exp. Biol. Med.* 75, 215, 1984.

48. Anderson, J. W. and Bridges, S. R., Plant fiber metabolites alter hepatic glucose and lipid metabolism, *Diabetes,* 30 (suppl. 1), 532A, 1981.

49. Illman, R. J., Topping, D. L., McIntosh, G. H., Trimble, R. P., Storer, G. B., Taylor, M. N., and Cheng, B.-Q., Hypocholesterolaemic effects of dietary propionate: studies in whole animals and perfused rat liver, *Ann. Nutr. Metab.*, 32, 97, 1988.

50. Topping, D. L., Propionate as a mediator of the effects of dietary fiber, *Dietary Fiber in Health and Disease*, Kritchevsky, D. and Bonfield, C., Eds., Eagan Press, St. Paul, 1995, 340.

51. Coleman, E., Update on carbohydrate: solid versus liquid, Int. *J. Sport Nutr.*, 4, 80, 1994.

52. Horowitz, J. F. and Coyle, E. F., Metabolic responses to preexercise meals containing various carbohydrates and fat, *Am. J. Clin. Nutr.*, 58, 235, 1993.

53. Ahlborg, G. and Felig, P., Influence of glucose ingestion on the fuel-hormone responses during prolonged exercise. *J. Appl. Physiol.*, 41, 683, 1976.

54. Ahlborg, G. and Bjorkman, O., Carbohydrate utilization by exercising muscle following preexercise glucose ingestion, *Clin Physiol.*, 7, 181, 1987.

55. Coyle, E.F., Substrate utilization during exercise in active people, *Am. J. Clin. Nutr.* 61(suppl), 968S, 1995.

56. Jarvis, J. K., Pearsall, D., Oliner, C. M. and Schoeller, D. A., The effect of food matrix on carbohydrate utilization during moderate exercise, *Med Sci. Sports Exerc.*, 24, 320, 1992.

57. Jenkins, D. J., Wolever, T. M., Taylor, R. H., Barker, H., Fielden, H., Baldwin, J. M., Bowling, A.C., Newman, H.C., Jenkins, A. L., and Goff, D.V., Glycemic index of foods: a physiological basis for carbohydrate exchange, *Am. J. Clin. Nutr.*, 34, 362, 1981.

58. Mourot, J., Thouvenot, P., Couet, C., Antoine, J. M., Krobicka, A. and Debry, G., Relationship between the rate of gastric emptying and glucose and insulin responses to starchy foods in young healthy adults, *Am. J. Clin. Nutr.*, 48, 1035, 1988.

59. Goddard M.S., Young, G., and Marcus, R., The effect of amylose content on insulin and glucose responses to ingested rice, *Am. J. Clin. Nutr.*, 39, 388, 1984.
60. Yoon, J.H., Thompson, L.U., and Jenkins, DJ., The effect of phytic acid on in vitro rate of starch digestibility and blood glucose response, *Am. J. Clin. Nutr.* 38, 835, 1983.
61. Thompson, L.U., Yoon, J.H., Jenkins, D.J., Wolever, T.M., and Jenkins, A.L., Relationship between polyphenol intake and blood glucose response of normal and diabetic individuals, *Am. J. Clin. Nutr.,* 39, 745, 1984.
62. Wood, P., Braaten, J., Scott. F., Riedel, D., and Poste, L., Comparisons of viscous properties of oat and guar gum and the effects of these and oat bran on glycemic index, *J. Agric. Food Chem.,* 38, 753, 1990.
63. Liebman, M., Smith, M. C., Iverson, J., Thye, F. W., Hinkle, D. E., Herbert, W. G., Ritchey, S. J. and Driskell, J. A., Effects of coarse wheat bran fiber and exercise on plasma lipids and lipoproteins in moderately overweight men, *Am. J. Clin. Nutr.* 36, 71, 1983.
64. Hough, D. O., Diabetes mellitus in sports, *Med. Clin. North. Am.,* 78, 423, 1994.
65. Nieman, D. C., Butler, J. V., Pollett, L. M., Dietrich, S. J., and Lutz, R. D., Nutrient intake of marathon runners, *J. Amer. Dietet. Assoc.,* 89, 1273, 1989.
66. Sutherland, W. H. F., Nye, E. R., Macfarlane, D. J., Robertson, M. C., and Williamson, S. A., Fecal bile acid concentration in distance runners, *Int. J. Sports Med.,* 12, 533, 1991.
67. Tanaka, J. A., Tanaka, H. and Landis, W., An assessment of carbohydrate intake in collegiate distance runners, *Int. J. Sport Nutr.,* 5, 206, 1995.
68. Peters, E. M. and Goetzsche, J. M., Dietary practices of South African ultradistance runners, *Int. J. Sport Nutr.,* 7, 80, 1997.
69. Boman, K., Hellsten, G., Bruce, Å, Hallmans, G., and Nilsson, T. K., Endurance physical activity, diet, and fibrinolysis, *Atherosclerosis,* 106, 65, 1994.
70. Rankinen, T., Fogelholm, M., Kujala, U., Rauramaa, R., and Uusitupa, M., Dietary intake and nutritional status of athletic and nonathletic children in early puberty, *Int. J. Sport Nutr.,* 5, 136, 1995.
71. Asp, N.-G., Sweden, *Dietary Fibre Intakes in Europe,* Cummings, J. H. and Frolich, W., Eds., Commission of the European Communities, Luxembourg, 1993, 77.
72. Thomas, D. E., Brotherhood, J. R., and Brand, J.C., Carbohydrate feeding before exercise: effect of glycemic index, *Int. J. Sports Med.,* 12, 180, 1991.
73. Thomas, D.E., Brotherhood, J.R., and Miller, J. B., Plasma glucose levels after prolonged strenuous exercise correlate inversely with glycemic response to food consumed before exercise, *Int. J. Sport Nutr.* 4, 361, 1994.
74. Paul, G. L., Rokusek, J.T., Dystra, G.L., Boileau, R.A., and Layman, D.K., Oat, wheat or corn cereal ingestion before exercise alters metabolism in humans, *J. Nutr.,* 126, 1372, 1996.
75. Kirwin, J. P., O'Gorman, D., and Evans, W. J., A moderate glycemic meal before endurance exercise can enhance performance, *J. Appl. Physiol.,* 84, 53, 1998.
76. MacLaren, D. P. M., Reilly, T., Campbell, I. T., and Frayn, K. N., Hormonal and metabolite responses to glucose and maltodextrin ingestion with or without the addition of guar gum, *Int. J. Sports Med.* 15, 466, 1994.

CHAPTER 6

Lipids in Exercise and Sports

J. Larry Durstine, Stephen F. Crouse, and Robert J. Moffatt

CONTENTS

0-8493-0755-4/00/$0.00+$.50

6.1 INTRODUCTION

Knowledge regarding the beneficial effects of physical activity on plasma lipid and lipoprotein metabolism has greatly expanded. In recent years both genetic and environmental factors have been found to influence the lipoprotein metabolic pathways. Factors such as gender, age, body composition, body fat distribution, cigarette smoking, medication use, physical activity, and dietary fat, cholesterol, carbohydrate, fiber and alcohol intake have been found to impact various aspects of lipid and lipoprotein metabolism. Abnormal lipid and lipoprotein profiles have been evaluated in regard to disease (e.g., coronary artery disease [CAD]) and to a lesser extent the use of dietary lipids as an aid to enhanced physical performance. This chapter 1) briefly defines and characterizes lipids, lipoproteins, and their metabolic pathways, 2) presents current information regarding lipids and CAD, 3) discusses the impact that exercise has on lipid and lipoprotein metabolism, and 4) addresses the issue of lipids as an ergogenic aid.

6.2 LIPID AND LIPOPROTEIN METABOLISM

6.2.1 Lipids

The primary blood lipids are free fatty acids (FFAs), triglyceride, and cholesterol. FFAs arise in the plasma from lipolysis of triglyceride in adipose tissue or as a result of the action of lipoprotein lipase (LPL) during uptake of plasma lipoprotein triglyceride into tissues. Triglyceride is the main storage form for FFAs (one triglyceride is made up of one glycerol molecule and three FFA molecules). Cholesterol is a lipid, an essential structural component of membranes, and the precursor of all other steroids in the body such as corticosteroid hormones, sex hormones, bile acids, and vitamin D.

FFAs are made available from triglyceride stores and provide an important energy source for the production of ATP during resting conditions, while increased FFA oxidation is characteristic of moderate intensity physical activity. Complete oxidation of FFA requires several metabolic steps (see Figure 6.1). The first step is the activation of the FFA by the action of the enzyme acyl-CoA synthetase. This reaction requires the expenditure of energy and results in an "active" fatty acid acyl-CoA. The long-chain acyl-CoA must then complex with carnitine before transport into the mitochondria where complete oxidation of the fatty acid can take place. Once inside the mitochondria, FFAs are sequentially oxidized by several enzymes collectively known as fatty acid oxidase to yield 2-carbon fragments referred to as acetyl-CoA, a process is known as β-oxidation. Each 2-carbon acetyl-CoA can then enter the Krebs Cycle. High energy compounds produced from β-oxidation and the Krebs Cycle will enter the electron-transport chain for a series of reactions coupled to the generation of ATP molecules. Because FFAs are very energy-dense, the net yield from the oxidation of a single molecule of palmitate, a commonly occurring 16 carbon fatty acid, is 130 ATP molecules.

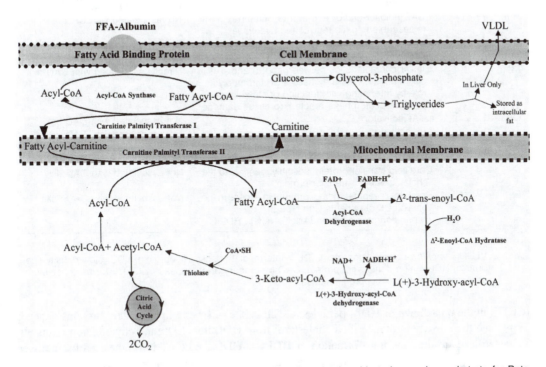

Figure 6.1   Free fatty acid transport into the cell and into the mitochondria to be used as substrate for Beta-oxidation.

6.2.2   Lipoproteins

Triglyceride and cholesterol alone are not water-soluble and must combine with apolipoproteins (apo) to form lipoprotein complexes in the blood. Lipoproteins have measurable dimensions, are water-soluble, and contain various amounts of cholesterol, triglyceride, phospholipid, and apolipoprotein. There are at least 17 different apolipoproteins, and in addition to making lipids soluble in an aqueous solution, they have various other functions (e.g., apo A-I will activate the enzyme lecithin:cholesterol acyltransferase (LCAT); see Table 6.1). Plasma lipoproteins form a complex transport system necessary for the movement of exogenous and endogenous lipids between the liver, the intestine, and peripheral tissues (see Figure 6.2). Essentially, four classes of lipoproteins exist: chylomicron, obtained from intestinal absorption of fatty acid; very-low-density-lipoprotein (VLDL or pre-β-lipoprotein), originates in the liver and is involved in the movement of triglyceride to peripheral tissue; low-density-lipoprotein (LDL or β-lipoprotein), the remaining constituent after the catabolism of VLDL; and high-density-lipoprotein (HDL or α-lipoprotein), involved in the reverse cholestrerol transport. Further, subfactions of each lipoprotein exist, including intermediate-density-lipoprotein (IDL), an intermediate step in VLDL catabolism; lipoprotein(a) [Lp(a)], a subfraction of LDL that is highly related to CAD, and two seperate HDL subfracions, HDL_2 and the more dense HDL_3[1] (see Table 6.2).

Plasma lipoprotein metabolism incorporates several key enzymes. LPL, an enzyme bound to capillary walls and found in various tissues (e.g., heart, adipose tissue, skeletal muscle), primary function is to hydrolyze the chylomicron and VLDL triglyceride core. Hepatic lipase (HL) is bound to the liver endothelial capillary lining and participates indirectly in the final conversion of chylomicron and VLDL remnants into LDL.[2–8] HL also works in conjunction with cholesterol ester transfer protein

Table 6.1 Major Human Apolipoproteins

Apolipoprotein	Major Function	CAD Risk Factor
A-I	LCAT activator	Inversely related with CAD risk
A-II	LCAT inhibitor and/or activator of heparin releaseable hepatic triglyceride hydrolase	Not associated with CAD risk
B-48	Required for synthesis of chylomicron	Directly associated with CAD risk
B-100	LDL receptor binding site	Directly associated with CAD risk
(a)	Similar characteristics between apo(a) and plasminogen, thus may have a prothrombolytic role by interfering with function of plasminogen, possible acute phase reactant to tissue damage	Directly associated with CAD risk
C-I	LCAT activator	Not associated with CAD risk
C-II	LPL activator	Not associated with CAD risk
C-III	LPL inhibitor, several forms depending on content of sialic acids	Not associated with CAD risk
D	Core lipid transfer protein, possibly identical to the cholesteryl ester transfer protein	Not associated with CAD risk
E	Remnant receptor binding, present in excess in the beta-VLDL of patients with type III hyperlipoproteinemia and exclusively in HDL-C	Not associated with CAD risk

VLDL = very-low-density lipoprotein, IDL = intermediate-density lipoprotein, LDL = low-density lipoprotein, HDL = high-density lipoprotein, CAD = coronary artery disease, LCAT = lecithin:cholesterol acyltransferase, LPL = lipoprotein lipase.

(CETP) in the breakdown of HDL_2 particles. CETP is one of several lipid transfer proteins believed to mediate the movement of esterified cholesterol from HDL_2 to VLDL and chylomicron remnants. This step leads to the final transformation of HDL_2 to HDL_3.[3-8] LCAT is synthesized by the liver, bound to plasma HDL_3, catalyzes the esterification of free cholesterol on the HDL surface, and eventually promotes the movement of esterified cholesterol into the HDL core forming the less dense HDL_2.[4]

6.2.3 Lipoprotein Metabolic Pathways

Foods that contain fat are digested in the small intestine and absorbed as fatty acids, free cholesterol, monoglycerides, and diglycerides.[9] The absorbed lipids combine with apolipoproteins (e.g., apo B-48, A-I, A-II, A-IV) to form lipid-rich chylomicrons that enter the blood from the lymphatic system by the thoracic duct.[6] LPL with apo C-II as an activator hydrolyzes the lipid core of blood chylomicrons, causing the release of FFAs, monoglycerides, and diglycerides.[8] During this process, surface remnants from the chylomicron are transferred to nascent HDL while the core remnants acquire other apolipoproteins such as apo C and apo E from interstitial fluid.[9] Lastly, receptors specific for apo E and apo B-48 on the surface of hepatic cells bind to core remnants and remove them from circulation.[9]

VLDL is synthesized by the liver and the intestine[19] and is the primary transport mechanism for endogenous synthesis by liver and dietary (absorbed from intestine) fatty acids.[9] Like chylomicron metabolism, the VLDL core is hydrolyzed by LPL, resulting in the release of triglyceride that is taken up by extra-hepatic tissue.[8] The remaining molecule, IDL, interacts with LPL and also HL to form LDL.[5,10] The remaining VLDL remnants bind to hepatic apo E receptors and are removed from the circulating blood.[10] The remaining LDL particles are the primary cholesterol transport mechanism to peripheral tissue cells where delivery is mediated by LDL receptors located on peripheral tissue cell surfaces.[11] Once recognition of the LDL molecule is achieved by the LDL-apo B-100 cellular receptor, LDL is moved inside the cell and exposed to lysomal digestion where cholesterol is released and used for cellular metabolic needs (see Figure 6.2).

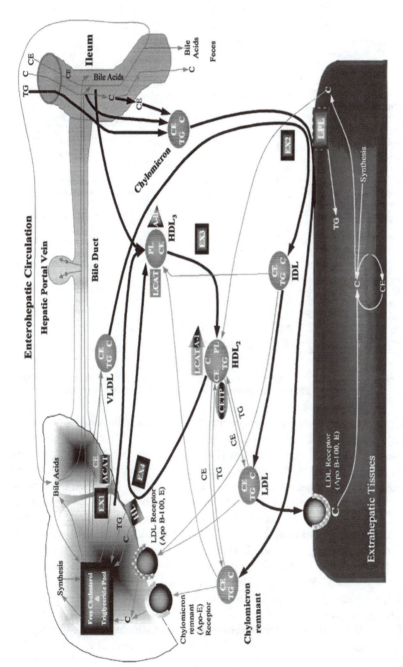
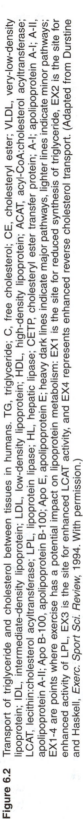

Figure 6.2 Transport of triglyceride and cholesterol between tissues in humans. TG, triglyceride; C, free cholesterol; CE, cholesteryl ester; VLDL, very-low-density lipoprotein; IDL, intermediate-density lipoprotein; LDL, low-density lipoprotein; HDL, high-density lipoprotein; ACAT, acyl-CoA:cholesterol acyltransferase; LCAT, lecithin:cholesterol acyltransferase; LPL, lipoprotein lipase; HL, hepatic lipase; CETP, cholesteryl ester transfer protein; A-I, apolipoprotein A-I; A-II, apolipoprotein A-II; Apo B-100, apolipoprotein B-100; Apo E, apolipoprotein E; heavy dark lines indicate major pathways, lighter lines indicate minor pathways; EX1-4 are points where exercise has a potential impact on lipoprotein metabolism: EX1 is the site for reduced synthesis of triglyceride, EX2 is the site for enhanced activity of LPL, EX3 is the site for enhanced LCAT activity, and EX4 represents enhanced reverse cholesterol transport. (Adapted from Durstine and Haskell, *Exerc. Sport Sci. Review*, 1994. With permission.)

Table 6.2. Characteristics of Plasma Lipoproteins and Lipids

Lipid/ Lipoprotein	Source	Protein %	Total Lipid %	TG	Chol	Phosp	Free Chol	Apolipoprotein
				Composition — Percentage of Total Lipid				
Chylomicron	Intestine	1–2	98–99	88	8	3	1	Major: A-IV, B-48, B-100, H Minor: A-I, A-II, C-I, C-II, C-III, E
VLDL	Major: Liver Minor: Intestine	7–10	90–93	56	20	15	8	Major: B-100, C-III, E, G Minor: A-I, A-II, B-48, C-II, D
IDL	Major: VLDL Minor: Chylomicron	11	89	29	26	34	9	Major: B-100 Minor: B-48
LDL	Major: VLDL Minor: Chylomicron	21	79	13	28	48	10	Major: B-100 Minor: C-I, C-II, (a)
HDL$_2$	Major: HDL$_3$	33	67	16	43	31	10	Major: A-1, A-II, D, E, F Minor: A-IV, C-I, C-II, C-III
HDL$_3$	Major: Liver and Intestine Minor: VLDL and Chylomicron Remnants	57	43	13	46	29	6	Major: A-1, A-II, D, E, F Minor: A-IV, C-I, C-II, C-III
Chol	Liver and Diet		100			70–75	25–30	
TG	Diet and Liver		100	100				

VLDL = very-low-density lipoprotein, IDL = intermediate-density lipoprotein, LDL = low-density lipoprotein, HDL = high-density lipoprotein, Chol = cholesterol, TG = triglyceride, Phosp = phospolipid.

The function of HDL is to transport cholesterol from peripheral tissue back to the liver for catabolism. This process has been termed reverse cholesterol transport. Several HDL pathways exist for cholesterol removal from HDL.[12] The first pathway involves nascent HDL particles that are secreted by the liver and/or small intestine and are derived from LPL catabolism of chylomicron and VLDL.[5,13] These HDL particles contain phospholipid and free cholesterol that will readily react with LCAT. Apo A-I in this case will serve as a co-factor.[14] This interaction results in free cholesterol being esterified and the ester being shifted into the HDL$_3$ core.[4] The shift of cholesterol toward the HDL$_3$'s core results in a chemical gradient that allows for continual supply of cholesterol for the LCAT reaction.[15] The cholesterol esters influx into the HDL$_3$'s core causes an expansion in the HDL$_3$ size and eventual conversion to the less dense, larger HDL$_2$ particle. During this particular removal process, two important series of reactions must occur. The first reaction is the CETP-facilitated movement of HDL$_2$ cholesterol esters from either chylomicron and/or VLDL remnants in exchange for triglyceride.[12] The remnants are delivered to the liver where they are metabolized and removed from the blood.[1] The second reaction relates to the triglyceride-enriched HDL$_2$ particles. The added triglyceride on the HDL$_2$ molecule provides the substrate necessary for HL to degrade the HDL$_2$ in the liver. Once triglyceride removal from the HDL$_2$ is completed, the end product of this reaction is HDL$_3$, which will return to the blood and continue the cycle. Two other potential pathways exist for the removal of cholesterol from the blood. One is the exit of HDL$_2$ from circulating blood through hepatic apo E LDL receptors. A second is the direct HDL$_2$ cholesterol exit from circulating blood through liver cells by phospholipase and HL activity.[16]

6.2.4   Implications

Lipids and lipoproteins do have valuable funtions as cellular components and as energy sources at rest and during exercise. Triglycerides are used to store energy, while cholesterol is used as a component for cellular membranes and in steroid hormones synthesis. When used as an energy source, FFAs are released from the triglyceride stores and undergo β-oxidation (see Figure 6.1) FFA oxidation provides the majority of the energy needs at rest and during low- to moderate-intensity exercise. Both triglyeride and cholesterol must combine with apolipoproteins in the blood for transport throughout the vascular compartment. This transport system is in part the lipoprotein metabolic pathway (see Figure 6.2).

6.3 LIPIDS, LIPOPROTEINS, AND ATHEROSCLEROSIS

Atherosclerosis has historically been defined as "the widely prevalent arterial lesion character-ized by patchy thickening of the intima. This thickening comprising accumulations of fat and layers of collagen-like fibers, both being present in widely varying proportions."[17] Atherosclerosis affecting the coronary vessels, often referred to as CAD, is the most prevalent cause of heart disease in Western societies. The genesis and growth of this thickening referred to as arterial plaque occur gradually by a process that involves endothelial injury, connective tissue proliferation, infiltration and retention of plasma-derived lipids, and tissue necrosis.[18]

6.3.1   Lipids and Lipoproteins as CAD Risk Factors

Epidemiologically, the association between blood cholesterol and atherogenesis is well-documented[19–21] and is reportedly both continuous and graded.[22] Early experimental studies designed to test the hypothesis that lowering blood cholesterol through drug treatment could reduce the incidence for new myocardial infarction were inconclusive.[23,24] However, recent clinical trials, particularly those employing the statin drugs to lower blood cholesterol concen-tration, provide convincing support for a causal relationship between blood cholesterol and CAD risk.[25,26] Added support for a reduced mortality is found in recently reported studies of patients who have experienced a previous coronary event. Lowering plasma cholesterol and LDL-C reduced the incidence of CAD death.[27] This was also true for patients with average pre-inter-vention blood LDL-C concentrations.[28] Furthermore, aggressive cholesterol-lowering therapy has been shown to be effective in reducing the rate of atherosclerotic disease progression in native coronary arteries[29,30] and in patients with venous coronary artery bypass grafts.[31] Desirable blood cholesterol concentrations for adults are now defined as less than 200 mg/dL.[32]

Emerging research has made clear that in addition to the atherogenic risk of elevated blood choles-terol, the manner that cholesterol is distributed among the various lipoproteins influences the pathoge-nicity of this lipid. The historical roots relating blood lipoproteins to atherosclerosis can be traced to Barr et al.[33] who stated that "the outstanding fact in our observations is the relative and absolute reduction of HDL in atherosclerosis." They noted that human infants carry a large proportion of plasma cholesterol in HDL. This observation is similar to that made in animals. Generally both infants and animals exhibit a high resistance to CAD. However, as humans age the HDL proportion will fall, and this is when humans develop CAD.[34] These findings lead Barr et al.[33] to the hypothesis that HDL exerts a protective effect on the heart. With rare exceptions,[35] these findings were virtually ignored for nearly two decades, and the majority of lipid and lipoprotein studies focused on serum total cholesterol and LDL-C. The early focus on LDL-C was most likely a logical outgrowth of the findings that in humans LDL, not HDL, is the major transport mechanism for the largest proportion of human blood cholesterol and plays a functional role in the movement of cholesterol to peripheral cells as well as to arterial plaque sites. Not surprisingly, LDL-C generally evinces a positive relationship with both total serum (or plasma) cholesterol and CAD. Thus, CAD risk cut-points are often defined in terms of LDL-C concentrations, and strategies to reduce LDL-C are generally employed in CAD risk management programs.[32,36]

Table 6.3   Plasma Lipids and Lipoproteins and Their Relationship to CAD Risk and the Effects of Physical Activity

Lipid/Lipoprotein	Relationship to CAD	Effect of Physical Activity
Chylomicron	Positive	None
VLDL	Somewhat positive	Decreased
IDL	Somewhat positive	Decrease or no change
LDL	Strong positive	Decrease or no change
Lp(a)	Strong positive	Presently, physical activity has no or little impact
HDL$_2$	Strong inverse	Increase
HDL$_3$	Inverse	Decrease
Cholesterol	Strong positive	No change
Triglyceride	Somewhat positive	Decrease

CAD = coronary artery disease, VLDL = very-low-density lipoprotein, IDL = intermediate-density lipoprotein, LDL = low-density lipoprotein, Lp(a) = lipoprotein(a), HDL = high-density lipoprotein.

Evidence also exists to show that the small, more-dense LDL particles are more atherogenic than the larger, more buoyant LDL.[37] Excess Lp(a), a subfraction of LDL containing the glycoprotein apo(a), is also a strong predictor of premature CAD[38] (see Table 6.3).

A resurgence of interest in HDL-C concentration and CAD risk occurred in the 1970s when the Framingham Heart Study lipoprotein results were first published. In 1968, 2815 men and women between the ages of 49 and 82 years from the Framingham cohort were recruited to undergo lipid and lipoprotein determinations. Following four years of follow-up, serum HDL-C concentration was found to be inversely related to CAD incidence and statistically the most potent lipid CAD risk marker. LDL-C concentration was only weakly associated with CAD incidence, and after this follow-up period, total cholesterol proved to be unrelated to CAD risk.[39] Later the Framingham Heart Study follow-up reports corroborated these earlier HDL-C findings. After 12 years of follow-up with the Framingham cohort, serum HDL-C concentration was found to be inversely associated with the incidence of myocardial infarction.[40] In a subsequent publication using this same data, men with the lowest serum HDL-C concentrations (≤ 46 mg/dL) compared with those with the highest (≥ 67 mg/dl) had a six-fold excess CAD risk. These findings presisted after adjusting for age and other factors. Similar HDL-C effects were found for women. Furthermore, low HDL-C concentrations have been shown to be predictive of myocardial infarction even in subjects with low total cholesterol concentrations.[41] On the basis of these data, an estimate of 1% lower HDL-C value was associated with a 3 to 4% increased CAD risk.[42] This strong inverse association between HDL-C and CAD has been confirmed in several other population based studies.[21,43,44–46] Either the ratios of total cholesterol or LDL-C concentration to HDL-C concentration (relates the anti-atherogenic aspects of HDL-C to the atherogenic potential of total cholesterol and LDL-C) are stronger predictors of CAD in both men and women than total cholesterol or HDL-C alone.[44,47]

Other information concerning atherogenic risk status as well as more precision in predicting future occurrences of atherosclerotic disease could be gained by measuring other blood lipoprotein-lipid constituents. In this regard, the HDL subfraction concentrations HDL$_2$-C and HDL$_3$-C may be useful in quantifying CAD risk. Women, who typically have lower rates of CAD, have serum HDL$_2$-C concentrations that are higher than men.[48] An inverse relationship between CAD and both HDL$_2$-C and HDL$_3$-C concentrations has been reported in prospective studies (see Table 6.3), and both are significantly associated with myocardial infarction.[37,44,49,50] High triglyceride concentration may be an independent predictor of CAD, especially when considered in light of low HDL-C values.[51,52] Apo A-I, the major protein found on HDL, is lower in patients who have suffered an acute myocardial infarction and is a good discriminator of angiographically documented CAD (see Table 6.1).[53,54] Similarly, apo B, the major protein associated with LDL, is elevated in individuals with CAD (see Table 6.1),[55] and the ratio of apo B to apo A-I has been shown to be a powerful discriminator for either the presence and/or severity of angiographically defined CAD.[56]

6.3.2 Lipids and the Injury Response Hypothesis

The morphological history of atherosclerotic lesions is generally thought to begin with the formation of the so-called fatty streak that is found in large elastic and muscular arteries. The fatty streak is characterized by the presence of sub-endothelial lipid-laden macrophage and T-lympho-cytes.[18,57,58] Necropsy data have shown fatty streaks in 43% of deceased children age ranging from one month to one year.[59] Some reports suggest that small blister-like elevations in the aortic intima, referred to as gelatinous lesions, constitute the next step in the formation of more fully developed arterial plaque. These lesions involve a separation of the connective tissue elements of the intima by interstitial edema, and they contain small amounts of lipid as well as increased amount of fibrinogen and LDL-C.[60,61] This intermediate lesion consists of layers of macrophages and smooth muscle cells. These lesions further develop into the more definitive atherosclerosis lesion known as a raised lesion or fibrolipid plaque that is characterized by connective tissue and smooth muscle cell "cap" covering a lipid-enriched area of necrotic tissue.[18,62] These raised plaques are associated with changes in the adventitial tissues that include an increase in fibrous tissue, an increase in vascularity, and the frequent presence of cellular aggregates consisting primarily of lymphocytes.[63] Necropsy results from the coronary arteries of 100 patients who died suddenly of heart disease show thrombi related to plaque fissures in 74% of the cases, while in 44% the thrombi occupied over half of the lumen diameter.[64] Thus, not only does the plaque cause a mechanical narrowing of the arterial lumen with obvious impairment in arterial flow, but plaque fissuring or rupture also appears to be related to thrombi formation and sudden death. Evidence suggests that elevated plasma LDL-C concentrations may contribute to plaque instability and rupture.[65]

Although there is disagreement, a considerable amount of evidence suggests that subtle injury to the endothelial cell can lead to functional arterial wall changes. These small changes are insufficient to cause cell retraction or loss of cell integrity, yet they likely lead to atherosclerosis.[18,66] CAD risk factors such as cigarette smoke and hypertension are thought to lead to altered endothelial cell ultrastructure function, resulting in the formation of microthrombi.[67–71] More pertinent is the fact that hypercholesterolemia has also been shown to contribute to ultrastructural changes in the endothelium, while LDL, particularly following oxidation, exhibits direct cytotoxic effects on endothelial tissue.[72–75] There is also evidence from animal research that viral infections (e.g., herpes virus) may either cause or accelerate the development of atherosclerosis.[66,67]

Following injury, the endothelium expresses adhesion molecules, chemoattractants, and cytokines to recruit mononuclear cells and T lymphocytes to the injury site. These cells attach to the endothelium and then migrate between endothelial cells, resulting in intimal cell proliferation and further subsequent lipid deposition. Monocytes become lipid-laden macrophages (foam cells) and together with phenotypically distinct, noncontractile smooth muscle cells (SMCs) that have migrated as immature SMC blasts into the intima from the media, constitute the major forms of cells comprising the active atheromatous lesion.[78] SMCs are capable of synthesizing collagen, elastin, and proteoglycans and dividing in response to mitogenic stimuli, thereby forming the matrix characteristic for atherosclerotic plaque.[79] Several other regulatory molecules, such as platelet-derived growth factor, epidermal growth factor, and transforming growth factor — all derived from platelets — are thought to act in concert to stimulate SMC growth and division.[80,81] Platelet-derived growth factor can also be synthesized and secreted by endothelial cells[82] and macrophages,[83] as well as SMCs.[84] In addition, lipoproteins,[85] particularly LDL[86,87] and hormones[88] are involved in the increased growth of mitogen-stimulated arterial SMCs. In contrast to the enabling influence of LDL, some evidence exists that suggests that HDL may play a role in restricting SMC growth and division[89] while other evidence suggests that lowering blood LDL-C concentration may help stabilize vulnerable plaque and improve vasomotor functional responsiveness.[65]

The weight of present evidence points to the circulating lipoproteins, particularly LDL-C, as the source of lipid that accumulates in the atherosclerotic lesion.[90] Most cells of the body, including macrophages[91] and arterial SMCs,[92] have tightly regulated surface LDL receptors that bind with plasma LDL. Once plasma LDL takes up the cell's LDL receptor, they are transported by endocytosis into the cell as a receptor-LDL complex. The resulting intracellular lipoprotein vacuole is subsequently digested by cellular lysosome and releases unesterified cholesterol[11,93] used by the cell or esterified for storage. Brown and Goldstein[11,94] have shown that cholesterol synthesis in the cell is normally inhibited when the cell's receptor is occupied by LDL. Inasmuch as normal concentrations of circulating blood LDL are generally enough to repress the rate of cellular cholesterol production, cellular cholesterol synthesis under normal circumstances is thought to contribute little to the massive cholesterol accumulation characteristically found in foam cell development. Excess cholesterol deposition from elevated circulating blood sources and inefficient removal of excess cholesterol are the most frequent contributing factors for the development of atherosclerosis. In theory, cellular accumulation of cholesterol could occur when LDL-C blood levels are high[95] and, conversely, when intracellular LDL-C degradation or removal is impaired.[93]

Macrophages also possess scavenger receptors capable of binding both acetylated and oxidatively modified LDL. In contrast to the LDL receptor, scavenger receptor activity is not regulated by cell cholesterol content and may, therefore, lead to massive cholesterol accumulation and foam cell formation, particularly in the presence of excess LDL.[11,96] The macrophage can also bind and ingest lipid through a chylomicron remnant receptor,[97] through a specialized receptor for VLDL,[98] and by the process of phagocytosis following the formation of aggregated LDL particles.[99] Additional evidence for the importance of receptor up-regulation comes from animal models for atherosclerosis in which mRNA for scavenger receptors and VLDL receptors were highly induced in atherosclerotic lesions.[100] Each process can contribute to macrophage and smooth muscle cell-derived foam cell formation and thereby to the development of the mature atherosclerotic lesion.

6.3.3. Smoking

Epidemiological studies suggest that cigarette smoking is modestly associated with elevated serum cholesterol, triglyceride and LDL-C levels,[101] while other studies report no change in these parameters due to smoking.[102–104] Decreases in blood HDL-C and HDL_2-C levels in association with cigarette smoking are more consistent. Reports of decreased levels relative to non-smokers of 15–20% for HDL-C and 40–50% for HDL_2-C are common.[102,103,105] However, cessation from cigarette smoking normalizes these levels[103,106,107] and in some cases as quickly as 17 days.[103] Furthermore, levels of HDL-C and HDL_2-C as well as apo A-1 levels are also depressed by exposure to environmental tobacco smoke.[108]

6.3.4 Implications

Cholesterol and the cholesterol present with the various lipoproteins are associated with increased CAD risk. The CAD and cholesterol relationship is well-documented by epidemiologic trials, and information suggests that the cholesterol distributed among the various lipoproteins is as important, if not more important, than knowing just the plasma cholesterol concentration. The morphology of atherosclerotic lesion is thought to begin with the formation of the fatty streak. Evidence suggests that elevated plasma LDL-C may contribute to arterial wall plaque accumulation, and HDL-C is involved in the reverse cholesterol transport process and may confer protection from plaque buildup.

6.4 PHYSICAL ACTIVITY, LIPIDS, AND LIPOPROTEINS

Physical activity can elicit changes in plasma lipids and lipoproteins (see Table 6.3).[1] This section summarizes the exercise-induced impact on intramuscular triglyceride stores, plasma lipids, lipoproteins, apolipoproteins, and lipoprotein enzymes.

6.4.1 Lipids

6.4.1.1 Intramuscular Triglyceride

Because blood chylomicron and VLDL concentrations, especially in the post-absorptive period, are generally low when exercise commences,[110] the main lipid sources used for muscular work come from the adipose tissue and intramuscular triglyceride stores.[111–115] Traditional views maintain that adipose tissue triglyceride supplies the majority of fatty acids for low to moderate intensity exercise (25–50% maximal oxygen consumption $\dot{V}O_{2\,max}$). When exercise intensity increases past 50–60% $\dot{V}O_{2\,max}$, carbohydrate oxidation increases exponentially.[111,112,116,117] However, studies conducted over the last decade have determined that a major substrate for moderate to heavy intensity (60–80% V.O2 max) is the endogenous muscle triglyceride store or intramuscular triglyceride (IMTG).[111,118–125] This is particularly true in trained subjects[111,112,119,121] when blood fatty acids have been shown to actually decrease during exercise.[111,122]

After exercise training, intramuscular triglyceride stores increase[112,120,121,126] and provide evidence that IMTG are indeed an important energy source during exercise. In fact, IMTG will respond to both diet[126–128] and exercise training, adding further support that IMTG are increased in the muscle similarly to muscle glycogen store changes after exercise training. Although there is considerable evidence for the use of IMTG during exercise, one investigation has dismissed the idea of IMTG as providing a significant and trainable energy source during exercise.[129]

6.4.1.2 Plasma FFAs

Plasma FFAs have long been considered the primary fuel for prolonged low- to moderate-intensity exercise.[111,112,117,122,130–132] Their importance during this type of work is supported by the fact that FFA uptake is concentration-dependent, with greater FFA uptake occurring with greater plasma FFA levels.[115,132] Fatty acid uptake responds positively to exercise training. Uptake of FFAs will increase linearly with increased supply in trained subjects, whereas saturation kinetics are displayed (e.g., a plateau effect) in inactive subjects.[116,132] These two facts indicate that FFA uptake from the blood is carrier-dependent.[115,132]

Because of their essentially unlimited supply, fatty acids derived from adipose tissue are an attractive fuel source for prolonged endurance activity.[117] However, evidence exists that shows a reduction in peripheral FFA mobilization following exercise training when the whole body fat oxidation capacity increases (due to increased mitochondrial volume and enzyme activity levels).[111,121,122] This discrepancy indicates that perhaps blood FFAs are diminished as a fuel source during moderate- to high-intensity exercise following exercise training.[111,112,120]

6.4.1.3 Plasma Triglyceride

Plasma triglyceride concentrations generally decrease after exercise training.[1] These changes are related to baseline concentrations. Persons with higher triglyceride concentrations before beginning a physical activity program may experience a greater reduction in triglyceride levels after exercise training intervention completion.[133,134] Starting a physical activity program in hypertriglyceridemic patients will result in lower plasma triglyceride concentrations.[135,136] Though the size of change was not as great, formerly inactive subjects with triglyceride concentrations of 130 mg/dL had approximately a 10–20% lower triglyceride concentration following exercise intervention of 3 to 12 months.[133,137,138] Whereas, subjects with lower triglyceride concentrations and completing exercise training programs with similar frequency, intensity, and duration had only small nonsignificant triglyceride concentration reductions.[139,140] Collectively, these studies suggest that exercise training can decrease triglyceride concentrations in most people, and individuals who have the highest initial triglyceride concentrations receive the greatest reductions.

6.4.1.4 Plasma Cholesterol

Physical activity studies employing exercise training and lasting between three weeks to one year have observed no change in plasma cholesterol concentration.[133,135,137,138,140–142] Infrequently, decreased cholesterol concentrations have been found after exercise training.[143–145] Such changes were not related to initial cholesterol concentration or length of the exercise training program. Cholesterol reductions up to 11% have been described after some physical activity intervention studies when statistical significance was not found.[135,137–139,142] Decreased body fat percentages were found in some studies reporting statistical significance cholesterol change,[144,145] whereas no change in body composition was also reported[143] when significant cholesterol change was also reported. Other investigations have not found a significant decrease in cholesterol, but they have found decreased percentage body fat.[137,138,140,141] Consequently, body composition change in response to exercise training is most likely not a cholesterol change determinant.

6.4.2 Plasma Lipoproteins

6.4.2.1 Chylomicron and VLDL

Blood chylomicrons and VLDLs are not thought to provide a very large supply of fatty acids for oxidation during exercise.[112,117] The reason for this is two-fold. One, chylomicron and VLDL concentrations are elevated only during the immediate postprandial period when most people don't exercise, and two, the caloric equivalent of these circulating blood lipoproteins is too small to supply a major portion of the energy supply during muscular work.[112] A small body of research indicates an increase in the clearance of lipids from the blood during exercise following acutely elevated circulating blood triglyceride levels (e.g., postprandial lipemia).[110,146] This fact supports the concept for the potential uptake and oxidation of triglyceride from chylomicron and VLDL during muscular work. However, Kiens et al.[147] demonstrated that muscle LPL activity in opposition to adipose tissue LPL is down regulated by physiologic concentrations of insulin and indicated that uptake of triglyceride from chylomicron and VLDL during exercise in the postprandial period will be limited.

6.4.2.2 Low Density Lipoprotein

LDL-C is increased in plasma in individuals who have high dietary fat intake, especially saturated fats.[1,146] LDL-C is a potent predictor of cardiovascular disease (see Table 6.3)[1,112,148,149] and is generally lower after regular endurance exercise participation,[1,146,150] although some studies have reported no changes.[133,140–142,151,152] Lower LDL-C in physically active individuals is due in part to the effect of HDL-C mediated reverse cholesterol transport.[1,153,154]

LDL has been divided into different density ranges, each carrying different CAD risk. The concentration of smaller denser LDL particles correlates positively with CAD incidence and may depend on high triglyceride concentration.[155] Williams et al.[156,157] has examined "small" LDL particle concentration in healthy and mildly overweight [mean body mass index (BMI) of 30] men one year after beginning a physical activity program. Small LDL concentrations were not significantly changed after exercise training, but both distance run per week and reduced fat mass correlated significantly with the decrease in small LDL concentrations in men of normal body fat percentages (22%).[156] BMI reduction in the mildly overweight subjects was related to decrease in small LDL.[157] Halle et al.[158] cross-sectionally evaluated physically active and inactive hypercholesterolemic (cholesterol > 240 mg/dL) men. Triglyceride and small LDL concentrations were lower in physically active men. Multivariate regression analysis revealed that the amount of "small" LDL particles present were influenced by $\dot{V}O_{2\,max}$ and not BMI.

6.4.2.3 Lp(a)

Lp(a) is a LDL subfraction. It contains the apolipoprotein apo(a)[148,149,159] and is highly homologous with plasminogen (80%). As a result, Lp(a) can inhibit fibrinolysis due to competitive binding with plasminogen for fibrin.[149,159,160] Thus, Lp(a) has the same negative effects of LDL-C in terms of lipid composition. In addition, it inhibits the blood clotting process.[159] Furthermore, individuals with elevated levels (>25 mg/dL) appear to have inherited this trait.[148,160] Moreover, Lp(a) levels greater than 25 mg/dL are positively correlated to the development of CAD (see Table 6.3).[148,160] Lp(a), unfortunately, does not appear to respond to regular exercise training and/or a single exercise session.[149,159,161,162]

6.4.2.4 *High-Density Lipoprotein*

HDL is generally responsive to aerobic training and increases in a dose-dependent manner with increased energy expenditure found during exercise.[1,153,163,164] Again, HDL-C is not thought to be an energetic substrate, but it has a role in determining CAD risk. Interventional studies often show that exercise training lasting 12 weeks or more will likely increase HDL-C concentrations,[133,136,139,141,142,145,165] but not always.[138,139,166] Exercise training-induced increases in HDL-C concentration range from 4% to 22%. However, the absolute increase in HDL-C was much more uniform ranging from 2 to 8 mg/dL. A meta-analysis by Tran et al.[167] reported a negative correlation between initial HDL-C concentrations and exercise training HDL-C change. Further, Williams et al.[168] found greater exercise-induced changes in HDL-C and HDL₂-C in overweight subjects (mean BMI of 29) with higher initial concentrations, and Thompson et al.[133] reported no relationship between exercise-induced change in HDL-C and baseline HDL-C concentration.

The length of the exercise intervention and exercise training volume (number of kcals spent during training) have a role for determining HDL-C change. Wood et al.[169] observed that 12 weeks of exercise training produced an increased HDL-C concentration, but when the intervention program length was ten weeks or less, the results were equivocal. Exercise training volume performed or the number of kcals expended may be a key factor in HDL-C change. Tran et al.[167] found a significant correlation between hours spent in exercise training and HDL-C change. Similarly, Wood et al.[140] observed a significant correlation between distance run per week and HDL-C change. In addition, Williams et al.[170] observed that weekly distance run correlated positively with baseline HDL-C concentrations. These results when considered together suggest that subjects with a better ability to metabolize lipids may choose to exercise more and, therefore, elicit increased plasma HDL-C.[170] An important concept to remember is that comparisons among studies is difficult because of different exercise frequencies, durations, and intensities and different study lengths. Therefore, exercise quantification by calories expended per exercise session throughout the training program would help correct this problem.

Furthermore, the time that blood samples are taken after exercise training intervention may also impact blood lipid profiles. Crouse et al.[171] found a rise in HDL-C and HDL₂-C during the 24- to 48-hour time period immediately after a single exercise session, whereas the overall effect after the exercise training intervention was an increased HDL₂-C and a decreased HDL₃-C concentration. Thus, both a single exercise session and exercise training can have independent effects on blood lipid profiles. These data support the notion that exercise should be performed at least every other day throughout a training period of several months to maximize the exercise effect.

Body composition is altered after exercise training and can contribute to increased HDL-C concentrations. Wood et al.[140] reported a negative relationship between change in body fat and HDL-C, but the addition of distance run per week to a multiple regression model did not improve the ability to predict HDL-C change. Using specific diets with supplemental calories to compensate for the extra energy expended during exercise training, Thompson et al.[133,151] was able to maintain body weight and body fat percentage while HDL-C increased 8 mg/dL in one study[151] and 3 mg/dL in another.[133] Wood et al.[172] employed weight-loss programs using caloric restriction alone or caloric restriction and exercise training. Body weight and body fat percentage were reduced in both experimental groups while HDL-C concentrations increased. More important, the group that combined caloric restriction and exercise had greater changes in body composition and HDL-C. Whereas, exercise training-induced increased HDL-C has been found both in the presence[137,138,141,144] and in the absence[139,151] of reduced body fat percentage. These findings collectively suggest that exercise training without altered body weight and/or body composition may increase HDL-C, but this increase may be augmented if body fat reduction occurs.

Some studies found increased concentrations of the HDL-C subfraction HDL_2-C[133,145,151] and HDL_3-C[145,151] after exercise training, and other studies have failed to find exercise-induced change in cholesterol associated with HDL subfractions.[138,139] These studies did not, however, correct lipoprotein concentrations for plasma volume change. Thompson et al.[151] found statistical change in HDL_2-C and HDL_3-C concentrations only after correcting for plasma volume expansion. Therefore, plasma volume correction after exercise training studies should be considered.

HDL subfractions are also studied by particle diameter. Although most reported literature indicate that the HDL_{3b} subfraction is related to CAD risk, some literature indicate an inverse relationship to CAD risk, whereas the HDL_{2a} and HDL_{2b} have generally been inversely related to CAD risk. Williams et al.[175] reported increased HDL_{2b} and decreased HDL_{3b} after a one-year exercise intervention program with moderately overweight men (20% to 60% above ideal weight). Nevertheless, when changes in BMI or body fat percentage were included as covariates, neither the concentrations of HDL_{2b} or HDL_{3b} were significantly different from initial pre-exercise training concentrations.

6.4.3   Plasma Apolipoproteins

Apolipoproteins are the protein portion of the circulating blood lipoproteins.[1,153] Their major functions appear to be enzymes regulation in the lipoprotein metabolic pathways and cellular recognition (see Table 6.1). Though apolipoproteins are necessary for the metabolism of lipoproteins, some apolipoproteins can also serve as CAD risk indicators (see Table 6.1).[1,153]

Apo A-I is associated with HDL_2-C and is an LCAT activator.[1] Individuals with high levels of apo A-I are at reduced CAD risk.[1,153] Apo A-II is associated with HDL_3-C and is thought to activate HL.[1] Some reports have found increases in Apo A-I from 1–10% after exercise training,[133,143,175] while other reports have not.[137,138–140,144,171] Thompson et al.[151] did not report a significant increase in apo A-I concentrations despite finding increased HDL_2-C concentrations, and Williams et al.[175] reported no statistical change in apo A-I levels when BMI change was included as a covariate. After exercise training, apo A-II changes are equivocal. Huttunen et al.[137] reported a 10% decrease in apo A-II after a 16-week low-intensity (40% heart rate reserve) exercise intervention program. No change[133] while a 5%[175] and a 21%[151] increase in apo A-II concentrations have been reported. Williams et al.[175] found a significant 7% increase in apo A-II after exercise training and correction for decreased BMI.

Apo B has two forms: B-48 and B-100. Apo B-48 is the major chylomicron protein[1,153] and is required for chylomicron synthesis.[1] Apo B-48 is synthesized by intestinal cells, and the ratio apo B-48 to apo A-I is thought to be a sensitive index of CAD risk (e.g., lower ratio means lower risk).[1,153] Apo B-100 is synthesized in the liver, is associated with plasma chylomicron, VLDL, and LDL, and is necessary for peripheral tissue LDL receptor binding.[1,153] Whether apo B concentrations significantly decrease[138,144,171] or not,[139,140,142] the changes in apo B after exercise training parallel those of LDL-C (e.g., apo B changes only if LDL-C changes). Wood et al.[140] found after a one-year exercise training program that there was no overall change in apo B, but there was a significant correlation between distance run and apo B concentration decrease.

Apo C has several forms: apo C-I, apo C-II, and apo C-III. These apolipoproteins are synthesized by the liver[1,153] and are necessary for activation of LCAT (apo C-I) and LPL (apo C-II). Though little is known about the impact that exercise has on these apolipoproteins, apo C has only been examined cross-sectionally with no differences reported between physically active and inactive groups of young and elderly male subjects.[139,176]

Apo E is synthesized in the liver, is necessary for recognition of chylomicron remnant removal by the liver,[1,153] and is involved with LDL receptor recognition.[1] Thus, apo E is necessary for the removal of triglyceride-rich chylomicron remnants by the liver.[1] Very few studies have been published regarding an exercise-induced effect on apo E. Marti et al.[139] found no apo E differences in current and former runners. Higher apo E concentrations were reported in young runners, but not in older runners.[177]

6.4.4 Enzymes

6.4.4.1 Lipoprotein Lipase

Following exercise of sufficient volume and intensity that depletes intramuscular triglyceride stores, increased secretion and/or synthesis of LPL is promoted by muscle cells.[178] Increased LPL activity, usually not found until 4 to 18 hours after exercise completion, will increase chylomicron and VLDL triglyceride core hydrolysis and decrease plasma triglyceride concentrations.[179-181] LPL increases catabolism of chylomicrons, and VLDLs cause, in part, an increased production of cholesterol ester remnants that can combine with HDL_3, yielding an increase in plasma HDL_2 concentrations.[182] After endurance exercise training, this process likely contributes to the increased HDL mass that occurs in the vascular compartments of adipose[157] and muscle tissue.[181]

Endurance athletes usually have elevated plasma LPL activity,[183-185] but not always.[186] Female endurance-trained runners have higher post-heparin LPL activity and higher triglyceride clearance when compared with sedentary controls.[183] Further, LPL activity was directly associated with HDL-C concentrations.[183] Seip et al.[138] found higher LPL activity after 9 to 12 months of endurance exercise training, whereas Cedermark et. al.[187] found increased LPL activity following 10 days of military training (12–32 km/day). Following endurance exercise training, sedentary men exhibit significantly higher adipose tissue and post-heparin LPL activity.[151,188] Kiens and Lithell[181] had subjects complete eight weeks of cycle ergometer training with one leg. Following the exercise training program, two hours of exercise was performed with both legs and blood samples were taken from each leg four hours after exercise. Higher LPL activity was found in the trained leg compared with the untrained leg. This suggested that LPL activity changes may be partially explained by skeletal muscle adaptations following exercise training.[181] Williams et al.[157] provided additional support for other anatomical sites for exercise-induced adaptations. Their results indicate that the weight loss associated with endurance exercise training may cause increased adipocyte LPL activity that results in modified blood lipid and lipoprotein profiles. Thus, several possible sites exist for exercise training-induced adaptations that could explain lipid and lipoprotein profile change.

After a short endurance exercise program and/or after a single exercise session, LPL activity was changed. LPL activity increased after one week of endurance training.[188] Kantor et al.[180] had trained and sedentary subjects complete a single cycling exercise session and found that both groups exhibited higher post-heparin LPL activity. Gordon et al.[189] found no significant differences in LPL activity following a single exercise session at either low intensity (60% $\dot{V}O_{2\,max}$) or high intensity (70% $\dot{V}O_{2\,max}$) exercise that elicited 800 kcal of energy expenditure. But the higher exercise intensity produced a trend for increased LPL activity. Shoup et al.[190] found increased LPL activity 24 hours after a single high-intensity resistance exercise session requiring 250 kcal energy expenditure. Ferguson et al.[191] found increased LPL activity 24 hours after several single endurance runs at 70% $\dot{V}O_{2\,max}$ requiring energy expenditures of more than 1100 kcal. Sady et al.[192] found that after a marathon run LPL activity and the clearance of an artificial lipid emulsion were increased.

6.4.4.2 Hepatic Lipase

HL has been negatively associated with HDL_2-C and positively with HDL_3-C.[193,194] When comparing active and inactive individuals, observational studies indicate that no difference in resting HL activity exist.[185,195] However, Peltonen et al.[188] found in middle-aged men decreased resting HL activity following 15 weeks of endurance exercise training. Similarly, resting HL activity was decreased following 9 to 12 months of endurance exercise training in elderly subjects[138] and in middle-aged men following weight loss by diet and/or exercise.[196] Nevertheless, when adjusted for plasma volume changes, no changes in resting HL were found following 14 and 32 weeks after endurance exercise training.[151] Further, a single exercise session was not associated with significant change in HL activity.[180,189,191,197]

6.4.4.3 Cholesterol Ester Transfer Protein (CETP)

The relationship between CETP and atherogenesis remain unclear. A decrease in CETP activity may be anti-atherogenic by slowing hepatic catabolism of HDL_2 and decreasing the amount of cholesterol-rich particles in the circulation,[198] though few exercise studies concerning CETP have been completed. One cross-sectional physical activity study found higher CETP activity in physically active persons;[199] however, the method used to measure CETP activity in this study was unusual because the transfer of cholesterol ester from the solid phase bound HDL to VLDL and LDL was assessed.[200] After 12 months of endurance exercise training, Seip et el.[138] found a significant decrease in CETP activity, whereas lower CETP mass[201] and activity[202] were observed in marathon runners. These values were associated with lowered plasma concentrations of VLDL-C and apo B and with elevated concentrations of HDL-C and apo A-I.[201,202] Notwithstanding, following one week of exercise cessation, CETP activity was elevated, suggesting a transient exercise effect.[201] In contrast, Föger et al.[203] found an increase in CETP mass 24 and 48 hours after a 230 km cycle race, but there was no significant CETP activity change.

6.4.4.4 Lecithin:Cholesterol Acyltransferase

Following endurance training programs, increased LCAT has been observed in young physically active individuals,[152] middle-aged men,[204] and endurance-trained athletes.[152,199] However, no change was found in LCAT activity following an exercise-induced weight loss program[157] or an 11-week interval training program.[205] After a single session exercise, LCAT has been reported to increase[206,207] or remain unchanged.[208,209] Because LCAT is not a rate limiting enzyme in the lipoprotein metabolic pathway, a change may simply reflect the availability of substrate for the reaction to occur.

6.4.5 Implications

Regular physical activity reduces circulating plasma triglyceride levels, particularly in those with high initial levels. Moreover, evidence suggests an increased clearance of triglycerides from the blood following a high-fat meal in endurance training individual. Because blood cholesterol concentrations (particularly LDL-C) are highly correlated to CAD, some evidence exists that reduced LDL-C levels sometimes follow exercise training. Additionally, the number of "small" atherogenic LDL-C particles have been shown to be reduced roughly in proportion to the increase in aerobic capacity. However, Lp(a), a potent predictor of CAD, does not appear to respond to regular physical exercise. HDL-C has been shown to increase in a dose-responsive manner with the increase in energy expenditure associated with endurance exercise training, but this increased HDL-C is not always seen. The HDL-C increase may be magnified if body fat is reduced and if the exercise training period is longer than 12 weeks. Both apo A and apo B have been reported to change following exercise training, with apo A-I sometimes increasing, and apo B decreasing. This decrease is related to the decrease in LDL-C. LPL is elevated following a single exercise session and is dependent upon exercise intensity and caloric expenditure. Changes in HL and LCAT following exercise training are equivocal, whereas the influence of regular physical activity on CETP has not been completely defined.

6.5 LIPIDS AND SPORTS PERFORMANCE

6.5.1 IMPACT OF LIPIDS ON PHYSICAL PERFORMANCE

Athletes have tried numerous ways to increase fat utilization and reduce carbohydrate oxidation during exercise. The rationale behind this attempt to increase fat utilization is to increase endurance performance for the competitive athlete[127,130,210,211,212] and to reduce total body adiposity[118,131,146,173] and/or improve blood lipid profiles[1,146,154,213] for the noncompetitive recreational exerciser. In fact, fats are the preferred substrate during rest and exercise up to 50% of $\dot{V}O_{2\,max}$.[111–114,118] However, most athletic events occur at much higher intensities, usually between 75 and 100% $\dot{V}O_{2\,max}$.[126] Because carbohydrates have superior ATP yield per unit $\dot{V}O_2$ at these exercise intensities, a greater reliance on carbohydrates is typically found.[111,112,116,117,119]

Thus, athletes are at a quandary as to how to increase fatty acid oxidation during competition and hard training. Although some published literature suggest that a high-fat diet will mandate increased fatty acid oxidation during exercise by such mechanisms as the glucose-fatty acid cycle,[214] other literature suggest that diet supplementation with such compounds as carnitine,[117,215] high-fat diets[117,127,130,173,211,216] and caffeine[217,218] will enhance fatty acid oxidation. Still other literature present data that muscle phosphorylation potential ultimately determines substrate utilization during exercise.[219,220] Thus, an increase in muscle oxidative potential is necessary to increase lipid utilization during vigorous exercise.[116,118,120,121,128]

6.5.2 Control of Lipolysis During Exercise

Adipose tissue lipolysis appears to be under both hormonal[111–114,131,221] and intracellular feedback control[222–226] during exercise and can be regulated at both the transcriptional[227,228] and post-transcriptional level.[228] Decreased blood insulin[112,147,228] and an increase in blood catecholamines[111,112,131] are necessary for an increase in lipolytic rate during exercise. Evidence suggests that increased exercise intensity is associated with an increased blood catecholamine concentration. Catecholamines in humans have a dual effect; lipolysis in adipose tissue is stimulated by β-adrenergic receptors or inhibited by stimulating α_2 receptors.[131] Thus, adrenergic receptor pathway in adipose tissue can both stimulate and inhibit lipolysis. At the same time, the hormones cortisol and growth hormone also have potent lipolytic properties and are increased with a single exercise session.[112]

Support for a dominant catecholamine β-adrenergic effect in stimulating lipolysis comes from the knowledge that lipolysis is increased by cold exposure,[229–231] caffeine ingestion,[217,218] and increased exercise intensity,[112–114] while lipolysis is completely inhibited by non-selective β-blockade (a pharmaceutical agent such as propranolol that has an impact on all β-receptors).[221] This last β-adrenergic effect is particularly evident for IMTG release.[112,221] Intramuscular lipolysis is also subject to local muscular control (e.g., Ca^{2+}).[117,124,232] Further, muscle malonyl-CoA level[222,226] and acetyl-CoA carboxylase activity[222,225] have a profound effect upon lipolysis. Malonyl-CoA is the first step in fatty acid synthesis.[222] High malonyl-CoA levels should inhibit lipolysis, and lower malonyl-CoA levels should promote lipolysis. Indeed, Winder et al.[226] have found a 64% decrease in malonyl-CoA and a 278% increase in circulating FFA during exercise. Therefore, at high exercise intensities when blood catecholamine levels are high, adipose tissue lipolysis will be inhibited while IMTG lipolysis is accelerated. This information is supportive for an increased exercise lipolytic rate.

Rasmussen and Winder[225] evaluated the effect of exercise intensity on malonyl-CoA and acetyl-CoA carboxylase (ACC) activity (ACC is the enzyme responsible for synthesizing malonyl-CoA from extramitochondrial acetyl-CoA).[222] They noted a progressive decrease in ACC activity and malonyl-CoA levels with increased exercise intensity particularly in the red vastus lateralis muscle (Type IIa) fibers. Their results indicate that ACC activity and malonyl-CoA content in oxidative muscle are reduced as a function of exercise intensity, thus facilitating increased skeletal muscle lipolysis.

Carnitine has a permissive effect upon lipolysis due to its ability to form acetylcarnitine esters in times of accelerated acetyl-CoA production.[223,224] This is especially important in oxidative fiber Type I and IIa and allows for pyruvate dehydrogenase activity to remain high[223,233] while facilitating oxidative ATP production from both lipids and carbohydrates.[224] Of interest are the several studies that have shown a 13–17% increase in muscle carnitine concentrations after exercise training.[215] Thus, exercise training adaptations (increased sensitivity to catecholamine and insulin, increased carnitine stores) allow both an accelerated lipolytic flux[111,112,114,118] and increased lipid utilization.[117,118,120,121]

6.5.3 Moderate-Intensity Exercise

Hurley et al.[121] used a 12-week period of endurance and intermittent exercise training to evaluate fat oxidation. Exercise training consisted of alternating three days of continuous running for 40 minutes at 75% $\dot{V}O_{2\,max}$ with three days of intermittent cycling using six exercise periods (each five minutes in length separated by two minutes of rest) at 90–100% $\dot{V}O_{2\,peak}$. Fat oxidation after the exercise training program using the same absolute cycling work rate (64% pre-training $\dot{V}O_{2\,peak}$) increased from 35 to 57%, IMTG use was increased by 105%,[121] and glycogen utilization was reduced by 41%. Furthermore, Hurley et al. concluded that all of the increase in fat oxidation after exercise training could be accounted for by the increase in IMTG utilization.[121]

Martin et al.[118] studied the effect of endurance training on plasma FFA oxidation during exercise by infusion of [1-^{13}C] palmitate. A 41% increase in total fat oxidation during the same absolute work rate (63% pre-training $\dot{V}O_{2\,peak}$) was found. Interestingly, blood FFA turnover was 33% less after exercise training due to a slower adipose tissue FFA release. Reduced FFA release following exercise training was attributed to the blunted sympathoadrenal "drive." Martin et al.[118] said the blunted sympathoadrenal "drive" obviates the increased utilization of IMTG during moderate intensity exercise following exercise training.

Romijn et al.[111] investigated the regulation of fat and carbohydrate metabolism during exercise at three different exercise intensities and durations. Five trained cyclists were evaluated at 25, 65, and 85% of $\dot{V}O_{2\,peak}$. Exercise duration was 120 minutes at 25% and 65% $\dot{V}O_{2\,peak}$ and 30 minutes at 85% $\dot{V}O_{2\,peak}$. Stable isotope tracers and indirect calorimetry were used to measure fat and carbohydrate metabolism at these intensities. Peripheral adipose tissue lipolysis was maximally stimulated at the lowest exercise intensity, and adipose tissue FFA release decreased with increasing exercise intensity. Also, IMTG use increased at only the two higher exercise intensities. This suggested that peripheral adipose tissue release is limited due to reductions in adipose tissue blood flow and possibly the capacity of albumin to transport FFAs.[111]

Jones et al.[122] noted that IMTGs provide energy even in inactive subjects during intensity exercise at 70% $\dot{V}O_{2\,max}$. Forty minutes of cycle exercise at 36% $\dot{V}O_{2\,peak}$ was sufficient for plasma FFA to supply energy for this low-intensity exercise session, whereas peripheral lipolysis was reduced by 40% during vigorous exercise at 70% $\dot{V}O_{2\,max}$. However, plasma glycerol levels during the vigorous exercise session were increased by 144% when compared with the light exercise session. This indicates that IMTG supplied a large percentage of the FFA utilized during vigorous exercise. In addition, plasma lactate concentration averaged 9.9 mM. When considered together, a high degree of non-oxidative glucose metabolism will not inhibit intramuscular lipolysis, as has been shown in adipose and cardiac tissues.[214,232]

Phillips et al.[120] studied the effects of exercise training on substrate turnover during exercise completed at 60% of pre-training $\dot{V}O_{2\,peak}$. Cycle ergometer tests lasting 90 minutes were performed at pre-training, and again at five and 31 days following endurance exercise training. Training consisted of consecutive days of exercise cycling at 60% of pre-training $\dot{V}O_{2\,peak}$. A 10% increase in total fat oxidation was found and attributed to an increased IMTG, with a further increase in total fat oxidation of 58% after 31 days. Oxidation of IMTG was increased twofold after 31 days of exercise training. This information supports the notion that even short-term training can increase the utilization of fat primarily from IMTG.

Kiens et al.[116] investigated skeletal muscle substrate utilization during sub-maximal quadriceps exercise (modified Krogh cycle ergometer). Healthy male subjects ($\dot{V}O_{2\,peak}$ ranging from 46 to 54 ml/kg/min) performed dynamic knee extension exercise after an eight-week period of one leg exercise training. This experimental design allowed for the comparison between trained and untrained legs in each subject. RQ values for the exercising leg (0.81 vs. 0.91) indicated that a shift toward higher fat oxidation took place following exercise training. Interestingly, no significant utilization of IMTG was found (e.g., almost all of the fat oxidation came from FFA and serum triglyceride). However, because only a small amount of active muscle was used, insulin, and blood catecholamine concentrations were not elevated and may explain why IMTG was not changed.

6.5.4   High-Intensity Exercise

McCartney et al. demonstrated that IMTG may provide the substrate for a supra-maximal exercise effort.[125] Eight inactive male subjects performed four 30 second maximal isokinetic cycling exercise periods with four minutes rest between each period. Muscle lactate (1.43 to 35.1 mM/kg) and plasma glycerol increased progressively (500%) across the four work periods while plasma FFA levels did not change. These results suggest that a large percentage of the energetic needs during repetitive maximal exercise cycling are provided by IMTG. This concept is also supported by the results of Hopp and Palmer[124] who noted that IMTG content was significantly reduced during one hour of intermittent stimulation (30 seconds of stimulation and 60 seconds of rest) of rat hind limb muscle at 5 Hz. Together these results support the concept that fats can be used as a fuel source even during high-intensity exercise.

Kanaley et al.[119] investigated fatty acid kinetics during running above and below the lactate threshold. Twenty-four moderately trained and elite marathon runners were infused with [1-^{14}C] palmitate while running at work rates just above the lactate threshold and at 10% below lactate threshold. Total FFA oxidation exceeded FFA availability and support significant IMTG use. Of interest, no statistical difference in fat oxidation was noted for the above or below lactate threshold tests and indicate that 1) significant FFA oxidation occurs above lactate threshold (67–77% $\dot{V}O_{2\,peak}$) and 2) IMTGs can supply a large portion (more than 50%) of total fat oxidation.

6.5.5   Fat Loading

Although enhancing exercise performance by lipid supplementation has been considered for many years, the systemic evaluation of lipid as an ergogenic aid is relatively new. Several recent reviews on this and related topics have been completed,[112,234–236] and at least one popular lay publication[237] has given this topic considerable commentary. In addition, Chapter 6 in this book addresses lipid supplements and exercise performance. The intent here is to briefly summarize present literature on fat loading.

6.5.5.1   Moderate Intensity Exercise

Vukovich et al.[212] demonstrated that fat feeding can improve performance by sparing glycogen during 60 minutes of exercise at 70% $\dot{V}O_{2\,peak}$ (no exercise was completed 48 hours prior to the performance test). Moderately trained subjects ($\dot{V}O_{2\,peak}$ of 57 ml/kg/min) ingested a 90% saturated fat shake 195 minutes before exercise. Significant increases in serum triglyceride, glycerol, and fatty acid levels during exercise were found while a 25% drop in glycogen utilization during exercise was reported. This would presumably have the effect of sparing glycogen use early in exercise and making glycogen available later in exercise.

Starling et al.[126] evaluated the effect of diet upon both IMTG and endurance performance. After completing a 120-minute period of exercise cycling at 65% $\dot{V}O_2$, seven trained cyclists received one of two treatments: an isocaloric high-carbohydrate (83%) diet or an isocaloric high-fat (68%) diet for 12 hours. Following a 12-hour overnight fast and after both the high-carbohydrate diet or again after the high-fat diet, the subjects completed a self-paced time trial of equal energy expenditure (1600 kJ). Muscle triglyceride level was significantly elevated (62%) following the high-fat diet, but time to complete the cycling time trial was 19% slower. This suggested that the high-carbohydrate diet was more beneficial in terms of performance.

6.5.5.2 High-Intensity Exercise

Helge et al.[128] investigated the interaction of high-fat and high-carbohydrate diets on endurance performance tests completed at 81% $\dot{V}O_{2\,max}$. Subjects performed the endurance test and ingested a high-fat (62%) or high-carbohydrate (65%) diet for seven weeks and then completed a second performance test. The high-fat group then changed to the high-carbohydrate diet for one week and then completed another endurance performance test. After the initial seven-week period, an increased performance time was noted in both groups, but the increase was greatest in the high-carbohydrate group when compared with the high-fat group (102 minutes vs. 65 minutes). Even after the high-fat group changed to the high-carbohydrate diet for one week, endurance performance time (77 minutes vs. 102 minutes) was still sub-optimal. Thus, a high-fat diet consumed for more than four weeks can have deleterious effects upon high-intensity performance. This damaging effect was attributed to an increase in membrane fluidity that increased the ATP cost for membrane transport.

Okano et al.[210] looked at the effect of ingestion of a high fat (61%) or high carbohydrate (79%) isocaloric meal four hours before exercise (120 minutes at 65% $\dot{V}O_{2\,peak}$ followed by exercise cycling to exhaustion at 80% $\dot{V}O_{2\,peak}$) in trained distance runners. Endurance capacity did not differ significantly between treatments; however, time to exhaustion was six minutes longer in the high carbohydrate trial (128 minutes vs. 122 minutes).

6.5.6 Implications

High-fat diets (more than 60% fat) or meals can increase fat oxidation and sometimes endurance performance, particularly in trained athletes at moderate work intensities. The effect of such meals or diets is not as evident when work intensity exceeds 75% $\dot{V}O_{2\,max}$ or in physically inactive subjects who do not have the capacity to oxidize FFAs at high work rates. Because the long-term health consequences of high fat diets are at best inconsequential and at worst detrimental, following such diets for longer than four weeks does not appear warranted.

6.6 PRACTICAL RECOMMENDATIONS

Lipids have important functions by providing for cellular components and steroid hormone synthesis and as an energy source at rest and during low to moderate exercise intensity. However, to reduce the risk of CAD, individuals should be strongly encouraged to attain desirable blood lipid and lipoprotein concentrations defined as (values in mg/dL): total cholesterol < 200; LDL-C < 130; HDL-C > 60; and triglyceride < 200 (32). Adopting a lifestyle of regular exercise, balanced nutrition, and weight management can often lead to the achievement of these goals. Blood lipid and lipoprotein concentrations can be beneficially altered by endurance training and by a single exercise session, even in those with high blood cholesterol.[171] Thus, one should exercise at least every other day to produce lipid changes consistent with a lowered CAD risk. Exercising regularly may increase and maintain LPL enzyme activity at a relatively high level. High LPL activity would increase the catabolism of chylomicron and VLDL particles that would result in the dual benefit for an increased blood HDL-C concentration and an increased FFA oxidation. Indeed, fat oxidation during exercise can be increased dramatically with endurance training. Adipose tissue can supply FFAs for low- to moderate-intensity exercise, but IMTGs appear to be the primary source of fats oxidized during more vigorous exercise. It is unclear whether high fat diets in trained individuals improves exercise performance, and any benefit may depend on the exercise intensity at which the exercise is performed. A high-fat diet may improve low-intensity exercise endurance performance but impair high-intensity exercise performance. When the goal is to maximize high-intensity endurance performance, a high-carbohydrate diet is best.

6.7 RESEARCH RECOMMENDATIONS

During the past 25 years we have gained a better understanding of dietary fat and its impact on health and disease and exercise performance. Regarding health and disease, future research investigations should attempt to develop a better understanding of the relationship between single exercise session response and exercise adaptations that occur because of regular daily physical activity participation (e.g., exercise training). Specifically, some exercise adaptations are really responses (e.g., triglycerides change very quickly after one starts to exercise regularly), and some exercise responses may occur several days after a single exercise session has occurred and after several months of regular daily physical activity are seen as adaptations. It has been established that a dose-response relationship for blood lipid and lipoprotein adaptations to regular physical activity exists, but little is known regarding the optimum exercise modality, intensity, frequency, and caloric expenditure required to elicit these beneficial responses and adaptations. Most important is an increased understanding of the mechanisms responsible for these exercise responses and adaptations. The relationship between changes in lipoprotein enzymes such as LPL, CETP, LCAT, and HL needs to be understood more completely. The greater concern is gaining understanding of the molecular changes responsible for these exercise responses and adaptations. Finally, there is a need to discern why some persons, in regard to exercise and lipid and lipoprotein change, may be referred to as responders while others are viewed as nonresponders.

Future directions concerning fat metabolism and exercise performance are necessary to better grasp the relationship between dietary fat intake, health and disease, and the use of fat as an erogenic aid. Along this line, dietary fat intake has been associated with increased risk for CAD and some forms of cancer. Thus, when one uses dietary fat as an ergogenic aid, a question that remains unanswered is what are the short- and long-term impacts of these dietary patterns and on disease processes? Further, the time course for dietary fat intake and its relationship with both exercise intensity and duration are yet to be determined. Mechanisms responsible for any enhanced performance are not completely understood. Most of this work has been completed with medium-chain triglyceride metabolism (see Chapter 8). Finally, little is know about the factor/s that limit the maximal rate of fat oxidation during exercise.

REFERENCES

1. Durstine J. L. and Haskell W. L., Effects of exercise training on plasma lipids and lipoproteins, in *Exerc. Sport. Sci. Rev.*, Holloszy, J. O., editor, Williams & Wilkins, Baltimore, 1994; 22: 447.

2. Sady, S. P., Cullinane, E. M., Saritelli, A., et al., Elevated high-density lipoprotein cholesterol in endurance athletes is related to enhanced plasma triglyceride clearance, *Metabolism*, 37(6): 568; 1988.

3. Brewer, H.B., Greg, R.E., Hoeg, J.M., and Fojo, S.s., Apolipo proteins and lipoproteins in human plasma: An overview, *Clin. Chem.*, 34 (Suppl. B) B4; 1988.

4. Tall, A. R. and Small, D. S., Plasma high-density lipoproteins, *N. Engl. J. Med.*, 299: 1232; 1978.

5. Shepherd, J., Lipoprotein metabolism: An overview, *Ann. Acad. Med.* 21: 106,1992.

6. Voutilainen, E. and Hietanen, E., Characterization of lipoproteins and their metabolism: Synthesis and catabolism, in *Regulation of Serum Lipids by Physical Exercise*, Hietanen, E, editor, CRC Press LLC, Boca Raton, FL, 1982; 1.

7. Lusis, A. J., Genetic factors affecting blood lipoproteins: The candidate gene approach, *J. Lipid. Res.*, 29: 397; 1988.

8. Nilsson, P. E., Garfunkel, A. S., and Schotz, M. C., Lipolytic enzymes and plasma lipoprotein metabolism, *Ann. Rev. Biochem.*, 49: 667; 1980.

9. Green, P. H. R., Glickman, R. M., Sandel, C. D., et al., Human intestinal lipoproteins: Studies in chyluric subjects, *J. Clin. Invest.*, 64: 233; 1979.

10. Nozaki, S., Kubo, M., Sudo, H., et al., The role of hepatic triglyceride lipase in the metabolism of intermediate-density lipoprotein-postheparin lipolytic activities determined by a sensitive, nonradio-isotopic method in hyperlipidemic patients and normals, *Metabolism*, 35(1): 53; 1986.

11. Brown, M. S. and Goldstein, J. L., A receptor-mediated pathway for cholesterol homeostasis, *Science*, 232: 34; 1986.

12. Tall, A. R., Plasma lipid transfer proteins, *J. Lipid. Res.*, 27: 361; 1986.

13. Tikkanen, M. J., Plasma lipoproteins and atherosclerosis, *J. Diabetes Complications*, 4(2): 35; 1990.

14. Levy, R. I. and Rifkind, B. M., The structure, function, and metabolism of high-density lipoproteins: a status report, *Circulation*, 62(supp. IV): 4; 1980.

15. Deckelbaum, R. J., Olivecrona, T., and Eisenberg, S., Plasma lipoproteins in hyperlipidemia: Roles of neutral lipid exchange and lipase, in *Treatment of Hyperlipoproteinemia*, Carlson, L. A. and Olsson, A. G., editors, Raven Press, New York, 1984; 85.

16. Tall, A. R. Plasma high density lipoproteins: Metabolism and relationship to atherogenesis, *J. Clin. Invest.*, 86: 379; 1990.

17. Crawford, T., Some aspects of the pathology of atherosclerosis, *Proc. R. Soc. Med.*, 53:9; 1960.

18. Ross, R., The pathogenesis of atherosclerosis: a perspective for the 1990s, *Nature*, 362:801; 1993.

19. Anderson, K. M., Castelli, W. P., and Levy, D., Cholesterol and mortality: 30 years of follow-up from the Framingham study, *J.A.M.A.*, 257:2176; 1987.

20. Gouldbourt, V., Holtzman, E., and Neufeld, H. N., Total and high density lipoprotein cholesterol in the serum and risk of mortality: Evidence of a threshold effect, *Br. Med. J.*, 290:1239; 1985.

21. Pekkanen, J., Linn, S., Heiss, G., Suchindran, C. M., Leon, A., Rifkind, B. M., and Tyoler, H. A., Ten-year mortality from cardiovascular disease in relation to cholesterol level among men with and without preexisting cardiovascular disease, *N. Engl. J. Med.*, 322:1700; 1990.

22. Stamler, J., Wentworth, D., and Neaton, J. D., Is relationship between serum cholesterol and risk of premature death from coronary heart disease continuous and graded?, *J.A.M.A.*, 256:2823; 1986.

23. The Coronary Drug Project Research Group. Clofibrate and niacin in coronary heart disease, *J.A.M.A.*, 231:360; 1975.

24. Report from the Committee of Principal Investigators. A cooperative trial in the primary prevention of ischemic heart disease using clofibrate, *Br. Heart J.*, 40:1069; 1978.

25. Lipid Research Clinics Program. The lipid research clinics coronary primary prevention trial results. I. Reduction in incidence of coronary heart disease. II. The relationship of reduction in incidence of coronary heart disease to cholesterol lowering, *J.A.M.A.*, 251:351; 1984.

26. Shepherd, J., Cobbe, S. M., Ford, I., Isles, C. G., Larimer, A. R., MacRarlane, P. W., McKillop, J. H., and Packard, C. J., Prevention of coronary heart disease with pravastatin in men with hypercholester-olemia, *N. Engl. J. Med.*, 333:1301; 1995.

27. Scandinavian Simvastatin Survival Study Group. Randomized trial of cholesterol lowering in 4444 patients with coronary heart disease: the Scandinavian Simvastatin Survival Study (4S), *Lancet*, 344:1383; 1994.

28. Sacks, F. M., Pfeiffer, M. A., Maye, L. A., Rouleau, J. L., Rutherford, J. D., Cole, T. G., Brown, L., Warnica, J. W., Arnold, J. M., Wun, C. C., Davis, B. R., and Braunwald, E., The effect of pravastatin on coronary events after myocardial infarction in patients with average cholesterol levels, *N. Engl. J. Med.*, 335:1001; 1996.

29. Blankenhorn, D. H., Azen, S. P., Kramsch, D. M., Mack, W. J., Cashin-Hemphill, L., Hadis, H. N., Deboer, L. W., Mohner, P. R., Masteller, M. J., and Vailas, L. I., Coronary angiographic changes with lovastatin therapy: The Monitored Atherosclerosis Regression Study (MARS), *Ann. Intern. Med.*, 119:969; 1993.

30. Waters, D., Higginson, L., Gladstone, P., Kimball, B., Le May, M., Boccuzzi, S. J., and Lesperance, J., Effects of monotherapy with HMG-CoA reductase inhibitor on the progression of coronary atherosclerosis as assessed by serial quantitative arteriography: The Canadian Coronary Atherosclerosis Intervention Trial, *Circulation*, 89:959; 1994.

31. The Post Coronary Artery Bypass Graft Trial Investigators. The effect of aggressive lowering of low-density lipoprotein cholesterol levels and low-dose anticoagulation on obstructive changes in saphenous-vein coronary-artery bypass grafts, *N. Engl. J. Med.*, 336:153; 1997.

32. Expert Panel on Detection, E., and Treatment of High Blood Cholesterol in Adults of the National Cholesterol Education Program Summary of the second report of the National Cholesterol Education Program (NCEP) expert panel on detection, evaluation, and treatment of high blood cholesterol in adults (adult treatment panel II), *J.A.M.A.*, 269(23):3015; 1993.

33. Barr, D. P., Russ, E. M., and Eder, H. A., Protein-lipid relationships in human plasma, *Am. J. Med.*, 11:480; 1951.

34. Barr, D. P., Some chemical factors in the pathogenesis of atherosclerosis, *Circulation*, 8:641; 1953.

35. Gofman, J., Young, W., and Tandy, R. Ischemic heart disease, atherosclerosis, and longevity, *Circulation*, 34:679; 1966.

36. Expert Panel on Population Strategies for Blood Cholesterol Reduction of the National Cholesterol Education Program Report of the expert panel on population strategies for blood cholesterol reduction, CVD, Hypercholesterol, Evaluation and Treatment. National Institutes of Health 90; 1990.

37. Lamarche, B., Tchernof, A., Moorjani, S., Cantin, B., Dagenais, G. R., Lupien, P. J., and Despres, J. P., Small, dense low-density lipoprotein particles as a predictor of the risk of ischemic heart disease in men, *Circulation*, 95:69; 1997.

38. Bostom, A. G., Cupples, L. A., Jenner, J. L., Ordovas, J. M., Seman, L. J., Wilson, P. W. F., Schaefer, E. J., and Castelli, W. P., Elevated plasma lipoprotein(a) and coronary heart disease in men aged 55 years and younger, *J.A.M.A.*, 276(7):544; 1996.

39. Gordon, T., Castelli, W. P., Hjortland, M. C., Kannel, W. B., and Dowber, T. R., High density lipoprotein as a protective factor against coronary heart disease: the Framingham study, *Am. J. Med.*, 62:707; 1977.

40. Castelli, W. P., Garrison, R. J., Wilson, P. W., Abbott, R. D., Kalousdian, S., and Kannel, W. B., Incidence of coronary heart disease and lipoprotein cholesterol levels: the Framingham Study, *J.A.M.A.*, 256:3835; 1986.

41. Abbott, R. D., Wilson, P. W., Kannel, W. B., and Castelli, W. P., High density lipoprotein cholesterol, total cholesterol screening, and myocardial infarction: the Framingham Study, *Arteriosclerosis*, 8:207; 1988.

42. Wilson, P. W., High-density lipoprotein, low-density lipoprotein and coronary artery disease, *Am. J. Cardiol.*, 66:7A; 1990.

43. Castelli, W. P., Doyle, J. T., Gordon, T., Hames, C. G., Hjortland, M. C., Hulley, S. B., Kagan, A., and Zukel, W. J., HDL-cholesterol and other lipids in coronary heart disease: the cooperative lipoprotein phenotyping study, *Circulation*, 55:767; 1977.

44. Stampfer, M. J., Sacks, F. M., Salvini, S., Willett, W. C., and Hennekens, C. H., A prospective study of cholesterol, apolipoproteins, and the risk of myocardial infarction, *N. Engl. J. Med.*, 325:373; 1991.

45. Jacobs, D. R., Mebane, I. L., Bongdiwala, S. L., Criqui, M. H., and Tyroler, H. A., High density lipoprotein cholesterol as a predictor of cardiovascular disease mortality in men and women: The follow-up study of the lipid research clinics prevalence study, *Am. J. Epidemiology*, 131:32; 1990.

46. Miller, N. E., Forde, O. H., Thelle, D. S., and Mjos, O. D., The Tromso Heart Study: High-density lipoprotein and coronary heart-disease: A prospective case-control study, *Lancet*, 1:965; 1977.

47. Manninen, V., Tenkanen, L., Koskinen, P., et al., Joint effects of serum triglyceride and LDL cholesterol and HDL cholesterol concentrations on coronary heart disease risk in the Helsinki Heart Study, *Circulation*, 85:37; 1992.

48. Wood, P. and Haskell, W., The effect of exercise on plasma high-density lipoproteins, *Lipids*, 14:417; 1979.

49. Buring, J. E., O'Connor, G. T., Goldhaber, S. Z., Rosner, B., Herbert, P. N., Blum, C. B., Breslow, J. L., and Hennekens, C. H., Decreased HDL_2 and HDL_3 cholesterol, Apo A-I and Apo A-II, and increased risk of myocardial infarction, *Circulation*, 85:22; 1992.

50. Lamarche, B., Moorjani, S., Cantin, B., Dagenais, G. R., Lupien, P. J., and Despres, J. P., Associations of HDL_2 and HDL_3 subfractions with ischemic heart disease in men, *Ateroscler. Thromb. Vasc. Biol.*, 17:1098; 1997.

51. Jeppesen, J., Hein, H. O., Suadicani, P., and Gyntelberg, F., Triglyceride concentration and ischemic heart disease An eight-year follow-up in the Copenhagen male study, *Circulation*, 97:1029; 1998.

52. Gaziano, J. M., Hennekens, C. H., O'Donnell, C. J., Breslow, J. L., and Buring, J. E., Fasting triglycerides, high-density lipoprotein, and risk of myocardial infarction, *Circulation*, 96:2520; 1997.

53. Fager, G., Wiklund, O., Olofsson, S., Wilhelmsson, C., and Bondjers, B., Serum apolipoprotein levels in relation to acute myocardial infarction and its risk factors, *Arteriosclerosis*, 36:67; 1980.

54. Maciejko, J. J., Holmes, D. R., Kottke, B. A., Zinsmeister, A. R., Dinh, D. M., and Mao, S. J. T., Apolipoprotein A-I as a marker of angiographically assessed coronary-artery disease, *N. Engl. J. Med.*, 309(7):385; 1983.

55. DeBacker, G., Rosseneu, M., and Deslypere, J. P., Discriminative value of lipids and apoproteins in coronary heart disease, *Atherosclerosis*, 42:197; 1982.

56. Noma, A., Yokosuka, T., and Kitamura, K., Plasma lipids and apolipoproteins as discriminators for presence and severity of angiographically defined coronary artery disease, *Atherosclerosis*, 49:1; 1983.

57. Faggiotto, A., Ross, R., and Harker, L., Studies of hypercholesterolemia in the nonhuman primate. I. Changes that lead to fatty streak formation, *Arteriosclerosis*, 4:323; 1984.

58. Rosenfeld, M. E., Tsukada, T., Chait, A., Bierman, E. L., Gown, A. M., and Ross, R., Fatty streak initiation in Wantanabe heritable hyperlipemic and comparably hypercholesterolemic fat-fed rabbits, *Arteriosclerosis*, 7:9; 1987.

59. Schwartz, C. J., Ardie, N. G., Carter, R. F., and Paterson, J. C., Gross aortic sudanophilia and hemosiderin deposition. A study on infants, children and young adults, *Arch. Pathol.*, 83:325; 1967.

60. Smith, E. B., Development of the athermatious lesion, *Adv. Exp. Med. Biol.*, 57:254; 1975.

61. Smith, E. B. and Smith, R. H., *Atherosclerosis reviews*, Raven Press, New York, pp 119; 1976.

62. Ross, R., Wight. T. N., Strandress, E., and Thiele, B., Human atherosclerosis. I. Cell constitution and characterization of advanced lesions of the superficial femoral artery, *Am. J. Pathol.*, 114:79; 1984.

63. Mitchell, J. R. A. and Schwartz, C. J., *Arterial Disease*, Blackwell Scientific Publications, Oxford 50; 1965.

64. Davis, M. J. and Thomas, A. C., Thrombosis in acute coronary artery lesions in sudden cardiac ischaemic death, *N. Eng. J. Med.*, 310:1137; 1984.

65. Libby, P., Schoenbeck, U., Mach, F., Selwyn, A. P., and Ganz, P., Current concepts in cardiovascular pathology: the role of LDL cholesterol in plaque rupture and stabilization, *Am. J. Med.*, 104(2A):14S; 1998.

66. Ross, R., The pathogenesis of atherosclerosis—an update, *N. Engl. J. Med.*, 314:485; 1986.

67. Asmussen, I. and Kjeldsen, K., Intimal ultrastructure of human umbilical arteries. Observations on arteries from newborn children of smoking and non-smoking mothers, *Circ. Res.*, 36:579; 1975.

68. Pittilo, R. M., Mackie, I. J., Rowles, P. M., Machin, S. J., and Woolf, N., Effects of cigarette smoking on the ultrastructure of rat thoracic aorta and its ability to produce prostacyclin, *Thromb. Haemost.*, 48:173; 1982.

69. Woolf, N. and Wilson-Holt, N., Cigarette smoking and atherosclerosis. In: Greenhalgh, R.M. (ed.), *Smoking and Arterial Disease*, Pitman Medical, Bath 46; 1981.

70. Gabbiani, G., Elemer, G., Guelpa, C., Vallotton, M. B., Badonnel, M. C., and Huttner, I., Morphological and functional changes of the aortic intima during experimental hypertension, *Am. J. Pathol.*, 96:399; 1979.

71. Schwartz, S. M. and Benditt, E. P., Aortic endothelial cell replication. I. Effects of age and hypertension in the rat,. *Circ. Res.*, 41:248; 1977.

72. Rosenfeld, M. E., Tsukada, T., Gown, A. M., and Ross, R., Fatty streak expansion and maturation in Wantanabe heritable hyperlipidemic and comparably hyercholesterolemic fat-fed rabbits, *Arteriosclerosis*, 7:24; 1987

73. Woolf, N., The pathology of atherosclerosis with particular reference to the effects of hyperlipidaemia, *Eur. Heart. J.*, 8(sppl E):3; 1987.

74. Cathcart, M. K., Morel, D. W., and Chisolm, G. M. 3d., Monocytes and neutrophils oxidize low density lipoprotein making it cytotoxic, *J. Leukocyte. Biol.*, 38:341; 1985.

75. Henriksen, T., Mahoney, E. M., and Steinber, D., Interactions of plasma lipoproteins with endothelial cells, *Ann. N.Y. Acad. Sci.*, 401:102; 1982.

76. Fabricant, C. G., Hajjar, D. P., Minick, C. R., and Fabricant, J., Herpesvirus infection enhances cholesterol and cholesteryl ester accumulation in cultured arterial smooth muscle cells, *Am. J. Pathol.*, 105:176; 1981.

77. Hajjar, D. P., Fabricant, C. G., Minick, C. R., and Fabricant, J., Virus-induced atherosclerosis. Herpesvirus infection alters aortic cholesterol metabolism and accumulation, *Am. J. Pathol.*, 122:62; 1986.

78. Schwartz, S. M., Reidy, M. R., and Clowes, A., Kinetics of atherosclerosis. A stem cell model, *Ann. N.Y. Acad. Sci.*, 454:301; 1985.

79. Chamley-Campbell, J. H. and Campbell, G. R., What controls smooth muscle phenotype?, *Atherosclerosis*, 40:347; 1981.

80. Assoian, R. K., Grotendarst, G. R., Miller, D. M., and Sporn, M. B., Cellular transformation by coodinated sction of three peptide growth factors from human platelets, *Nature*, 309:804; 1984.

81. Bowen-Pope, D. F., Ross, R., and Seifert, R. A., Locally acting growth factors for vascular smooth muscle cells: endogenous synthesis and release from platelets, *Circulation*, 72:735; 1985.

82. DiCorleto, P. E., Gajdusek, C. M., Schwartz, S. M., and Ross, R., Biochemical properties of the endothelium-derived growth factor: comparison to other growth factors, *J. Cell. Physiol.*, 114:339; 1983.

83. Shimokado, K., Raines, E. W., Madtes, D. K., Barrett, T. B., Benditt, E. P., and Ross, R., A significant part of macorphage-derived growth factor consists of at least two forms of PDGF, *Cell*, 43:277; 1985.

84. Seifert, R. A., Schwartz, S. M., and Bowen-Pope, D. F., Developmentally regulated production of platelet-derived growth factor-like molecules, *Nature*, 311:669; 1984.

85. Libby, P., Miao, P., Ordovas, J. M., and Schaefer, E. J., Lipoproteins increase growth of mitogen-stimulated arterial smooth muscle cells, *J. Cell Physiol.*, 124:1; 1985.

86. Fisher-Dzoga, K., Chen, R., and Wissler, R. W., Effects of serum lipoproteins on the morphology, growth, and metabolism of arterial smooth muscle cells, *Adv. Exp. Med. Biol.*, 43:299; 1974.

87. Seewald, S., Nickenig, G., Ko, Y., Vetter, H., and Sachinidis, A., Low density lipoprotein enhances the thrombin-induced growth of vascular smooth muscle cells, *Cardiovasc. Res.*, 36:92; 1997.

88. Stout, R. W., Bierman, E. L., and Ross, R., Effect of insulin on the proliferation of cultured primate arterial smooth muscle cells, *Circ. Res.*, 36:319; 1975.

89. Tammi, M., Ronnemaa, T., Vihersaari, T., Lehtonen, A., and Viikari, J., High density lipoproteinemia due to vigorous physical work inhibits the incorporation of (3H) thymidine and the synthesis of glycosaminoglycans by human aortic smooth muscle cells in culture, *Atherosclerosis*, 32:23; 1979.

90. Portman, O. W., Arterial composition and metabolism: esterified fatty acids and cholesterol, *Adv. Lipid. Res.*, 8:41; 1970.

91. Fogelman, A. M., Haberland, M. E., Seager, J., Hokom, M., and Edwards, P. A., Factors regulating the activities of low density lipoprotein receptor and the scavenger receptor on human monocyte-macrophages, *J. Lipid. Res.*, 22:1131; 1981.

92. Bierman, E. L. and Albers, J. J., Regulation of low density lipoprotein receptor activity by cultured human arterial smooth muscle cells, *Biochem. Biophys. Acta.*, 488:152; 1977.

93. Peters, T. J. and DeDuve, C., Lysosomes of the arterial wall. II. Subcellular fractionation of aortic cells from rabbits with experimental atheroma, *Exp. Mol. Pathol.*, 20:228; 1974.

94. Goldstein, J. L. and Brown, M. S., The low-density lipoprotein pathway and its relation to atherosclerosis, *Annu. Rev. Biochem.*, 46:897; 1977.

95. Smith, E. B. and Slater, R. S., Relationship between low density lipoprotein in aortic intima and serum lipid levels, *Lancet*, 1:463; 1972.

96. Goldstein, J. L., Ho, Y. K., Basu, S. K., and Brown, M. S., Binding site on macrophages that mediates uptake and degradation of acetylated low density lipoprotein, producing massive cholesterol deposition, *Proc. Natl. Acad. Sci. U.S.A.,* 76:333; 1979.

97. Van Lenten, B. J., Fogelman, A. M., Jackson, R. L., Shapiro, S., Haberland, M. E., and Edwards, P. A., Receptor-mediated uptake of remnant lipoprotiens by cholesterol-loaded human monocyte-macrophages, *J. Biol. Chem.,* 260:8783; 1985.

98. Gianturco, S. H., Lin A. Y., Hwand, S. L., Young, J., Brown, S. A., Via, D. P., and Bradley, W. A., Distinct murine macrophage receptor pathway for human triglyceride-rich lipoproteins, *J. Clin. Invest.,* 82:1633; 1988.

99. Suits, A. G., Chait, A., Aviram, M., and Heinecke, J. W., Phagocytosis of aggregated lipoproteins by macrophages: low density lipoprotein receptor dependent foam cell formation, *Proc. Natl. Acad. Sci. U.S.A.,* 86:2713; 1989.

100. Hiltunen, T. P., Luoma, J. S., Nikkari, T., and Yla-Herttuala, S., Expression of LDL receptor, VLDL receptor, LDL receptor-related protein, and scavenger receptor in rabbit atherosclerotic lesions, *Circulation,* 97:1079; 1998.

101. Craig, W. Y., Palomaki, G., and Haddow, J. E., Cigarette smoking and lipid and lipoprotein concentration: An analysis of published data, *Br. Med. J.,* 298:784; 1989.

102. Moffatt, R. J., Effects of cessation of smoking on serum lipids and high density lipoprotein-cholesterol, *Atherosclerosis,* 74:85; 1988.

103. Moffatt, R. J., Stamford, B. A., Owens, S. G., et al., Cessation from cigarette smoking: lipoprotein changes in men and women, *J. Smoking-Related Dis.,* 3:11; 1992.

104. Muscat, J. E., Harris, R. E., Haley, N. J., et al., Cigarette smoking and plasma cholesterol, *Am. Heart. J.,* 121:141; 1991.

105. Freeman, D. J., Griffin, B. A., Murray, E., et al., Smoking and plasma lipoproteins in man: effects on low density lipoprotein subfraction distributions, *Eur. J. Clin. Invest.,* 23:630; 1993.

106. Moffatt, R. J., Normalization of high density lipoprotein cholesterol following cessation from cigarette smoking, *Adv. Exp. Med. Biol.,* 267; 1990.

107. Stamford, B. A., Matter, S., Fell, R. D., and Papanek, P., Effects of smoking cessation on weight gain, metabolic rate, caloric consumption, and blood lipids, *Am. J. Clin. Nutr.,* 43:486; 1986.

108. Moffatt, R. J., Stamford, B. A., and Biggerstaff, K. D., Influence of worksite environmental tobacco smoke on serum lipoprotein profiles of female nonsmokers, *Metabolism,* 44:1536; 1995.

109. Karlsson, J., Lipoidic Structures, Lipophilic Antioxidants, and Clinical Interpretations, in *Antioxidants and Exercise,* Washburn, R., Smith, N., and Woosley, H., Eds., Human Kinetics, Champaign, Il., 1967; Ch. 10.

110. Terjung, R. L., Mackie, B. G., Dudley, G. A., et al., Influence of exercise on chylomicron triacylglycerol metabolism: plasma turnover and muscle uptake, *Med. Sci. Sports Exerc.,* 15(4):340; 1983.

111. Romijn, J. A., Coyle, E. F., Sidossis, L. S., et al., Regulation of endogenous fat and carbohydrate metabolism in relation to exercise intensity and duration, *Am. J. Physiol.,* 265(28)(Endocrinology and Metabolism): E380; 1993.

112. Martin, W. H., Effects of acute and chronic exercise on fat metabolism, in *Exerc. and Sport Sci. Rev.,* Holloszy J.O., Ed., Williams and Wilkins, Baltimore, 1996; 24:203.

113. Oscai, L. B. and Palmer, W. K., Muscle lipolysis during exercise: an update, *Sports Med.,* 6:23; 1988.

114. Martin, W. I., Effect of endurance training on fatty acid metabolism during whole body exercise, *Med. Sci. Sports Exerc.,* 29(5):635; 1997.

115. Kiens, B., Effect of endurance training on fatty acid metabolism: local adaptations, *Med. Sci. Sports Exerc.,* 29(5):640; 1997.

116. Kiens, B., Essen-Gustavsson, B., Christensen, N. J., et al., Skeletal muscle substrate utilization during submaximal exercise in man: effect of endurance training, *J. Physiol.,* 469:459; 1993.

117. Brouns, F. and Van der Vusse, G. J., Utilization of lipids during exercise in human subjects: metabolic and dietary constraints, *Br. J. Nutr.,* 79:117; 1998.

118. Martin, W. H., Dalsky, G. P., Hurley, B.F., et al., Effect of endurance training on plasma free fatty acid turnover and oxidation during exercise, *Am. J. Physiol.,* 265(28):E708; 1993.

119. Kanaley, J. A., Mottram, C. D., Scanlon, P. D., et al., Fatty acid kinetic responses to running above or below lactate threshold, *J. Appl. Physiol.,* 79(2):439; 1995.

120. Phillips, S. M., Green, H. J., Tarnopolsky, M. A., et al. Effects of training duration on substrate turnover and oxidation during exercise, *J. Appl. Physiol.*, 81(5):2182; 1996.

121. Hurley, B. F., Nemeth, P. M., Martin, W. H., et al., Muscle triglyceride utilization during exercise: effect of training, *J. Appl. Physiol.*, 60(2):562; 1986.

122. Jones, N. L., Heigenhauser, G. J., Kuksis, A., et al., Fat metabolism in heavy exercise, *Clin. Sci.*, 59:469; 1980.

123. Spriet, L. L., Heigenhauser, G. J. F., and Jones, N. L., Endogenous triacylglycerol utilization by rat skeletal muscle during tetanic stimulation, *J. Appl. Physiol.*, 60(2):410; 1986.

124. Hopp, J. F. and Palmer W. K., Effect of electrical stimulation on intracellular triacylglycerol in isolated skeletal muscle, *J. Appl. Physiol.*, 68(1):348; 1990.

125. McCartney, N., Spriet, L. L., Heigenhauser, G. J., et al., Muscle power and metabolism in maximal intermittent exercise, *J. Appl. Physiol.*, 60(4):1164; 1986.

126. Starling, R. D., Trappe, T. A., Parcell, A. C., et al., Effects of diet on muscle triglyceride and endurance performance, *J. Appl. Physiol.*, 82(4):1185; 1997.

127. Lapachet, R. A. B., Miller W. C., and Arnall D. A., Body fat and exercise endurance in trained rats adapted to a high-fat and/or high-carbohydrate diet, *J. Appl. Physiol.*, 80(4):1173; 1996.

128. Helge, J. W., Richter, E. A., and Kiens, B., Interaction of training and diet on metabolism and endurance during exercise in man, *J. Physiol.*, 492(1):293; 1996.

129. Helge, J. W., Wulff, B., and Kiens, B., Impact of a fat-rich diet on endurance in man: role of the dietary period, *Med. Sci. Sports Exerc.*, 30(3):456; 1998.

130. Pendergast, D. R., Horvath, P. J., Leddy, J. J., et al., The role of dietary fat on performance, metabolism, and health, *Am. J. Sports Med.*, 24(6):S53; 1996.

131. Nicklas, B. J., Effects of endurance exercise on adipose tissue metabolism, *Exerc. Sport Sci. Rev.*, 25:77; 1997.

132. Turcotte, L. P., Richter, E.A., and Kiens, B., Increased plasma FFA uptake and oxidation during prolonged exercise in trained vs. untrained humans, *Am. J. Physiol.*, 262(25):E791; 1992.

133. Thompson, P. D., Yurgalevitch, S.M., Flynn, M.M., et al., Effect of prolonged exercise training without weight loss on high-density lipoprotein metabolism in overweight men, *Metabolism*, 46: 217; 1997.

134. Gyntelberg, F., Brennan, R., Holloszy, J., et al., Plasma triglyceride lowering by exercise despite increased food intake in patients with Type-IV hyperlipoproteinemia, *Am. J. Clin. Nutr.*, 30: 716; 1977.

135. Holloszy, J. O., Skinner, J. S., Toro, G., et al., Effects of a six month program of endurance exercise on lipids of middle-aged men, *Am. J. Cardiol.*, 14: 753; 1964.

136. Lavie, C. J. and Milani, R. V., Effects of nonpharmacological therapy with cardiac rehabilitation and exercise training in patients with low levels of high-density lipoprotein cholesterol, *Amer. J. Cardiol.*, 78: 1286; 1996.

137. Huttunen, J. K., Länsimies, E., Voutilainen, E., et al., Effect of moderate physical exercise on serum lipoproteins: A controlled clinical trial with special reference to serum high-density lipoproteins, *Circulation*, 60(6): 1220; 1979.

138. Seip, R. L., Moulin, P., Cocke, T., et al., Exercise training decreases plasma cholesteryl ester transfer protein, *Arterioscler. Thromb.*, 13: 1359; 1993.

139. Marti, B., Suter, E., Riesen, W. F., et al., Effects of long-term, self-monitored exercise on the serum lipoprotein and apolipoprotein profile in middle-aged men, *Atherosclerosis*, 81: 19; 1990.

140. Wood, P. D., Haskell, W. L., Blair, S. N., et al., Increased exercise level and plasma lipoprotein concentrations: A one-year randomized, controlled study in sedentary middle-aged men, *Metabolism*, 32(1): 31; 1983.

141. Leon, A. S., Conrad, J., Hunninghake, D. B., et al., Effects of a vigorous walking program on body composition, and carbohydrate and lipid metabolism of obese young men, *Am. J. Clin. Nutr.*, 32: 1776; 1979.

142. Després, J-P., Moorjani, S., Tremblay, A., et al., Heredity and changes in plasma lipids and lipoproteins after short-term exercise training in men, *Arteriosclerosis*, 8: 402; 1988.

143. Kiens, B., Jörgenson, I., Lewis, S., et al., Increased plasma HDL-cholesterol and apo A-I in sedentary middle-aged men after physical conditioning, *Eur. J. Clin. Invest.*, 10: 203; 1980.

144. Després, J-P., Tremblay, A., Moorjani, S., et al., Long-term exercise training with constant energy intake: Effects on plasma lipoprotein levels, *Int. J. Obes.*, 14: 85; 1990.

145. Wood, P. D., Stefanick, M. L., Dreon, D. M., et al., Changes in plasma lipids and lipoproteins in overweight men during weight loss through dieting as compared with exercise, *N. Engl. J. Med.*, 319(18): 1173; 1988.

146. Ziogas, G. G., Thomas, T. R., and Harris W. S., Exercise training, postprandial hypertriglyceridemia, and LDL subfraction distribution, *Med. Sci. Sports Exerc.*, 29(8):986; 1997.

147. Kiens, B., Lithell, H., Mikines, K. J., et al., Effects of insulin and exercise on muscle lipoprotein lipase activity in man and its relation to insulin action, *J. Clin. Invest.*, 84:1124; 1989.

148. Israel, R. G., Sullivan, M. J., Marks, R. H., et al., Relationship between cardiorespiratory fitness and lipoprotein(a) in men and women, *Med. Sci. Sports Exerc.*, 26(4):425; 1994.

149. Hubinger, L. and Mackinnon, L. T., The effect of endurance training on lipoprotein(a) [LP(a)] levels in middle-aged males, *Med. Sci. Sports Exerc.*, 28(6):757; 1996.

150. Gaesser, G. A. and Rich, R. G., Effects of high- and low-intensity exercise training on aerobic capacity and blood lipids, *Med. Sci. Sports Exerc.*, 16(3):269; 1984.

151. Thompson, P. D., Cullinane, E. M., Sady, S. P., et al., Modest changes in high-density lipoprotein concentrations and metabolism with prolonged exercise training, *Circulation*, 78(1): 25; 1988.

152. Marniemi, J., Dahlstrom, S., Kvist, M., et al., Dependence of serum lipid and lecithin: cholesterol acyltranferase levels on physical training in young men, *Eur. J. Appl. Physiol.*, 49: 25; 1982.

153. Brewer, H. B., Gregg, R. E., Hoeg, J. M., et al., Apolipoproteins and lipoproteins in human plasma: an overview, *Clin. Chem.*, 34(8B):B4; 1988.

154. Crouse, S. F., O'Brien, B. C., Rohack, J. J., et al., Changes in serum lipids and apolioproteins after exercise in men with high cholesterol: influence of intensity, *J. Appl. Physiol.*, 79(1):279; 1995.

155. Coresh, J. and Kwiterovich, P. O. Jr., Small, dense low-density lipoprotein particles and coronary heart disease risk: a clear association with uncertain implications, *J.A.M.A.*, 276(11): 914; 1996.

156. Williams, P. T., Krauss, R. M., Vranizan, K. M., et al., Effects of exercise-induced weight loss on low density lipoprotein subfractions in healthy men, *Arteriosclerosis*, 9(5): 623; 1989.

157. Williams, P. T., Krauss, R. M., Vranizan, K. M., et al., Changes in lipoprotein subfractions during diet-induced weight lost in moderately overweight men, *Circulation*, 81: 1293; 1990.

158. Halle, M., Berg, A., König, D., et al., Differences in the concentration and composition of low-density lipoprotein subfraction particles between sedentary and trained hypercholesterolemic men, *Metabolism*, 46(7): 186; 1997.

159. MacKinnon, L. T., Hubinger, L., and Lepre, F., Effects of physical activity and diet on lipoprotein(a), *Med. Sports Sci. Exerc.*, 29(11):1429; 1997.

160. Halle, M., Berg, A., von Stein, T., et al., Lipoprotein(a) in endurance athletes, power athletes, and sedentary controls, *Med. Sci. Sports Exerc.*, 28(8):962; 1996.

161. Durstine, J. L., Ferguson, M. A., and Szymanski, L. M., Effect of a single session of exercise on lipoprotein(a), *Med. Sci. Sports Exerc.*, 28(10):1277; 1996.

162. Szymanski, L. M., Durstine, J. L., Davis, P. G., et al., Factors affecting fibrinolytic potential: Cardiovascular fitness, body composition, lipoprotein(a), *Metabolism*, 45: 1427; 1996.

163. Durstine, J. L., Pate, R. R., Sparling, P. B., et al., Lipid, lipoprotein, and iron status of elite women distance runners, *Int. J. Sports Med.*, 8: 119; 1987.

164. Kokkinos, P. F., Holland, J. C., Narayan, P., et al., Miles run per week and high-density lipoprotein cholesterol levels in healthy, middle-aged men: A dose response relationship, *Arch. Intern. Med.*, 155: 415; 1995.

165. Stein, R. A., Michielli, D. W., Glantz, M. D., et al., Effects of different exercise training intensities on lipoprotein cholesterol fractions in healthy middle-aged men, *Am. Heart J.*, 119: 277; 1990.

166. Stefanick, M. L., Mackey, S., Sheehan, M., et al., Effects of diet and exercise in men and postmenopausal women with low levels of HDL cholesterol and high levels of LDL cholesterol, *N. Eng. J. Med.*, 339(1): 12; 1998.

167. Tran, Z. V., Weltman, A., Glass, G. V., et al., The effects of exercise on blood lipids and lipoproteins: A meta-analysis of studies, *Med. Sci. Sports Exerc.*, 15(5): 393; 1983.

168. Williams, P. T., Stefanick, M. L., Vranizan, K. M., et al., Effects of weight loss by exercise or by dieting on plasma high-density lipoprotein (HDL) levels in men with low, intermediate, and normal-to-high HDL at baseline, *Metabolism*, 43(7): 917; 1994.

169. Wood, P. D., Williams, P. T., Haskell, W. L., et al., Physical activity and high density lipoproteins, in: *Clinical and Metabolic Aspects of High-Density Lipoproteins*, Amsterdam, Elsevier 1984; 133.

170. Williams, P. T., Wood, P. D., Haskell, W. L., et al., The effects of running mileage and duration on plasma lipoprotein levels, *J.A.M.A.*, 247(19): 2674; 1982.

171. Crouse, S. F., O'Brien, B. C., Grandjean, P. W., et al., Effects of training and single session of exercise on lipids and apolipoproteins in hypercholesterolemic men, *J. Appl. Physiol.*, 83(6): 2019; 1997.

172. Wood, P. D., Stefanick, M. L., Williams, P. T., et al., The effects on plasma lipoproteins of a prudent weight-reducing diet, with or without exercise in overweight men and women, *N. Eng. J. Med.*, 325: 461; 1991.

173. Leddy, J., Horvath, P., Rowland, J., et al., Effect of a high or a low fat diet on cardiovascular risk factors in male and female runners, *Med. Sci. Sports Exerc.*, 29(1):17; 1997.

174. Moffatt, R. J., Wallace, M. B., and Sady, S. P., Effects of anabolic steroids on lipoprotein profiles of female weightlifters, *Phys and Sports Med.*, 18(9):106; 1990.

175. Williams, P. T., Krauss, R. M., Vranizan, K. M., et al., Effects of weight-loss by exercise and by diet on apolipoproteins A-I and A-II and the particle-size distribution of high-density lipoproteins in men, *Metabolism*, 41(4): 441; 1992.

176. Tamai, T., Nakai, T., Takai, H., et al., The effects of physical exercise on plasma lipoproteins and apoliproteins metabolism in elderly men, *J. Gerontol.*, 43(4): M75; 1988.

177. Tamai, T., Higuchi, M., Oida, K., et al., Effects of exercise on plasma lipoprotein metabolism, in: Sato, Y., Poortmans J, Hashimoto I, Oshida Y, editors. Integration of Sports Sciences, *Medicine and Sports Science*, Vol 37. Basel: Karger, 1992; 430.

178. Cullinane, E., Siconolfi, S., Saritelli, A., et al., Acute decrease in serum triglycerides with exercise: Is there a threshold for an exercise effect? *Metabolism*, 1982; 31(8): 844.

179. Borensztajn, J., Rone, M. S., Babirak, S. P., et al., Effect of exercise on lipoprotein lipase activity in rat heart and skeletal muscle, *Am. J. Physiol.*, 229(2): 394; 1975.

180. Kantor, M. A., Cullinane, E. M., Sady, S. P., et al., Exercise acutely increases high density lipoprotein-cholesterol and lipoprotein lipase activity in trained and untrained men, *Metabolism*, 36(2): 188; 1987.

181. Kiens, B. and Lithell, H., Lipoprotein metabolism influenced by training-induced changes in human skeletal muscle, *J. Clin. Invest.*, 83: 558; 1989.

182. Thompson, P. D., What do muscles have to do with lipoproteins?, *Circulation*, 81(4): 1428; 1990.

183. Podl, T. R., Zmuda, J. M., Yurgalevitch, S. M., et al., Lipoprotein lipase and plasma triglyceride clearance are elevated in endurance-trained women, *Metabolism*, 43(7): 803; 1994.

184. Nikkilä, E. A., Taskinen, M. R., Rehunen, S., et al., Lipoprotein lipase activity in adipose tissue and skeletal muscle of runners: Relation to physical training, *Metabolism*, 27(11): 1661; 1978.

185. Thompson, P. D., Cullinane, E. M., Sady, S. P., et al., High density lipoprotein metabolism in endurance athletes and sedentary men, *Circulation*, 84(1): 140; 1991.

186. Sady, S. P., Cullinane, E. M., Saritelli, A., et al., Elevated high-density lipoprotein cholesterol in endurance athletes is related to enhanced plasma triglyceride clearance, *Metabolism*, 37(6): 568; 1988.

187. Cedermark, M., Froberg, J., Lithel,l H., et al., Effects of long term heavy exercise on skeletal muscle metabolism in man, in: Poortmans, J, and Niset, G, editors, *Biochemistry of Exercise IV-B*, Baltimore, University Park Press, 1981; 117.

188. Peltonen, P., Marniemi, J., Hietanen, E., et al., Changes in serum lipids, lipoproteins and heparin releasable lipolytic enzymes during moderate physical training in man: A longitudinal study, *Metabolism*, 30(5): 518; 1981.

189. Gordon, P. M., Gross, F. L., Visich, P. S., et al., The acute effects of exercise intensity on HDL-C metabolism, *Med. Sci. Sports*, 26(6): 671; 1994.

190. Shoup, E. E., Durstine, J. L., Davis, J. M., et al., Effects of a single session of resistance exercise on plasma lipoproteins and postheparin lipase activity, in review.

191. Ferguson, M. A., Durstine, J. L., Alderson, N. L., et al., Effects of four different single exercise sessions on lipids, lipoproteins, and lipoprotein lipase, *J. Appl. Physiol.*, 85(3) 1169; 1998.

192. Sady, S. P., Thompson, P. D., Cullinane, E. M., et al., Prolonged exercise augments plasma triglyceride clearance, *J.A.M.A.*, 256(18): 2552; 1986.

193. Ehnholm, C. and Kuusi, T., Preparation, characterization, and measurement of hepatic lipase, *Methods Enzymol.*, 129: 716; 1986.

194. Lokey, E. A. and Tran, Z. V., Effects of exercise training on serum lipid and lipoprotein concentrations in women: A meta-analysis, *Int. J. Sports Med.*, 10(6): 424; 1989.

195. Marniemi, J., Peltonen, P., Vuori, I., et al., Lipoprotein lipase of human postheparin plasma and adipose tissue in relation to physical training, *Acta. Physiol. Scand.*, 110: 131; 1980.

196. Stefanick, M.L., Terry, P.B., Haskell, W.L., et al., Relationships of changes in postheparin hepatic and lipoprotein lipase activity to HDL-cholesterol changes following weight loss achieved by dieting versus exercise, in: Gallo, L, editor, *Cardiovascular Disease: Molecular and Cellular Mechanisms, Prevention, and Treatment*, New York, Plenum Press, 1984; 61.

197. Kantor, M.A., Cullinane, E.M., Herbert, P.N., et al., Acute increase in lipoprotein lipase following prolonged exercise, *Metabolism*, 33(5): 454; 1984.

198. Quintao, E., Is reverse cholesterol transport a misnomer for suggesting its role in the prevention of atheroma formation?, *Atherosclerosis*, 116: 1; 1995.

199. Gupta, A. K., Ross, E. A., Myers, J. N., et al., Increased reverse cholesterol transport in athletes, *Metabolism*, 42(6): 684; 1993.

200. Lagrost, L., Regulation of cholesteryl ester transfer protein (CEPT) activity: Review of in vitro and in vitro studies, *Biochim. Biophys. Acta.*, 1215: 209; 1994.

201. Ritsch, A., Auer, B., Foger, B., et al., Polyclonal antibody-based immunoradiometric assay for quantification of cholesteryl ester transfer protein, *J. Lipid Res.*, 34: 673; 1993.

202. Serrat-Serrat, S. J., Ordóñez-Llanos, J., Serra-Grima, R., et al. Marathon runners presented lower serum cholesteryl ester transfer activity than sedentary subjects, *Atherosclerosis*, 101: 43; 1993.

203. Föger, B., Wohlfarter, T., Ritsch, A., et al., Kinetics of lipids, apolipoproteins, and cholesteryl ester transfer protein in plasma after a bicycle marathon, *Metabolism*, 43(5): 633; 1994.

204. Marniemi, J. and Hietanen, E., Response of serum lecithin: cholesterol acyltranferase activity to exercise training In: Hietanen, E, editor, *Regulation of Serum Lipids by Physical Exercise*, CRC Press LLC, Boca Raton, FL, 1982; 116.

205. Thomas, T. R., Adeniran, S. B., Iltis, P. W., et al., Effects of interval and continuous running on HDL-Cholesterol, apoproteins, A-I and B, and LCAT, *Can. J. Appl. Spt. Sci.*, 10(1): 52; 1985.

206. Dufaux, B., Order, U., Muller, R., et al., Delayed effects of prolonged exercise on serum lipoproteins, *Metabolism*, 35(2): 105; 1986.

207. Frey, I., Baumstark, M. W., Berg, A., et al., Influence of acute maximal exercise on lecithin: cholesterol acyltransferase activity in healthy adults of differing aerobic performance, *Eur. J. Appl. Physiol.*, 62: 31; 1991.

208. Berger, G. M. B. and Griffiths, M. P., Acute effects of moderate exercise on plasma lipoprotein parameters, *Int. J. Sports. Med.*, 8(5): 336; 1987.

209. Griffin, B. A., Skinner, E. R., Maughan, R. J., The acute effect of prolonged walking and dietary changes on plasma lipoprotein concentrations and high-density lipoprotein subfractions, *Metabolism*, 37(6): 535; 1988.

210. Okano, G., Sato, Y., Takumi, Y., et al., Effect of 4h pre-exercise high carbohydrate and high fat meal ingestion on endurance performance and metabolism, *Int. J. Sports Med.*, 17:4 530; 1996.

211. Muoio, D. M., Leddy, J. J., Horvath, P. J., et al., Effect of dietary fat on metabolic adjustments to maximal and VO_2 endurance in runners, *Med. Sci. Sports Exerc.*, 26(1):81; 1994.

212. Vukovich, M. D., Costill, D. L., Hickey, M. S., et al., Effect of fat emulsion infusion and fat feeding on muscle glycogen utilization during cycle exercise, *J. Appl. Physiol.*, 75(4):1513; 1993.

213. Wallace, M. B., Moffatt, R. J., Haymes, E. M., et al., Acute effects of resistance exercise on parameters of lipoprotein metabolism, *Med. Sci. Sports Exerc.*, 23(2):199; 1991.

214. Randle, P. J., Newsholme, E. A., and Garland, P. B., Regulation of glucose uptake by muscle. Effect of fatty acids, ketone bodies and pyruvate, and of alloxan diabetes and starvation, on the uptake and metabolic fate of glucose in rat heart and diaphragm muscles, *Biochem. J.*, 93:652; 1964.

215. Heinonen, O. J., Carnitine and physical exercise, *Sports Med.*, 22(2):109; 1996.

216. Schrauwen, P., van Marken Lichtenbelt, W. D., Sarius, W. H., et al., Changes in fat oxidation in response to a high-fat diet, *Am. J. Clin. Nutr.*, 66:276; 1997.

217. Trice, I. and Haymes E. M., Effects of caffeine ingestion on exercise-induced changes during high-intensity, intermittent exercise, *Int. J. Sport Nutr.*, 5:37; 1995.

218. Spriet, L. L., Maclean, D. A., Dyck, D. J., et al., Caffeine ingestion and muscle metabolism during prolonged exercise in humans, *Am. J. Physiol.*, 262(25):E891; 1992.

219. Krisanda, J. M., Moerland, T. S., and Kushmerick M. J., ATP supply and demand during exercise, *Exercise, Nutrition, and Energy Metabolism,* 1st ed., Horton, E. S. and Terjung, R. L. Eds., MacMillan Publishing Company, New York, 27; 1988.

220. Sahlin, K., Metabolic Changes Limiting Muscle Performance, *Symposium on the Biochemistry of Exercise*, Copenhagen, Denmark, Human Kinetics, 1986.

221. Cleroux, J., Van Nguyen, P., Taylor, A. W., et al., Effects of b_1- vs.b_1+ b_2- blockade on exercise endurance and muscle metabolism in humans, *J. Appl. Physiol.*, 66(2):548; 1989.

222. Winder, W. W., Malonyl-CoA-regulator of fatty acid oxidation in muscle during exercise, *Exerc. Sport Sci. Rev.*, 26:117; 1998.

223. Constantin-Teodosiu, D., Carlin, J. J., Cederblad, G., et al., Acetyl group accumulation and pyruvate dehydrogenase activity in human muscle during incremental exercise, *Acta. Physiologica. Scandinavica.*, 143:367; 1991.

224. Spriet, L. L., Dyck, D. J., Cederblad, G., et al., Effects of fat availability on acetyl-CoA and acetyl-carnitine metabolism in rat skeletal muscle, *Am. J. Physiol.*, 263(32):C653; 1992.

225. Rasmussen, B. B. and Winder, W. W., Effect of exercise intensity on skeletal muscle malonyl-CoA and acetyl-CoA carboxylase, *J. Appl. Physiol.*, 83(4):1104; 1997.

226. Winder, W. W., Arogyasami, J., Barton, R. J., et al., Muscle malonyl-CoA decreases during exercise, *J. Appl. Physiol.*, 67(6):2230; 1989.

227. Ladu, M. J., Kaspas, H., and Palmer, W. K., Regulation of lipoprotein lipase in muscle and adipose tissue during exercise, *J. Appl. Physiol.*, 71(2):404; 1991.

228. Seip, R. L. and Semenkovich, C. F., Skeletal muscle lipoprotein lipase: molecular regulation and physical effects in relation to exercise, *Exerc. Sport Sci. Rev.*, 26:191; 1998.

229. Vallerand, A. L. and Jacobs, I., Rates of energy substrates utilization during human cold exposure, *Eur. J. Appl. Physiol.*, 58:873; 1989.

230. Vallerand, A. L. and Jacobs, I., Energy metabolism during cold exposure, *Int. J. Sports Med.*, 13(suppl1):S191; 1992.

231. Hurley, B. F. and Haymes, E. M., The effects of rest and exercise in the cold on substrate mobilization and utilization, *Aviat. Space Environ. Med.*, 53(12):1193; 1982.

232. Gorski, J., Muscle triglyceride metabolism during exercise, *Can. J. Physiol. Pharmacol.*, 70:123; 1992.

233. Putman, C. T., Jones, N. L., Lands, C. L., et al., Skeletal muscle pyruvate dehydrogenase activity during maximal exercise in humans, *Am. J. Physiol.*, 269(32):E458; 1995.

234. Coyle, E. F. and Hodgkinson, B. J., Influence of dietary fat and carbohydrate on metabolic and performance responses, in *Metabolic Basis of Performance in Sport and Exercise*, vol. 12, Hargreaves, M. and Lamb, D. R., eds., Brown & Benchmark, Dubuque, IA, 1999; in press.

235. Sherman, M. W. and Leenders, N., Fat loading: the next magic bullet?, *Int. J. Sport Nutr.*, Supplement to V 5: s1; 1994.

236. Coggan, A. R. and Mendenhall, L. A., Effect of diet on substrate metabolism during exercise, in *Energy Metabolism in Exercise and Sport*, vol. 5. Lamb, D. R. and Gisolfi, C. V., eds., Brown and Benchmark, Dubuque, IA, 1992; Ch.10.

237. Bodary, P., Fat-loading: dietary strategy for the 21st century, in *Peak Running Performance*, vol. 7 num. 3. McMillan, G., ed., Road Runner Sports, 1998; pg. 1.

CHAPTER 7

Proteins and Amino Acids in Exercise and Sport

Mauro G. Di Pasquale

CONTENTS

7.1 INTRODUCTION

Of the three macronutrients — carbohydrates, fats, and protein — that make up our food, protein is the most important and versatile. Not only do proteins make up three quarters of body solids[1] (including structural and contractile proteins, enzymes, nucleoproteins, and proteins that transport oxygen), but protein and amino acids also have potent biological effects on the body that involve all tissues in the body and extend to almost all metabolic processes.

There is a vast body of research on the effects of protein and the individual amino acids on athletic performance. The results of this research has shown not only that athletes need more protein than their sedentary counterparts but also that protein and amino acids have profound effects on athletic performance, primarily on muscle size and strength, energy metabolism and immune function.

There has recently been an increased interest in determining the ergogenic effect of specific amino acids. Numerous studies have indicated that various amino acids are involved in the metabolic and physiological responses to both acute and chronic exercise. Because of a perceived need for protein, athletes have increased both their dietary protein consumption and the use of commercial protein and amino acid supplements.

This chapter examines the available scientific and medical information to determine the physiological and pharmacological effects of protein and amino acids on lean body mass, body fat, strength, and endurance.

7.2 THE STRUCTURE AND PROPERTIES OF PROTEIN

7.2.1 Structural, Contractile, Enzymes, and Other Proteins

The word protein comes from the Greek word proteios, which means of the first rank or importance. Protein is indeed important for life and is involved in every biological process within the body. The average human body is approximately 18% protein. Proteins are essential components of muscle, skin, cell membranes, blood, hormones, antibodies, enzymes, genetic material and almost all other body tissues and components. They serve as structural components, biocatalysts (enzymes), antibodies, lubricants, messengers (hormones), and carriers.

7.2.2 Free Amino Acid Pool

Of the body's vast content of amino acids, only a small amount is not bound up in protein structures of one sort or another. Only .5 to 1% of the amino acids in the body is present as free amino acids and make up the body's free amino acid pool.

The free amino acid pool represents the most bioactive part of the body's proteins and amino acid content. This pool is made up of free amino acids in plasma and in the intracellular and extracellular space. This relatively small amount of free amino acids, in equilibrium with the body's much larger amounts of proteins and amino acids, is responsible for the all the metabolic and substrate protein and amino acid interactions that take place in the body.

Various amino acids are represented in this pool with the nonessential or conditionally essential amino acids, glutamine, glycine, and alanine making up the highest concentrations. Of the essential amino acids, lysine, threonine, and the branched-chain amino acids (BCAA), valine, leucine, and isoleucine are present in the highest concentrations.

The amino acids present in the plasma portion and extracellular portions of the pool are in a sort of equilibrium with the amino acids in the intracellular portion. Because this equilibrium between the intracellular and extracellular portions of the amino acid pool is due in most cases to active transport of the amino acids, it is not a true equilibrium but a sort of steady state that is based on both concentrations of amino acids and the existing metabolic state. Measuring one portion of the pool without the other can give a false impression of the movement or flux of amino acids through the free pool.

The small free amino acid pool, while highly active, is relatively stable in size and content. However, there are some relatively small but important changes that take place in amino acid concentrations in response to various stimuli such as exercise, food intake, and various diseases.

7.2.3 Protein Balance

Protein balance is a function of intake relative to output (utilization and loss). Body proteins are in a constant state of flux, with both protein degradation and protein synthesis constantly going on. Normally, these two processes are equal with no net loss or net gain of protein taking place. Protein intake usually equals protein lost.

However, if protein synthesis (anabolism) is greater than protein degradation (catabolism), the overall result is anabolic with a net increase in body protein. If protein degradation is greater than protein synthesis, then the overall result is catabolic with a net decrease in body protein.

Although the end result may be the same, protein balance and protein turnover are not synonymous. Protein turnover is a measure of the rate of protein metabolism, and it involves both protein synthesis and catabolism.

7.2.3.1 Factors Affecting Protein Synthesis and Catabolism

Accelerated protein breakdown and a net protein loss occur secondary to exhaustive exercise and in injury and various diseases. The negative nitrogen balance observed in such cases represents the net result of breakdown and synthesis, with breakdown increased and synthesis either increased or diminished. Under certain conditions, protein catabolism can also be decreased. In addition, protein synthesis can be increased or decreased under certain conditions. The net result depends on the conditions present and the effects on both synthesis and catabolism.

For example, to have a net increase in protein synthesis so that there is an increase in the concentration of a protein in a cell, its rate of synthesis would have to increase or its breakdown decrease or both. There are several ways the concentration of protein in a cell could be increased, including the four outlined below:

1. The rate of synthesis of the mRNA that codes for the particular protein(s) could be increased (known as transcriptional control).
2. The rate of synthesis of the polypeptide chain by the ribosomal-mRNA complex could be increased (known as translational control).
3. The rate of degradation of the mRNA could be decreased (also translational control).
4. The rate of degradation of the protein could be decreased.

The following table outlines some of the conditions or factors that affect protein synthesis. Many of these conditions and factors are inter-related. Keep in mind that protein synthesis is increased as the result of a net positive change secondary to changes in both (or less commonly one of) synthesis and catabolism.

Table 7.1 Conditions and Factors That Affect Protein Synthesis

Condition or Factor	Effect on rate of protein synthesis
Decreased protein intake	Decreased
Increased protein intake	Increased
Decreased energy intake	Decreased
Increased cellular hydration	Increased
Decreased cellular hydration	Decreased
Increased intake of leucine in presence of sufficiency of other amino acids	Increased
Increased intake of glutamine in presence of sufficiency of other amino acids	Increased
Lack of nervous stimulation	Decreased
Muscle stretch, or exercise	Increased
Overtraining	Decreased
Testosterone (and anabolic steroids)	Increased
Growth hormone	Increased
Insulin-like growth factor one (IGF-I)	Increased
Normal Thyroxine levels	Increased
Excess Thyroxine	Decreased
Catecholamines (including synthetic β-adrenergic agonist such as clenbuterol)	Increased
Glucocorticoids	Decreased
Physical trauma, infection	Decreased

Table from *Amino Acids and Proteins for the Athlete: The Anabolic Edge*. Mauro G. Di Pasquale, CRC Press, 1997.

7.2.4 Energy Metabolism

Unlike the fats and carbohydrates that can be stored in the form of triglycerides and glycogen, there is no storage form of protein or amino acids. All of the protein and amino acids (except for the free amino acid pool) serve either a structural or metabolic function. Excess amino acids from protein are transaminated and the nonnitrogenous portion of the molecule is transformed into glucose and used directly or transformed into fat or glycogen. The unneeded nitrogen is converted to urea and excreted in the urine.

7.2.4.1 Oxidation of Amino Acids

Proteins contribute 10 to 15% to the energy value of most well-balanced diets and seldom exceed 20%. For some athletes in power sports and in bodybuilders who may be on very high-protein diets, the contribution can be as high as 50%. And in selective cases it can be even more.

Once the needed proteins are synthesized and the amino acid pools replenished, additional amino acids are degraded and used for energy or stored mainly as fat and to a lesser extent as glycogen. The primary site for degradation of most amino acids is the liver. The liver is unique because of its capacity to degrade amino acids and synthesize urea for elimination of the amino nitrogen.

The first step in the degradation of amino acids begins with deamination — the removal of the alpha-amino group from the amino acid to produce an oxoacid, which may be a simple metabolic intermediate (e.g., pyruvate) or be converted to a simple metabolic intermediate via a specific metabolic pathway. The intermediates are either oxidized via the citric acid cycle or converted to glucose via gluconeogenesis. For instance, deaminated alanine is pyruvic acid. This can be converted into glucose or glycogen. Or it can be converted into acetyl-CoA, which can then be polymerized into fatty acids. Also, two molecules of acetyl-CoA can condense to form acetoacetic acid, which is one of the ketone bodies.

The larger the body muscle mass, the more transamination of amino acids occurs to fulfill energy needs. Each kilocalorie needed for basal metabolism leads to the excretion of 1 to 1.3 mg of urinary nitrogen. For the same reason, nitrogen excretion increases during exercise and heavy work.

7.2.4.2 Gluconeogenesis

Certain processes such as glycogenolysis, gluconeogenesis, increasing fatty acid oxidation, utilization of ketones, and proteolysis ensure that the body has a continuous supply of available energy and substrates for its metabolic needs.

The rise in blood glucose and the subsequent rise in insulin that occur after a meal promote glycogen storage in liver and muscle and fat deposition in adipose tissue and liver. After a meal, both glucose and insulin levels fall and liver glycogen through the process of glycogenolysis becomes the primary source of available glucose.

Maintenance of plasma glucose concentrations within a narrow range despite wide fluctuations in the demand (e.g., vigorous exercise) and supply (e.g., large carbohydrate meals) of glucose results from coordination of factors that regulate glucose release into and removal from the circulation.[2]

The liver and kidneys use lactate, pyruvate, glycerol and certain amino acids to form glucose. Under normal conditions, amino acids, especially alanine and glutamine, serve as major substrates for gluconeogenesis.[3]

In one study, the contribution under various nutritional regimens of several amino acids and lactate to gluconeogenesis was estimated by measuring the glucose formation from 14C-labeled substrates.[4] Isolated rat hepatocytes were incubated for 60 minutes in a Krebs-Ringer bicarbonate buffer pH 7.4 containing lactate, pyruvate, and all the amino acids at concentrations similar to their physiological levels found in rat plasma, with one precursor labeled in each flask. In all conditions, lactate was the major glucose precursor, providing more than 60% of the glucose formed. Glutamine and alanine were the major amino acid precursors of glucose, contributing 9.8% and 10.6% of the glucose formed, respectively, in hepatocytes isolated from starved rats. Serine, glycine, and threonine also contributed to gluconeogenesis in the starved liver cells at 2.6, 2.1, and 3.8%, respectively, of the glucose formed.

This study showed that the availability of dietary carbohydrates varies the gluconeogenic response. The rate of glucose formation from the isolated hepatocytes of the starved rats and those fed either high protein or high fat was higher than that from rats fed a nonpurified diet.

The low insulin and the high glucagon output that characterizes the post-absorptive phase and fasting (the lower the glucose level the lower the insulin and higher the glucagon output) stimulates both glycogenolysis and gluconeogenesis. Initially approximately 70 to 75% of the hepatic glucose output is derived from glycogenolysis and the remainder from gluconeogenesis.

Starvation is associated initially with an increased release of the gluconeogenic amino acids from muscles and an increase in gluconeogenesis.[5] In one study that looked at amino acid balance across forearm muscles in postabsorptive (overnight fasted) subjects, fasting significantly reduced basal insulin and increased glucagon, and increased muscle release of the principal glycogenic amino acids (alanine, glutamine, glycine, threonine, serine, methionine, tyrosine, and lysine).[6] Alanine release increased 59.4%. The increase in release for all amino acids averaged 69.4% and was statistically significant for threonine, serine, glycine, alanine, alpha-aminobutyrate, methionine, tyrosine, and lysine. In the same study, seven subjects also fasted for 60 hours. In these subjects there was a reduction of amino acid release as the fasting continued.

Because these changes reproduce those observed after a few days of total fasting, it has been suggested that it is the carbohydrate restriction, and the subsequent decrease in insulin and increase in glucagon, that is responsible for the metabolic and hormonal adaptations of brief fasting.[7] A reduction in the release of substrate amino acids from skeletal muscle largely explains the decrease in gluconeogenesis characterizing prolonged starvation.

A similar response, an initial increase in gluconeogenesis followed in time by a decrease is seen in trauma such as burn injury[8] and in prolonged exercise.[9]

During prolonged mild exercise that increases the hepatic glucose output twofold, the relative contribution of gluconeogenesis to the overall hepatic output increases from 25% to 45%, indicating a threefold rise in the absolute rate of gluconeogenesis. After 12 to 13 hours of fasting, hepatic gluconeogenesis replaces glycogenolysis as the main source of glucose.[10]

7.3 DIETARY PROTEIN

Every cell in the body is partly composed of proteins that are subject to continuous wear and replacement. Carbohydrates and fats contain no nitrogen or sulphur, two essential elements in all proteins. Whereas the fat in the body can be derived from dietary carbohydrates and the carbohydrates from proteins, the proteins of the body are inevitably dependant for their formation and maintenance on the proteins in food. Protein from food is digested and the resultant amino acids and peptides are absorbed and used to synthesize body proteins.

Proteins consist of large molecules with molecular weights ranging from 1000 to over 1,000,000. In their native state, some are soluble and some insoluble in water. Although there are a great variety of proteins that can be subdivided into various categories, they are all are made up of the same building blocks called amino acids.

Every species of animal has its characteristic proteins — the proteins of beef muscle, for instance, differ from those of pork muscle. It is the proteins that give each species its specific immunological characters and uniqueness.

Plants can synthesize all the amino acids they need from simple inorganic chemical compounds, but animals are unable to do this because they cannot synthesize the amino (NH_2) group. To obtain the amino acids necessary for building protein, animals must eat plants or other animals that have lived on plants.

The human body has certain limited powers of converting one amino acid into another. This is achieved in the liver, at least partly by the process of transamination, whereby an amino group is shifted from one molecule across to another under the influence of aminotransferase, the co-enzyme of which is pyridoxal phosphate. However, the body's ability to convert one amino acid into another is restricted. There are several amino acids that the body cannot make for itself and so must obtain from the diet. These are termed essential amino acids.

Under normal circumstances, the adult human body can maintain nitrogenous equilibrium on a mixture of eight pure amino acids as its sole source of nitrogen. These eight are isoleucine, leucine, lysine, methionine, phenylalanine, threonine, tryptophan, and valine. Some consider several amino acids, including arginine, histidine, and glutamine, to be conditionally essential. That is, under certain conditions such as growth, these amino acids are not able to be synthesized in adequate amounts and thus need to be supplied in the diet.

Synthesis of the conditionally essential and nonessential amino acids depends mainly on the formation first of appropriate alpha-keto acids, the precursors of the respective amino acids. For instance, pyruvic acid, which is formed in large quantities during the glycolytic breakdown of glucose, is the keto acid precursor of the amino acid alanine. Then, by the process of transamination, an amino radical is transferred from certain amino acids to the alpha-keto acid while the keto oxygen is transferred to the donor of the amino radical. In the formation of alanine, for example, the amino radical is transferred to the pyruvic acid from one of several possible amino acid donors including asparagine, glutamine, glutamic acid, and aspartic acid.

Transamination is promoted by several enzymes among which are the aminotransferases, which are derivatives of pyridoxine (B6), one of the B vitamins. Without this vitamin, the nonessential amino acids are synthesized poorly and, therefore, protein formation cannot proceed normally. Other vitamins, minerals and nutrients can also affect the formation of protein.

All proteins are made up of varying numbers of amino acids attached together in a specific sequence and having a specific architecture. The sequence of the amino acids and form of the protein differentiates one protein from another and gives the protein special physiological and biological properties.

7.3.1 Slow and Fast Dietary Proteins

We know there are differences in carbohydrate — high glycemic, low glycemic, simple sugars, starches, etc. And we know that different carbohydrates are absorbed in the gut and appear in the blood at different rates depending on various factors — for example, simple sugars are absorbed quickly and more complex ones, depending on how quickly they can be broken down, are absorbed more slowly. This makes up the basis for the Glycemic Index of not only foods but also whole meals because the presence of protein and fat with the carbohydrates usually slows down the absorption over the whole digestive process. Fast and slow carbohydrates have different metabolic effects on the hormones and various metabolic processes.

We also have slow and fast dietary proteins. The speed of absorption of dietary amino acids by the gut varies according to the type of ingested dietary protein. This could affect postprandial (after meals) protein synthesis, breakdown, and deposition. A recent study looked at both casein and whey protein absorption and the subsequent metabolic effects.[11]

It has been shown that the postprandial amino acid levels differ a lot depending on the mode of administration of a dietary protein. A single protein meal results in an acute but transient peak of amino acids, whereas the same amount of the same protein given in a continuous manner, which mimics a slow absorption, induces a smaller but prolonged increase.

Because amino acids are potent modulators of protein synthesis, breakdown, and oxidation, different patterns of postprandial amino acidemia (the level of amino acids in the blood) might well result in different postprandial protein kinetics and gain. Therefore, the speed of absorption by the gut of amino acids derived from dietary proteins will have different effects on whole body protein synthesis, breakdown, and oxidation, which in turn control protein deposition.

To test this hypothesis, two labeled milk proteins, casein (CAS) and whey protein (WP), of different physicochemical properties were ingested as one single meal by healthy adults and postprandial whole body leucine kinetics were assessed. WP induced a dramatic but short increase of plasma amino acids. CAS induced a prolonged plateau of moderate hyperaminoacidemia, probably because of a slow gastric emptying. Whole body protein breakdown was inhibited by 34% after CAS ingestion but not after WP ingestion. Postprandial protein synthesis was stimulated by 68% with the WP meal and to a lesser extent (+31%) with the CAS meal.

Under the conditions of this study, i.e., a single-protein meal with no energy added, two dietary proteins were shown to have different metabolic fates and uses. After WP ingestion, the plasma appearance of dietary amino acids is fast, high, and transient. This amino acid pattern is associated with an increased protein synthesis and oxidation and no change in protein breakdown. By contrast, the plasma appearance of dietary amino acids after a CAS meal is slower, lower, and prolonged with a different whole body metabolic response: Protein synthesis slightly increases, oxidation is moderately stimulated, but protein breakdown is markedly inhibited.

This study demonstrates that dietary amino acid absorption is faster with WP than with CAS. It is very likely that a slower gastric emptying was mostly responsible for the slower appearance of amino acids into the plasma. Indeed, CAS clots into the stomach, whereas WP is rapidly emptied from the stomach into the duodenum. The results of the study demonstrate that amino acids derived from casein are indeed slowly released from the gut and that slow and fast proteins differently modulate postprandial changes of whole body protein synthesis, breakdown, oxidation, and deposition.

After WP ingestion, large amounts of dietary amino acids flood the small body pool in a short time, resulting in a dramatic increase in amino acid concentrations. This is probably responsible for the stimulation of protein synthesis. This dramatic stimulation of protein synthesis and absence of protein breakdown inhibition is quite different from the pattern observed with classic feeding studies and with the use of only one protein source.

The study demonstrated that the speed of amino acid absorption after protein ingestion has a major impact on the postprandial metabolic response to a single protein meal. The slowly absorbed CAS promotes postprandial protein deposition by an inhibition of protein breakdown without excessive increase in amino acid concentration. By contrast, a fast dietary protein stimulates protein synthesis as well as oxidation. This impact of amino acid absorption speed on protein metabolism is true when proteins are given alone, but as for carbohydrate, this might be blunted in more complex meals that could affect gastric emptying (lipids) and/or insulin response (carbohydrate).

7.3.2   The Recommended Daily Allowance (RDA)

The minimum daily requirement, that is the minimum amount of dietary protein that provides the needed amounts of amino acids to optimally maintain the body, is impossible to determine for each individual without expending a good deal of time and effort for each person.

To eliminate the necessity of determining individual nutrient requirements, a system called the recommended daily allowance (RDA) has been devised. As research accumulates for each of the many essential nutrients, its associated RDA is revised. How is the RDA established? Ideally, sufficient research is conducted to show 1) that a given nutrient is needed by the human, 2) that certain deficiency signs can be produced, 3) that these signs can be avoided or reversed if the missing nutrient is administered, and 4) that no further improvement is observed if the nutrient is administered at levels above that which reversed the deficiency symptoms.

Next, studies are conducted on a variety of subjects to determine their minimal need. Because humans vary so much, it is not possible to measure the requirements over a broad range of human variability. To allow for this variability, a safety factor is added on to the determined minimum needs of the group of subjects studied. As more subjects are studied and more data accumulated, the added safety factor becomes smaller.

In the case of protein and amino acid requirements, the RDA was set at twice the minimum value of the subject who required the most protein and/or amino acid in all the studies conducted. By greatly increasing the recommended intake figure over that experimentally determined, it was hoped that the protein and amino acid needs of the majority or 95% of the U.S. population would be met. The RDA for protein was originally quite high. For many years, it was set at 1 g/kg body weight for the average adult male. The average adult male was assumed to weigh 70 kg (about 155 pounds), so the RDA was 70 g/day. With an ever-increasing database that the Nutrition Board of the National Research Council can use for its recommendations, the RDA for protein has been adjusted downward every five years.

As of 1993, the protein RDA for an adult male was set at 56 g/day. This presumes that the dietary protein is coming from a mixed diet that contains a reasonable amount of good-quality proteins. For persons subsisting on mixtures of poor-quality proteins, this RDA may not be adequate.

RDAs are set not only for the individual nutrients but also for age groups within each nutrient. For some age groups, the database is very poor, e.g., preadolescents, toddlers, young children, and pregnant females; there is a continual revision as data become available.

Guidelines of nutritional requirements in health have been formulated in the reports, updated periodically, of the Food and Nutrition Board of the National Research Council of the United States.[12] These Recommended Dietary Allowances, expressed for age and sex and modified for such conditions as pregnancy and lactation, are designed to cover the requirements of virtually all healthy individuals. With the exception of energy, the allowances are not average requirements but rather a recommended intake sufficient to meet the needs of all healthy individuals.

Proper nitrogen balance studies are laborious and are performed over a period of several days. A shortcut is often taken and an estimate of nitrogen balance is made by collecting and measuring nitrogen in the urine, because the end products of protein metabolism leave the body mainly via this route, and estimating other losses.

Estimations are made of the nitrogen lost in the feces and the small losses of protein from skin, hair, fingernails, perspiration, and other secretions.

About 90% of the nitrogen in urine is urea and ammonia salts — the end products of protein metabolism. The remaining nitrogen is accounted for by creatinine (from creatine), uric acid (products of the metabolism of purines and pyrimidines), porphyrins, and other nitrogen-containing compounds.

Urinary nitrogen excretion is related to the basal metabolic rate (BMR). The larger the muscle mass in the body, the more calories are needed to maintain the BMR. Also, the rate of transamination is greater as amino acids and carbohydrates are interconverted to fulfill energy needs in the muscle. One to 1.3 mg of urinary nitrogen is excreted for each kilocalorie required for basal metabolism. Nitrogen excretion also increases during exercise and heavy work.

Fecal and skin losses account for a significant amount of nitrogen loss from the body in normal conditions, and these may vary widely in disease states. Thus, measurement of urinary nitrogen loss alone may not provide a predictable assessment of daily nitrogen requirement when it is most needed. Fecal losses are due to the inefficiency of digestion and absorption of protein (93% efficiency). In addition, the intestinal tract secretes proteins in the lumen from saliva, gastric juice, bile, pancreatic enzymes, and enterocyte sloughing.

Taking all these losses into consideration and using nitrogen balance as a tool, the minimum daily dietary allowance for protein may be derived on the following basis:

1. Obligatory urinary nitrogen losses of young adults amount to about 37 mg/kg of body weight.
2. Fecal nitrogen losses average 12 mg/kg of body weight.
3. Amounts of nitrogen lost in the perspiration, hair, fingernails, and sloughed skin are estimated at 3 mg/kg of body weight.
4. Minor routes of nitrogen loss such as saliva, menstruation, and seminal ejaculation are estimated at 2 mg/kg of body weight.
5. The total obligatory nitrogen lost — that which must be replaced daily — amounts to 54 mg/kg, or in terms of protein lost this is 0.34 g/kg (.054*6.25).
6. To account for individual variation, the daily loss is increased by 30%, or 70 mg/kg. In terms of protein, this is 0.45 g/kg of body weight.
7. This protein loss is further increased by 30% to 0.6 g/kg of body weight to account for the loss of efficiency when consuming even a high-quality protein such as egg.
8. The final adjustment is to correct for the 75% efficiency of utilization of protein in the mixed diet of North Americans. Thus, the RDA for protein becomes 0.8 g/kg of body weight for normal healthy adult males and females, or 63 g of protein per day for a 174 lb (79 kg) man and 50 g per day for a 138 lb (63 kg) woman.

The need for dietary protein is influenced by age, environmental temperature, energy intake, gender, micronutrient intake, infection, activity, previous diet, trauma, pregnancy, and lactation.

7.3.3 Recommended Daily Allowances (RDA) for Athletes

The RDAs make little provision for changes in nutrient requirements for the athlete. Energy requirements increase with exercise as the lean (muscle) mass increases and as resting metabolic energy expenditure increases. Increased physical activity at all ages promotes the retention of lean muscle mass and requires increased protein and energy intake.

7.3.3.1 Historical Overview

The history of protein requirements for athletes is both interesting and circular. In the mid-1800s, the popular opinion was that protein was the primary fuel for working muscle.[13] This was an incentive for athletes to consume large amounts of dietary protein.

In 1866, a paper based on urinary nitrogen excretion measures (in order for protein to provide energy its nitrogen must be removed and subsequently excreted primarily in the urine), suggested that protein was not an important fuel and contributed about 6% of the fuel used during a 1956 m climb in the Swiss Alps.[14] This paper and others led to the perception that exercise does not increase one's need for dietary protein. This view has persisted to the present.

Recently, however, there is some evidence to show that protein contributes more than is generally believed. The data in the 1866 study likely underestimated the actual protein use for several methodological reasons. For example, the subjects consumed a protein-free diet before the climb, post-climb excretion measures were not made, and other routes of nitrogen excretion may have been substantial.

However, based largely on these data, this belief has persisted throughout most of the 20th century. This is somewhat surprising because Cathcart[15] in an extensive review of the literature prior to 1925 concluded that "the accumulated evidence seems to me to point in no unmistakable fashion to the opposite conclusion that muscle activity does increase, if only in small degree, the metabolism of protein." Based on results from several separate experimental approaches, the conclusions of several more recent investigators support Cathcart's conclusion.[16]

Current dietary protein recommendations are insufficient for athletes and those wishing to maximize lean body mass and strength. These athletes may well benefit from protein supplementation. With exercise and under certain conditions, the use of protein and amino acid supplements may have significant anabolic and anticatabolic effects.

In a recent paper, Peter Lemon, of the Applied Physiology Research Laboratory at Kent State University, addressed the issue of the protein requirements of athletes.[17] Lemon remarked that current recommendations concerning dietary protein are based primarily on data obtained from sedentary subjects. However, both endurance and strength athletes, he says, will likely benefit from diets containing more protein than the current RDA of 0.8 g/kg/day, though the roles played by protein in excess of the RDA will likely be quite different between the two sets of athletes.

For strength athletes, Lemon states that protein requirements will probably be in the range of 1.4–1.8 g/kg/day, whereas endurance athletes need about 1.2–1.4 g/kg/day. There is no indication that these intakes will cause any adverse side effects in healthy humans. On the other hand, there is essentially no valid scientific evidence that protein intakes exceeding about 1.8–2.0 k/kg day will provide an additional advantage, he adds.

7.3.4 Effects of Exercise on Dietary Protein Requirements

High protein intake has been the mainstay of most athletes' diets. Athletes in general and strength athletes and bodybuilders in particular consume large amounts of protein.[18] One reason for their increased protein consumption is their increased caloric intake. Another is that most athletes deliberately increase their intake of protein-rich foods and often use protein supplements.

Many scientific and medical sources say protein supplementation and high protein diets are unnecessary and that the Recommended Allowance, suggested by government research committees, supplies more than adequate amounts of protein for the athlete.[19] In fact, overloading on protein is considered detrimental because of the increased load to the kidneys of the metabolic breakdown products formed when the excess protein is used as an energy source.

In recent years, the results of several investigations involving both strength and endurance athletes indicate that, in fact, exercise does increase protein/amino acid needs.[20–24] In a recent review, the overall consensus has been that all athletes need more protein than sedentary people and that strength athletes need the most.[25]

Recently, a group of researchers at McMaster University in Hamilton, Ontario concluded that the current Canadian Recommended Nutrient Intake for protein of 0.86 g/kg/day is inadequate for those engaged in endurance exercise.[26] Moreover, their results indicated that male athletes may have an even higher protein requirement than females.

Butterfield performed a review of the literature and recommended high protein intakes (up to 2–3 g/kg) for physically active individuals.[27] She found evidence for the existence of an intricate relationship between protein and energy utilization with exercise. "When energy intake is in excess of need, the utilization of even a marginal intake of protein will be improved, giving the appearance that protein intake is adequate. When energy intake and output are balanced, the improvement in nitrogen retention accomplished by exercise seems to be fairly constant at protein intakes greater than 0.8 g/kg/d, but falls off rapidly at protein intakes below this. When energy balance is negative, the magnitude of the effect of exercise on protein retention may be decreased as the activity increases, and protein requirements may be higher than when energy balance is maintained."

Somewhat in agreement with Butterfield's conclusions are the results of another study by Piatti et al.[28] They investigated the effects of two hypocaloric diets (800 kcal) on body weight reduction and composition, insulin sensitivity and proteolysis in 25 normal obese women. The two diets had the following composition: 45% protein, 35% carbohydrate, and 20% fat (high-protein diet); and 60% carbohydrate, 20% protein, and 20% fat (high-carbohydrate diet). The results, said the authors, suggest that 1) a hypocaloric diet providing a high percentage of natural protein can improve insulin sensitivity, and 2) conversely, a hypocaloric high-carbohydrate diet decreases insulin sensitivity and is unable to spare muscle tissue.

In another study, it was shown that a protein intake as high as four times the recommended RDA (3.3 g per kilogram of bodyweight per day vs. RDA of 0.8 g per kilogram per day) resulted in significantly increased protein synthesis even when compared with a protein intake that was almost twice the RDA.[29] This observation that a protein intake of approximately four times the RDA, in combination with weight training, can promote greater muscle size gains than the same training with a diet containing what is considered by many to be more than adequate protein, is in tune with what many bodybuilders and other weight training athletes believe.

In another study, the effects of two levels of protein intake (1.5 g/kg/day or 2.5 g/kg/day) on muscle performance and energy metabolism were studied in humans submitted to repeated daily sessions of prolonged exercise at moderate altitude.[30] The study showed that the higher level of protein intake greatly minimized the exercise-induced decrease in serum branched chain amino acids.

Thus the protein needs of athletes are substantially higher than those of sedentary subjects because of the oxidation of amino acids during exercise and gluconeogenesis, as well as the retention of nitrogen during periods of muscle building.[31] Intense muscular activity increases both protein catabolism and protein utilization as an energy source.[32] Therefore, a high-protein diet may decrease the catabolic effects of exercise by several means, including the use of dietary protein as an energy substrate, thus decreasing the catabolism of endogenous protein during exercise.

Athletes have for years maintained that a high-protein diet is essential for maximizing lean body mass. And even though there have been attempts to discourage it, the popularity of high-protein diets has not waned. Athletes seem to feel intuitively that they need higher levels of protein than the average sedentary person. This intuitive feeling is backed up by their claims of the ergogenic effects of high-protein diets. Are these effects simply psychological?

Not according to studies that have shown the anabolic effects of increased dietary protein intake. For example, in one study done in rats,[33] dietary energy had no identifiable influence on muscle growth. In contrast, increased dietary protein appeared to stimulate muscle growth *directly* by increasing muscle RNA content and inhibiting proteolysis, as well as increasing insulin and free T3 levels.

Supplements that may work through a placebo effect but have no intrinsic effects, although perhaps popular for a while, eventually fall by the wayside and are abandoned by the majority.

High-protein diets are used because they work. The use of protein supplements is also popular because of their effectiveness above and beyond a whole food high protein diet.

Although there has been some concern about the effects of a high-dietary protein intake on the kidney, there seems to be no basis for these concerns in healthy individuals.[34,35] In fact, some animal studies have pointed to a beneficial effect of high protein diets on kidney function.[36]

There has also been some concern about the adverse effects of high-protein diets on the serum lipid profile. However, it would seem that these concerns also have little basis in facts. In one study, a diet higher in lean animal protein, including beef, was found to result in more favorable HDL ("good" cholesterol) and LDL ("bad" cholesterol) levels.[37] The study involved ten moderately hypercholesterolemic subjects (six women, four men). They were randomly allocated to isocaloric high- or low-protein diets for four to five weeks, after which they switched over to the other. Protein provided either 23% or 11% of energy intake; carbohydrate provided 65% or 53%; and fats accounted for 24%. During the high-protein diet, mean fasting plasma total cholesterol, LDL and triglycerides were significantly lower, HDL was raised by 12%, and the ratio of LDL to HDL consistently decreased.

Intense muscular activity increases protein catabolism (breakdown) and protein use as an energy source. The less protein available, the less muscle one will be able to build. A high-protein diet protects the protein to be turned into muscle by, among other things, providing another energy source for use during exercise. The body will burn this protein instead of the protein inside the muscle cells.

In fact, studies have shown that the anabolic effects of intense training are increased by a high-protein diet. When intensity of effort is at its maximum and stimulates an adaptive, muscle-producing response, protein needs to accelerate to provide for that increased muscle mass. It is also well known that a high protein diet is necessary for anabolic steroids to have full effect.

Once a certain threshold of work intensity is crossed, dietary protein becomes essential in maximizing the anabolic effects of exercise. Exercise performed under that threshold, however, may have little anabolic effect and may not require increased protein. As a result, although serious athletes can benefit from increased protein, other athletes who do not undergo similar, rigorous training may not.

Whether you need to supplement your diet with extra protein depends on your goals. For those who do not have to worry about gaining some fat along with the muscle (traditionally athletes in sports without weight classes or those in the heavyweight classes in sports that do, where mass is an advantage — for example, in the shotput and in weightlifting), high-caloric diets will usually supply all the protein you need provided you include plenty of meat, fish, eggs, and dairy products. With the increased caloric intake and including high-quality protein foods, you will get extra protein at the dinner table without thinking about it.

Most athletes, however, need the economy of maximizing lean body mass and minimizing body fat. These athletes, both competitive and recreational, are on a moderate, or at times a low caloric intake. To increase their protein intake, they need to plan their diets carefully and in many cases use protein supplements because they cannot calorically afford to eat food in the volume necessary to get enough protein.

On average, I recommend a minimum of 1 g of high-quality protein per pound of bodyweight every day for any person involved in competitive or recreational sports who want to maximize lean body mass but does not wish to gain weight or have excessive muscle hypertrophy. This would apply to athletes who wish to stay in a certain competitive weight class or those involved in endurance events.

However for those athletes involved in strength events such as the Olympic field and sprint events, those in football or hockey, or weightlifters, powerlifters, and bodybuilders, I recommend between 1.2 to 1.6 g of high-quality protein per pound of total bodyweight. That means that if you weigh 200 lb and want to put on a maximum amount of muscle mass, you will have to take in as much as 320 g of protein daily. There are several competitive weightlifters, powerlifters and bodybuilders who take in 2 to 3 g of high quality protein per pound of bodyweight.

If you are trying to lose weight and/or body fat its important to keep your dietary protein levels high. That is because the body oxidizes more protein on a calorie deficient diet than it would in a diet that has adequate calories. The larger the body muscle mass, the more transamination of amino acids occurs to fulfill energy needs. Thus, for those wishing to lose weight but maintain or even increase lean body mass in specific skeletal muscles, at least 1.5 g of high quality protein per pound of bodyweight is needed. The reduction in calories needed to lose weight should be at the expense of the fats and carbohydrates, not protein.

7.3.5   Essential, Conditionally Essential, and Nonessential Amino Acids

The requirement for dietary protein consists of two components:

1. The requirement for the nutritionally essential amino acids (isoleucine, leucine, lysine, methionine, phenylalanine, threonine, tryptophan, and valine) under all conditions and for conditionally essential amino acids (arginine, cysteine, glutamine, glycine, histidine, proline, taurine and tyrosine) under specific physiological and pathological conditions.
2. The requirement for nonspecific nitrogen for the synthesis of the nutritionally dispensable amino acids (aspartic acid, asparagine, glutamic acid, alanine, serine) and other physiologically important nitrogen-containing compounds such as nucleic acids, creatine, and porphyrins.

With respect to the first component, it is usually accepted that the nutritive values of various food protein sources are to a large extent determined by the concentration and availability of the individual indispensable amino acids. Hence, the efficiency with which a given source of food protein is utilized in support of an adequate state of nutritional health depends on the physiological requirements for the indispensable amino acids and total nitrogen and on the concentration of specific amino acids in the source of interest.

7.3.5.1   Essential Amino Acids

Essential amino acids, also called indispensable amino acids, must be supplied in the diet either as free amino acids or as constituents of dietary proteins. By this criterion, the following eight amino acids are essential in man:

Table 7.2 Essential Amino Acids

**Isoleucine	Phenylalanine
**Leucine	Threonine
Lysine	Tryptophan
Methionine	**Valine

** Branched Chain Amino Acids—Leucine, Isoleucine, Valine

7.3.5.2   Conditionally Essential Amino Acids

Several amino acids are considered conditionally essential because they are rate-limiting for protein synthesis under certain conditions. Individual amino acids are often described as conditionally essential based on requirements for optimal growth and maintenance of positive nitrogen balance. In extreme circumstances, such as in the absence of certain nonessential amino acids from the diet and the presence of limited amounts of essential amino acids from which to synthesize the non essential amino acids, any of the amino acids might be considered conditionally essential, including arginine, citrulline, ornithine, proline, cysteine, tyrosine, histidine, taurine, etc.[38–42] However, only seven other amino acids can be considered essential under certain conditions.

The following amino acids can be considered to be conditionally essential (dispensable) based on the body's inability to synthesize them from other amino acids under certain conditions. By this criterion, the following seven amino acids are conditionally essential in man:

Table 7.3 Conditionally Essential Amino Acids

Arginine	Proline
Cysteine, Cystine	Taurine
Glutamine	Tyrosine
Histidine	

7.3.5.3 Nonessential or Dispensable Amino Acids

Dispensable amino acids, also called nonessential amino acids, can be synthesized by the body from other amino acids. The following eight amino acids can be considered nonessential in man based on the body's ability to synthesize them from other amino acids under almost all conditions, although as discussed above, there is likely no amino acid that is nonessential because limiting amounts of the precursors of these amino acids in a diet that does not contain adequate amounts of these amino acids will limit the body's ability to synthesize them.

Table 7.4 Nonessential Amino Acids

Alanine	Glutamic Acid
Asparagine	Glycine
Aspartic Acid	Serine
Citrulline	

7.4 EXERCISE AND PROTEIN METABOLISM

Exercise has profound effects on skeletal muscle. Skeletal muscle increases its contractile protein content, resulting in muscular hypertrophy as it successfully adapts to increasing work loads. Studies have shown that certain stimuli produce muscle hypertrophy.

In a review on the effects of exercise on protein turnover in man, Rennie et al. concluded the following:[43]

1. Exercise causes a substantial rise in amino acid catabolism.
2. Amino acids catabolized during exercise appear to become available through a fall in whole-body protein synthesis and a rise in whole-body protein breakdown.
3. After exercise, protein balance becomes positive through a rise in the rate of whole-body synthesis in excess of breakdown.
4. Studies of free 3-methylhistidine in muscle, plasma, and urine samples suggest that exercise decreases the fractional rate of myofibrillar protein breakdown, in contrast with the apparent rise in whole-body breakdown.

In contrast to exercise, most of the increased proteolysis during fasting is due to the degradation of myofibrillar proteins (contractile proteins) in skeletal muscle.[44,45]

Several studies have examined the influence of exercise on protein synthesis and protein degradation. In general, it seems that exercise suppresses protein synthesis and stimulates protein degradation in skeletal muscle proportional to the level of exertion. In one early study using rats, mild exercise decreased protein synthesis by 17%. More intense treadmill running reduced synthesis by 30%, and an exhaustive three hour run inhibited synthesis by 70%.[46]

Another study by the same author examined the effects of exhaustive running on protein degradation and found that exhaustive running stimulates protein degradation in skeletal muscle.[47] Other studies have also shown that exercise produces a catabolic condition. In one study looking at aerobic exercise in humans, six male subjects were exercised on a treadmill for 3.75 hours at 50% $\dot{V}O_{2\,max}$, and the rates of protein synthesis and degradation were measured.[48] During exercise there was a 14% decrease in protein synthesis and a 54% increase in the rate of degradation.

This study is one of the few studies to make measurements during recovery after exercise. The authors found that after exercise, protein synthesis increased above the initial resting levels while protein degradation decreased returning eventually to pre-exercise levels. Any gains in the recovery phase seem, therefore, to be due to increases in protein synthesis rather than to decreases in protein catabolism.

In another study, multiple amino acid tracers were used to further elucidate the changes in protein synthesis and degradation that occur during prolonged, aerobic exercise.[49,50] Male subjects exercised on a bicycle ergometer at 30% $\dot{V}O_{2\,max}$ for 105 minutes. The results of the study showed that although exercise inhibited protein synthesis, the degree of inhibition varied depending on the amino acid tracer used. For example, the authors found decreases in protein synthesis of 48% using labeled leucine and 17% using lysine. With the relatively light work loads used in these studies, there were no changes in protein degradation or increases in urea production.

Even though the acute effect of exercise on protein turnover is catabolic, the long-term effects are an overall increase in protein synthesis and lean body mass. Routine exercise produces maintenance or hypertrophy of muscle mass. Few studies have looked at the post-exercise recovery of protein turnover. The above report and a later report by Devlin et al.[51] suggest that recovery occurs through stimulation of protein synthesis.

Preliminary studies reported in the second edition of *Nutrition in Exercise and Sport* provide additional support for this recovery pattern.[52] The authors found that after a two-hour bout of running on a motor-driven treadmill at 26 m per minute, protein synthesis in the gastrocnemius muscle was suppressed by 26 to 30% in fasted male rats. Recovery of protein synthesis occurred during the next 4 to 8 hours even if the animals were withheld from eating. These data suggest that muscles have a very high capacity for recovery even during conditions of food restriction. Thus, exercise training and food intakes before and after exercise are likely to be important to the effects of exercise on muscle protein synthesis and on subsequent recovery.

Just what factors control protein synthesis during exercise remain largely unknown, although some general trends and associations have been recognized. For example, high-intensity, exhaustive bouts of exercise produce a transient catabolic effect on protein synthesis. This effect is controlled presumably at the translation level of protein synthesis. Transcription is depressed but RNA concentrations are unchanged during the relatively brief period of the exercise bout. At the level of translation, potential regulatory controls include 1) availability of substrates, 2) hormones, 3) energy states, and 4) initiation factors.[27]

7.4.1 Exercise Induced Amino Acid Flux

The changes that occur in the BCAAs, alanine and glutamine in the liver, plasma, and muscle during exercise suggest that individual amino acids may be limiting as substrates for protein synthesis. And that they may be an important source of energy for various tissues and organs in the body. In general, decreases in protein synthesis and increases in protein degradation produce a net release of amino acids into the intracellular free pool, which may or may not be reflected by increased plasma levels.

Exercise is accompanied by changes in anabolic and catabolic hormones. It would appear that the molecular mechanism for the action of these hormones on translation remains equivocal, but most evidence points to changes in the initiation phase of translation. The next chapter examines the hormonal response to exercise.

The availability of energy may also limit muscle protein synthesis. Studies have found that decreases in protein synthesis that occur in proportion to the number of contractions induced by electrical stimulation were in proportion to the decline in the level of ATP in muscle cells.[53]

7.4.2   The Timing of Nutrient and Protein Intake in Relation to Exercise

Nutrient intake, protein intake, and the use of individual amino acids and certain combinations of amino acids in and around exercise have specific physiological and pharmacological effects that can increase muscle glycogen storage, protein synthesis and the anabolic effects of exercise.

One study compared carbohydrate, protein, and carbohydrate-protein supplements to determine their effects on muscle glycogen storage during recovery from prolonged exhaustive exercise and on protein synthesis.[54] Nine male subjects cycled for two hours on three separate occasions to deplete their muscle glycogen stores. Immediately and two hours after each exercise bout, they ingested 112.0 g carbohydrate (CHO), 40.7 g of whey protein (PRO), or 112.0 g carbohydrate and 40.7 g protein (CHO-PRO). Blood samples were drawn before exercise, immediately after exercise, and throughout recovery. Muscle biopsies were taken from the vastus laterals immediately and four hours after exercise.

Interestingly enough during recovery the plasma glucose response of the CHO treatment was significantly greater than that of the CHO-PRO treatment, but the plasma insulin response of the CHO-PRO treatment was significantly greater than that of the CHO treatment. Both the CHO and CHO-PRO treatments produced plasma glucose and insulin responses that were greater than those produced by the PRO treatment. The results of the study suggest that post-exercise protein and carbohydrate supplementation increases muscle glycogen storage and enhances protein synthesis likely secondary to the interaction of carbohydrate and protein on insulin secretion.

It would appear that the post-exercise intake of carbohydrates and protein is important to maximize protein synthesis. In an as yet unpublished study, post-exercise net skeletal muscle protein balance, normally negative without nutrient supplementation, was increased by the provision of amino acids and glucose.[55] The authors of the study state that earlier nutrient administration may be more effective to increase skeletal muscle protein synthesis during recovery compared with a later administration. Although the mechanisms for these effects are not entirely clear, increased insulin responsiveness earlier in the recovery period may be involved.

In another unpublished study, six normal untrained men were studied during the intravenous infusion of a balanced amino acid mixture at rest and after a leg resistance exercise routine to test the influence of exercise on the regulation of muscle protein kinetics by hyperaminoacidemia.[56] Leg muscle protein kinetics and transport of selected amino acids (alanine, phenylalanine, leucine, and lysine) were isotopically determined using a model based on arteriovenous blood samples and muscle biopsy.

The intravenous amino acid infusion resulted in comparable increases in arterial amino acid concentrations at rest and after exercise, whereas leg blood flow was greater after exercise than at rest. During hyperaminoacidemia, the increases in amino acid transport above basal were 30% to 100% greater after exercise than at rest. Increases in muscle protein synthesis were also greater after exercise than at rest.

Muscle protein breakdown was not significantly affected by hyperaminoacidemia either at rest or after exercise. The authors concluded that the stimulatory effect of exogenous amino acids on muscle protein synthesis is enhanced by prior exercise, perhaps in part due to enhanced blood flow. The results imply that protein intake immediately after exercise may be more anabolic than when ingested at some later time.

And yet another recent study looked at the effect of the timing of glucose supplementation upon fractional muscle protein synthetic rate (FSR), urinary urea excretion, and whole body and myofibrillar protein degradation (WBPD and MPD, respectively) following resistance exercise.[57] Eight healthy males performed unilateral knee extensor exercise (8 sets /10 reps/85% 1RM). They received a carbohydrate (CHO) supplement (1g/kg) or placebo (PL) immediately (t = 0h) and 1 h (t = + 1h) post-exercise. The results suggests that CHO supplementation (1g/kg) immediately and 1 hour following resistance exercise can decrease myofibrillar protein breakdown and urinary urea excretion, resulting in a more positive body protein balance.

A later study by the same research group showed that both carbohydrate and protein carbohydrate and fat nutritional supplements can increase glycogen resynthesis in both men and women.[58]

A study published this year examined the association of the mRNA cap binding protein eIF4E with the translational inhibitor 4E-BP1 in the acute modulation of skeletal muscle protein synthesis during recovery from exercise.[59] In this study, fasting male rats were run on a treadmill for two hours at 26 m/min and were realimented immediately after exercise with either saline, a carbohydrate-only meal, or a nutritionally complete meal (54.5% carbohydrate, 14% protein, and 31.5% fat). Exercised animals and nonexercised controls were studied one hour after exercise. Muscle protein synthesis decreased 26% after exercise and was associated with a fourfold increase in the amount of eIF4E present in the inactive eIF4E.4E-BP1 complex and a concomitant 71% decrease in the association of eIF4E with eIF4G.

Refeeding the complete meal, but not the carbohydrate meal, increased muscle protein synthesis equal to controls, despite similar plasma concentrations of insulin. Additionally, eIF4E.4E-BP1 association was inversely related, and eIF4E.eIF4G association was positively correlated to muscle protein synthesis. This study demonstrates that recovery of muscle protein synthesis after exercise is related to the availability of eIF4E for 48S ribosomal complex formation, and postexercise meal composition influences recovery via modulation of translation initiation.

It seems, therefore, from looking at the above studies that taking a combination of carbohydrate, protein, and some fat right after exercise is the best way to reverse the decreased protein synthesis seen with exercise and to replenish muscle glycogen and increase protein synthesis and decrease protein catabolism post exercise.

7.5 PROTEIN AND AMINO ACID SUPPLEMENTS

7.5.1   Protein Foods vs. Protein and Amino Acid Supplements

The source of dietary protein can be from whole foods, especially eggs, meat, fish, soy and dairy products; whole protein supplements that usually are inexpensive and contain one or more of soybean, milk and egg protein; hydrolyzed protein containing variable amounts of di-, tri- and polypeptides; and amino acid mixtures.

The usual consensus is that there are no valid scientific or medical studies to show that supplements of intact protein have an anabolic advantage over high-quality protein foods. The advantages usually cited for the use of whole protein supplements include the following:

1. Convenience of preparation and storage, and long shelf life.
2. Replacement of dietary protein for those wishing to decrease dietary fat.
3. Ability to raise protein intake by those who wish to minimize caloric intake.
4. Increasing dietary protein by those who cannot eat the volume of food necessary to insure adequate or increased protein intake.
5. In some cases, the cost of protein supplements is lower than corresponding high protein foods.

Although these are valid points, protein supplements have other distinct advantages over whole food protein in hypocaloric, isocaloric, and hypercaloric diets.

For example, several studies involving Refit (a milk powder containing about 90% proteins and 5% mineral salts—Ca, P, K, Na) have shown the ergogenic effects of this protein supplement.[60,61] In one study, nine male and eight female top Olympic athletes were given 1.2 to 1.5 g of milk protein daily, per kg of body weight, during a period of six months.[62] The milk proteins were consumed in addition to 2.2 to 2.5 of proteins per kg body weight in their diet. A control group with the same number of athletes and the same sports was fed on the same diet but without extra addition of milk protein.

The effects of the addition of extra milk proteins were monitored by estimating some parameters such as lean body mass, fat mass, muscle strength, protein and lipid composition in the blood serum, calcium metabolism, urinary mucoproteins, liver and kidney functional tests. All the athletes had been under medical supervision during the experiment and no side effects were registered. The results indicated that extra milk proteins significantly improved physiological condition and led to better sports performance, even when compared with the controls.

In another study, 66 Romanian Olympic endurance athletes (30 kayak-canoe, 36 rowing; 45 males and 21 females) participated in a trial to determine the possible biological effects of an isolated soy protein supplement given at 1.5 g/kg/day, for eight weeks.[63] A control group was used that did not receive the supplemental protein. The soy protein supplementation resulted in significant increases of lean body mass and strength. The same author also found significant effects from the use of a combination vitamin supplement compound that contained amino acids.[64]

A recent study examined the effects of food supplements designed to foster muscular gains when combined with weight training.[65] The study included 28 weight-training subjects who took any of three supplements daily: 190 g of maltodextrin, a carbohydrate source that acted as a source of calories only (about 760 calories); Gainer's Fuel 1000, a weight-gain powder that provides both calories and protein (just over 1400 calories and 60 g of protein per day); and Phosphagain, a powder advertised to help increase muscle gains without gaining excess bodyfat, providing fewer calories and more protein in the form of whole food protein and high levels of creatine monohydrate and of certain amino acids such as glutamine and taurine (about 600 calories and 80 grams of whole food protein and amino acids per day).

Results showed that those on either Phosphagain and Gainer's Fuel gained more lean mass compared with those who consumed maltodextrin, showing that increasing dietary protein and other nutrients resulted in a superior gain in muscle as compared to those who simply took in the equivalent amount of calories. In addition, those on Phosphagain gained more lean body mass and less fat than those on Gainer's Fuel. Why the difference?

Phosphagain contains nutrients not found in the Gainer's Fuel product. These nutrients include creatine monohydrate, taurine, and L-glutamine. These three nutrients may have, along with the differences in the macronutrients, made the difference. Besides having more protein (due mainly to the large amounts of taurine and glutamine), Phosphagain also had a much lower carbohydrate content — 69 g vs. 290 g per daily serving. Both had low levels of fat. The increased carbohydrate and subsequent calorie content is likely responsible in the increased fat gain seen with Gainer's Fuel, a problem that is also seen when whole foods are used to increase protein intake and other nutrients.

Gainer's Fuel, Phosphagain, and others such as Met-Rx and Hot Stuff contain many nutrients and can be used as meal replacements or as a source of extra nutrients beyond the three square meals a day. Some of these products are advertised as weight gainers, while others are more specific and claim to be lean body mass weight gainers. Although the difference in products may not be as extreme as the advertiser's claim, there is some validity to the differentiation of the two product types and their effect on fat accretion and gains in lean body mass.

The meal-replacement products, whether for weight loss of for weight gain, provide the standard macro and micronutrients at different calorie levels. They may be convenient and either more or less costly than whole foods, but as an all-in-one package they are usually more convenient and provide better nutrition than many people get with junk food meals and calorie-full but nutrient-deficient snacks. But on the whole, if you are conscientious about what you buy and eat and willing to put in the time and energy, you can do as well or better by buying the whole foods and planning your own diet for weight gain or weight loss.

However, some of the newer complete nutrient supplements, such as Met-Rx and Myoplex Plus, definitely have an edge over even the most meticulously prepared diets. To get pharmacological levels of some of the nutrients present in these products, one would have to consume an unrealistic amount of certain foods, resulting in a much larger than desired calorie intake and increase in body fat.

7.5.2 Amino Acids

Athletes' use of commercial amino acid supplements has increased dramatically in the past decade. Although a certain amount of research has been done to determine the amount of dietary protein needed by strength and endurance athletes (see above), less is known about how the quality of protein or specific amino acid supplements affects metabolic and physiological responses to strength and endurance training.

Amino acids serve two rather different functions. Dietary amino acids are metabolized many ways and are used to replenish the free amino acid pools in tissues and plasma. Oxidative losses of free amino acids occur both during and after feeding. The oxidative losses occur during feeding because they are consumed at a rate that is usually in excess of the rate in which net protein synthesis can occur so that oxidation occurs as part of the process of maintaining the relatively small but important tissue-free amino acid pools. Any excess amino acids, that is above the amounts needed for immediate protein synthesis and replenishment of the free amino acid pool, are oxidized, transformed, or metabolized and stored as glycogen or fat.

Amino acids also exert an important regulatory influence on growth, development, and protein turnover through their activation of various hormonal and metabolic responses. This effect is primarily aimed at the stimulation of growth but also includes the stimulation of oxidative losses. These anabolic influences may be exerted for short periods after feeding and/or under the influence of specific hormones. With the manipulation of diet and of the hormonal milieu, the anabolic influences can be prolonged.

7.5.2.1 Physiological and Pharmacological Actions of Amino Acids

Amino acids are the building blocks of body proteins. They include structural and contractile proteins, enzymes, and certain hormones and neurotransmitters. They also function in many other metabolic activities, are used as substrates for energy production, are involved in immune function — ammonia detoxification, the synthesis of nucleic acids — and also function as antioxidants. Amino acids, either free form or in the form of small peptides, are potent physiological and pharmacological agents.

For example, amino acid availability rapidly regulates protein synthesis and degradation. In one recent study, endogenous leucine flux, reflecting proteolysis, decreased while leucine oxidation increased in protocols where amino acids were infused.[66] Nonoxidative leucine flux reflecting protein synthesis was also stimulated by amino acids.

Increasing amino acid concentrations stimulates protein synthesis in a dose-dependent manner at the level of mRNA translation-initiation and inhibits protein degradation by inhibiting lysosomal autophagy. Supplying energy alone (i.e., carbohydrate and lipids) cannot prevent negative nitrogen balance (net protein catabolism) in animals or humans; only the provision of certain amino acids allows the attainment of nitrogen balance.[67]

Certain neurotransmitters (i.e., acetylcholine, catecholamines, and serotonin) are formed from dietary constituents (i.e., choline, tyrosine, and tryptophan). Changing the consumption of these precursors alters release of their respective neurotransmitter products. Also, many amino acids have been shown to act as CNS neurotransmitters.[68–84]

Acute dietary indispensable amino acid deficiency may increase vulnerability to seizures by repeated activation of the anterior piriform cortex of the brain.[85]

Glutamine[86] and taurine[87] have hepatoprotective and antihepatotoxic effects.

Several amino acids, such as cysteine (decreases cross linkage of proteins) and histidine[88] ha significant antioxidant effects.

Several amino acids, including the essential BCAAs, especially leucine, are used directly as oxidizable fuels during exercise. Depending on the duration and intensity of exercise and other factors such as glycogen stores and energy intake, amino acids can provide from a few to approximately 10% of the total energy for sustained exercise.[89]

Arginine, glycine, and methionine are amino acids that are required for the hepatic synthesis of creatine. Creatine is taken up by skeletal muscle, where it is phosphorylated to form phosphocreatine (PC), a high-energy phosphate compound and an important energy source for cellular energy and muscular contraction.

Lysine has been shown useful for treating herpes infections in some patients, although there is considerable controversy on its effectiveness, perhaps because other factors, such as dietary intake, have not been taken into account.[90]

Cysteine, a precursor for reduced glutathione, may be of some use in reducing hepatotoxicity secondary to drugs (such as alcohol and anabolic steroids) and infections.[91,92]

Studies have shown that muscle wasting post-operatively can be countered by the use of enteral or parenteral glutamine, alpha-ketoglutarate and the BCAAs.

Intravenous or oral feedings rich in branched-chain amino acids are said to improve nutrition in chronic liver disease and to exert anticatabolic effects on protein degradation, thus sparing muscle protein.[93]

All amino acids have the capacity to accept or release hydrogen ions. Only glutamate, aspartate, histidine, and perhaps arginine serve as buffers with respect to regulation of hydrogen ions in the body. Glutamine is especially important as a buffer in the kidney.

Studies have shown a dose-related suppression of food intake by phenylalanine and an anorexic effect of aspartame.[94]

Some of the amino acids may also be effective for the treatment and prevention of certain diseases. For example, a study in rabbits has shown that L-arginine, the precursor of endothelium-derived relaxing factor (EDRF), decreases atherosclerosis in hypercholesterolemic animals.[95]

It has even been shown that certain amino acids may have protective effects on lactational performance against toxic compounds.[96] In this study, glycine, which increases growth hormone release, and tryptophan, which enhances and mimics prolactin secretion negate the harmful effects of 7,12-dimethylbenzanthracene by stimulating mammary gland growth and secretion.

Apart from acting as a protein supplement, amino acids alone or in various combinations can have specific and different pharmacological and physiological effects, including effects on immunomodulation, neurotransmitters, hormones, control of protein turnover, renal function, and maintenance of gut trophicity.[97] Certain amino acids exert pharmacological effects similar to hormones and drugs. Thus amino acids (and their metabolites and analogues) can transcend their roles of being just the building blocks of protein and can regulate protein synthesis by acting as anabolic and anticatabolic agents and affecting hormonal functions.

For example, in one study examining the effects of certain amino acid groups on renal hemodynamics, glomerular filtration rate and renal plasma flow were increased by infusion of mixed gluconeogenic amino acids (arginine, glycine, proline, cysteine, methionine, serine) but not by either alanine, another gluconeogenic amino acid, or the BCAAs.[98]

In another study, synthesis and degradation of globular and myofibrillar proteins across arm and leg muscles were examined during stepwise increased intravenous infusion of amino acids (0.1, 0.2, 0.4, and 0.8 g of nitrogen/kg/day) to healthy volunteers.[99] Protein dynamics were measured by a primed constant infusion of L-phenylalanine and the release of 3-methylhistidine from skeletal muscles. Amino acid infusion caused a significant uptake of the majority of amino acids across arm and leg tissues, except tyrosine, tryptophan, and cysteine, probably due to low concentrations of these amino acids in the formulation. The balance of globular proteins improved significantly due to stimulation of synthesis and attenuation of degradation across arm and leg tissues, despite significant uptake of tyrosine, tryptophan, and cysteine. Degradation of myofibrillar proteins was influenced by provision of amino acids.

Arterial concentrations and flux of glucose, lactate and free fatty acids were unchanged despite increasing concentrations of plasma amino acids from 2.6 to 5.8 mM. Plasma insulin, IGF-I and plasma concentrations of IGF-I binding proteins-1 and 3 remained at fasting levels throughout the investigation. The results of this study demonstrate that neither insulin nor circulating IGF-I explained improved protein balance in skeletal muscles following elevation of plasma amino acids. *Rather, some amino acids trigger cellular reactions that initiate peptide formation.* In this study, the limited availability of some extracellular amino acids was overcome by increased reutilization of the intracellular amino acid.

There is evidence that specific amino acids play a role in the etiology of fatigue and the overtraining syndrome in athletes because of their flux during exercise causes a change in certain metabolic kinetics. The metabolism of BCAAs, glutamine and tryptophan, may be the key to understanding some aspects of central fatigue and some aspects of immunosuppression that are very relevant to athletic endeavor.[100]

Complex amino acid mixtures do not give the same pharmacological effects as the use of individual or combinations of a few or more select amino acids. In the case of the effects on the central nervous system (CNS) (in regulating hypothalamic and pituitary function, and in affecting the level of certain neurotransmitters), the reason is partly due to the nature of the transport mechanism that carries the amino acids across the blood brain barrier into the specific CNS neurons.

The large neutral amino acids (LNAA) such as tryptophan, tyrosine, the BCAAs (valine, leucine, isoleucine), phenylalanine and methionine, compete with one another for the same available transport molecules. Thus the presence in plasma of several of these amino acids in any significant amounts results in a decrease in the amounts of each amino acid that is transported into the body and the CNS.[101] On the other hand, if only one or a small number of specific amino acids were ingested, then serum levels of these acids would rise appreciably over the serum levels of the other amino acids so that more of the ingested amino acids would enter the CNS.

It follows that individual or selectively combined amino acids should be taken on an empty stomach by themselves. If taken with food, the amino acids derived from natural sources compete with any individual or combination of specific amino acids, diluting their physiological and pharmacological effects.

7.5.2.2 *The Branched Chain Amino Acids: Isoleucine, Leucine, and Valine*

The branched-chain amino acids (BCAAs) are named because they have a carbon chain that deviates or branches from the main linear carbon backbone.

The BCAAs isoleucine, leucine, and valine have been investigated for their anticatabolic and anabolic effects. In heart and skeletal muscle *in vitro*, increasing the concentration of the three BCAAs or of leucine alone reproduces the effects of increasing the supply of all amino acids in stimulating protein synthesis and inhibiting protein degradation.[102]

Several studies have indicated that leucine is an *in vivo* regulator of protein metabolism by decreasing protein degradation and increasing protein synthesis. In one study, leucine infusion decreased plasma concentrations of several amino acids.[103] The authors concluded that leucine decreases protein degradation in humans and that this decreased protein degradation during leucine infusion contributes to the decrease in plasma essential amino acids.

In another study, excessive intake of a single BCAA led rapidly to elevated plasma concentration of both the amino acid administered and its corresponding alpha-keto acid. And if the rats had previously been fed a low-protein diet, it led to an increase in liver branched-chain alpha-keto acid dehydrogenase activity.[104] Leucine caused decreased plasma isoleucine, valine, alpha-keto-beta-methylvaleric acid, and alpha-keto isovaleric acid concentrations. These decreases were not caused by increased degradation of these metabolites to carbon dioxide, because branched-chain amino acid oxidation rates *in vivo* were unchanged by leucine loading and the degradative enzymes were unchanged in adequately fed rats. The authors suggest that the decreased concentrations of these amino and keto acids may be the result of decreased protein degradation or increased protein synthesis, possibly mediated by insulin.

Another study still to be published investigated the mechanisms of protein gain during protein feeding using a combination of oral and intravenous labeled leucine in healthy young men.[105] The oral labeled leucine was administered either as a free oral tracer (13C- or 2H3-leucine) added to unlabeled whey protein or as whey protein intrinsically labeled with L-[1-13C] leucine. When the oral tracer was free leucine, it appeared in the plasma more rapidly than the unlabeled leucine derived from the whey protein, and this resulted in an artifactual 88% decrease of protein breakdown. When the oral tracer was protein bound, protein breakdown did not change significantly after the meal. By contrast, non-oxidative leucine disposal (i.e., protein synthesis) was stimulated by 63% by the meal.

The authors concluded the following:

1. An intrinsically labeled protein is more appropriate than an oral free tracer to study post-prandial leucine kinetics under non-steady state conditions.
2. Protein gain after a single whey protein meal solely results from an increased protein synthesis with no modification of protein breakdown.

Louard et al. examined the effects of infused BCAAs on whole-body and skeletal muscle amino acid kinetics in ten post-absorptive normal subjects.[106] Ten control subjects received only saline. Infusion of BCAAs caused a fourfold rise in arterial BCAA levels and a twofold rise in BCAA keto acids. Plasma insulin levels were unchanged from basal levels. Their results implied that BCAA infusion results in a suppression of whole-body and forearm muscle proteolysis. Because insulin levels were unaffected by the infusion of BCAAs, the observed alterations in muscle and whole-body amino acid kinetics appear to be independent of insulin and are probably mediated by the elevated BCAA concentrations.

A recent study looked at the effects of long-term BCAA administration on metabolic and respiratory parameters.[107] The authors concluded that the physical fitness of BCAA-treated subjects was improved and that BCAAs seemed to promote protein synthesis in the fat-free body mass.

Leucine has also been shown to increase the release of acetoacetate and 3-hydroxybutyrate (as a result of the partial oxidation of leucine).[108] The ketone bodies, beta-hydroxybutyrate and acetoacetate, are known to be a useful source of energy and show a glucose-sparing effect.[109] It has been shown experimentally that oral or parenteral intake of beta-hydroxybutarate decreases the amount of protein catabolized in obese people on starvation diets.[110] Both Alpha-Ketoisocaproate (KIC) and Beta-Hydroxy-Beta-Methylbutyrate (HMB) (see below) also seem to have some ketone-like anticatabolic effects.

In a review of the metabolic effects of ketone bodies the authors concluded the following:[111]

1. The ketone bodies, D-beta-hydroxybutyrate and acetoacetate, inhibit glycolysis, thereby reducing pyruvate availability, which leads to a marked inhibition of branched-chain amino acid metabolism and alanine synthesis in skeletal muscles from fasted mammalian and avian species.
2. The rate of glutamine release from skeletal muscles from fasted birds is increased at the expense of alanine in the presence of elevated concentrations of ketone bodies because of an increase in the availability of glutamate for glutamine synthesis.
3. Ketone bodies inhibit both protein synthesis and protein degradation in skeletal muscles from fasted mammalian and avian species *in vitro*. The mechanisms involved remain unknown.
4. Inhibition of amino acid metabolism and protein turnover in skeletal muscle by ketone bodies may be an important survival mechanism during adaptation to catabolic states such as prolonged fasting.

Alvestrand et al.[112] found leucine to decrease the net degradation of muscle protein even in normal resting subjects, something Blomstrand and Newsholme[113] suggested might aid repair and recovery and be of importance for athletes doing regular physical training. Alvestrand found that approximately 40% of the leucine taken up by muscle was accumulated in the intracellular free pool, some 20% could have been incorporated into protein and 40% was probably oxidized.

Studies using BCAAs have found these acids to have a beneficial effect on the synthesis of proteins under special circumstances. For example, one study showed that BCAAs have a specific effect on the synthesis of plasma proteins by cultured hepatocytes.[114] Another study found a positive benefit from BCAAs as the protein component of total parenteral nutrition in cancer cachexia.[115]

On the other hand, the role of the BCAAs in protein synthesis is not completely clear. Current concepts for explaining the effects of BCAAs on protein turnover in skeletal muscle are based on the assumption that the BCAA or leucine alone might become rate-limiting for protein synthesis in muscle under catabolic conditions. However, in one study using suckling rats, the use of the leucine analogue norleucine was found to stimulate protein synthesis even though norleucine cannot replace any of the BCAA in protein.[116]

Several amino acids show changes in intracellular and extracellular concentrations in response to exercise, suggesting that skeletal protein and amino acid catabolism, and gluconeogenesis is increased by exercise.[117] The BCAAs (leucine, isoleucine, valine) are specifically utilized by muscle metabolism, although some evidence indicates their use by other organ tissues.[118]

Leucine and other BCAAs, unlike most other amino acids, are oxidized (used as energy) by muscle cells and are a source of cellular energy in the form of ATP and PC. They are also involved in the glucose-alanine cycle (see section on alanine). There is a significant activation of BCAA metabolism with prolonged exercise, and current studies indicate that this is more pronounced in endurance-trained subjects than in untrained controls.[119]

Plasma concentrations of the BCAAs (leucine, isoleucine, and valine) are more prominently affected than the concentrations of other amino acids by changes in dietary-caloric, protein, fat, and carbohydrate-intake in man.[120]

BCAA administration before exercise affects the response of some anabolic hormones, mainly growth hormone, insulin and testosterone.[121] A study conducted by Carli et al.[122] examined the effects of BCAA administration on the hormonal response in male marathon runners to a one-hour running test at constant speed.

In this study using 14 male long-distance runners, two trials were carried out at one-week intervals. In each trial, athletes ran one hour at a predetermined speed. In the first trial (E), the athletes were given a commercial diet product containing BCAAs (5.14 g leucine, 2.57 g isoleucine, 2.57 g valine), milk proteins (12 g), fructose (20 g), other carbohydrates (8.8 g), and fats (1.08 g), the total energy content being 216 kcal. In the second trial (P), the athletes received a similar mixture with the same energy content but without BCAAs, which were replaced by additional milk proteins (10 g). In both trials, the mixture was taken approximately 90 minutes before the running test.

The BCAA mixture ingested by the athletes in the E trial elicited, in resting conditions, a sustained elevation in plasma BCAA levels, which lasted several hours. In the whole milk protein without the BCAAs trial, there was a decrease in serum free testosterone (as measured by the decreased testosterone:SHBG ratio) and sex hormone binding globulin (SHBG). This was thought to have been an indication of increased metabolic clearance of testosterone.

In the E trial, testosterone was unchanged at the end of the exercise period, and it increased in the following rest period. The authors concluded, "We would suggest that exogenous administration of BCAAs and their uptake by muscle fibers could limit endogenous amino acid oxidation and indirectly prevent testosterone muscle clearance. This suggestion is also supported by the direct anabolic effect of BCAAs, mainly leucine, on muscle proteins."[123] The authors suggest that BCAAs may be rate-limiting for muscle protein synthesis.

An anticatabolic effect of BCAA administration was also indicated by the values of the testosterone:cortisol ratio, an indicator of changes in the anabolic-androgenic activity of the body,[124] in the last sample.

The study showed that the hormone response to exercise was modified by BCAA ingestion and that the anabolic hormones insulin and especially testosterone were favorably affected when BCAAs were substituted for equivalent amounts of whole milk proteins. These findings are extremely important and point out the advantages of BCAA supplementation over the use of whole food proteins and even whole food protein supplements.

Of the BCAAs, leucine appears to be the most important for athletes. Leucine affects various anabolic hormones and has anabolic and anticatabolic effects. It is also involved in nitrogen metabolism and ammonia removal. A study last year found that leucine infusion depressed muscle proteolysis.[125] The use of large amounts of leucine and not valine and isoleucine, while decreasing the serum levels of valine and isoleucine, does not adversely affect the rate of protein synthesis.[126]

In another, study the plasma and muscle concentrations of tyrosine, phenylalanine, and BCAAs were measured before and after two types of sustained intense exercise during which the subjects were given a mixture of BCAAs or a placebo.[127] An increase in the muscle concentration of tyrosine and/or phenylalanine could be an indication of net protein degradation in skeletal muscle because these amino acids are neither taken up nor metabolized by this tissue. The investigation comprised two separate studies, both involving male subjects.

In one aspect of the study, 26 subjects participated in a 30-km cross-country race. In a second aspect, 32 subjects participated in a full-length marathon race (42.2 km). All subjects were well-trained. In both races, the subjects were randomly divided into two groups. One group, the test group, was given a drink containing a mixture of BCAAs in a 5% (cross-country) or 6% (marathon) carbohydrate solution. The other group (placebo) was given 5% and 6% carbohydrate solutions in the cross-country and marathon races, respectively. The total amount of BCAAs given to each subject in the cross-country race was 7.5 g (2.6 g leucine, 3.8 g valine, 1.1 g isoleucine) and in the marathon race 12 g (4.2 g leucine, 4.8 g valine, 3.0 g isoleucine).

The results of the study showed that an intake of the BCAA mixture prevented an exercise-induced increase in the muscle concentration of tyrosine and phenylalanine which was found in the placebo groups. This, the authors remarked, might indicate an inhibitory effect of BCAAs on the net rate of protein degradation in the working muscles during exercise. Furthermore, they added "… a decreased net rate of protein degradation during exercise might improve physical performance and would probably aid repair and recovery after such intense exertion. Hence, this finding could be of some importance for athletes doing regular physical training."

The authors suggest that the intake of BCAAs during exercise might decrease protein degradation that occurs in human skeletal muscle during that exercise.

The intake of BCAAs during exercise might also alleviate some of the fatigue seen in prolonged exercise. Plasma levels of free tryptophan have been shown to increase during exercise and the levels of BCAAs to decrease. Thus the ratio of free tryptophan to BCAAs increases markedly with some forms of exercise. It is thought that this increased ratio may lead to an increase in the transport of tryptophan across the blood-brain barrier and hence to an increase in the synthesis of 5-hydroxytryptophan (5-HT or serotonin) in specific areas of the brain and thus may be responsible for the development of some of the physical/mental fatigue seen during prolonged exercise.[128]

There are several compounds that potentially may have more of an anticatabolic and anabolic effect than the BCAA but at present are not generally commercially available. For example, one study on amino acid metabolism with exercise[129] found that plasma concentration of glutamine, the branched-chain keto acids (BCKA) and short-chain acyl carnitines were elevated with exercise. Utilization of these compounds may spare muscle glutamine and BCAAs and thus may have a greater muscle-sparing effect than any other amino acid combination.

The significance of the serum changes of amino acids with exercise has not been fully explored. Serum amino acid levels can change for many reasons. For example, increases in the serum level of any amino acid could be due to decreased use, increased release, or increased formation of that amino acid and might be associated with increased use of that amino acid by other tissues. Thus in some instances of increased levels of an amino acid, such as glutamine, supplementation of that amino acid might be necessary to decrease protein catabolism and increase protein synthesis. In other instances, increased levels of an amino acid might simply show decreased use of that amino acid and supplementation would not be of any value.

In one study, the quantitative relationship between insulin and plasma amino acid levels were characterized in five healthy young men during several euglycemic insulin infusions.[130] While eight of ten amino acids measured decreases in a dose-responsive pattern to increasing levels of insulin, alanine and glycine concentrations remained unaffected. In this instance, the use of exogenous alanine would not affect protein metabolism, whereas the use of some of the other amino acids, such as the BCAA, would be. Alanine supplementation (because it is a major gluconeogenic precursor) might be useful before and/or during exercise because alanine flux would increase as exercise time and intensity increased.

Effects of BCAA on Exercise Time and VAT — Several recent studies have shown the usefulness of BCAA. In one study the use of BCAAs prior to exercise significantly increased the exercising time to exhaustion in rats compared to placebo.[131] In a study of wrestlers wanting to lose weight, the use of BCAAs along with a restricted caloric intake resulted in a decrease in percent body fat and a significant reduction in abdominal visceral adipose tissue (VAT — the stuff that most pot bellies are made of) above those who dieted but who did not use the BCAAs. The authors concluded that the combination of moderate energy restriction and BCAA supplementation induced significant and preferential losses of VAT and allowed maintenance of a high level of performance.

Another recent study also shows that BCAAs also prolongs exercise during heat stress in both men and women.[132] This study was set up to assess the effect of BCAA supplementation on endurance performance in the heat. Six women and seven men participated in two trials of rest in the heat followed by 40% $\dot{V}O_{2\,peak}$ exercise to exhaustion. Subjects ingested 5-mL•kg-1 of a placebo (PLAC) or BCAAs drink every 30 minutes. Cycle time to exhaustion increased during BCAA for men and women. The results of this study indicate BCAA supplementation prolongs moderate exercise performance in the heat.

So, along with all the other indications, it makes sense to use supplemental BCAAs if you are going to be training in the heat, whether outdoors or in a gym that is not adequately air-conditioned. One of the best and easiest ways to supplement your diet is to use whey protein as one of the main protein sources for increasing your dietary protein. During training one might also take a BCAA break and take some BCAA-fortified drink. Depending on your preference, you can use a shake containing whey or some powder or capsules containing BCAAs along with some water.

Overall, it seems that BCAAs can positively affect athletic performance, protein metabolism and decrease body fat, especially VAT.

7.5.2.3 Glutamine

Glutamine, a neutral amino acid, is the most abundant amino acid in human muscle and plasma and is found in relatively high levels in many human tissues. Glutamine constitutes over 50% of the total amino acid pool, making it the most highly concentrated amino acid in the plasma. Whole blood concentration of glutamine is higher than any other amino acid concentration.[133] Eighty percent of the free amino acids of the body reside within the intracellular compartment of skeletal muscle cells, of this pool, glutamine constitutes over 60% of the total intramuscular amino acids.

Glutamine plays fundamental physiological roles as a precursor of hepatic ureagenesis and renal ammoniagenesis (see above); in the maintenance of the acid-base balance during acidosis, as a nitrogen precursor for the synthesis of nucleotides; as cellular fuel in certain tissues such as muscle, intestine, skin, and in the immune system; and as a direct regulator of protein synthesis and degradation.[134–138]

From a review of the extensive literature on glutamine it would appear that the release and utilization of glutamine is a response to physiological and pathological stressors. In respect to glutamine, it also seems that all forms of stress, including trauma, surgery, burns, infections, fasting, malnutrition and exercise, all deplete muscles of glutamine.[139–142] During catabolic stress, reductions up to 50% have been documented.[143]

This drop in glutamine occurs in spite of the effect of stress hormones in increasing the production of glutamine secondary to muscle catabolism and de novo synthesis. In these cases, the production of glutamine cannot keep up to the demand. Also, because of the use of other amino acids (especially BCAAs) to produce glutamine and the relative need for glutamine by other tissues, less glutamine and other amino acids are available for protein synthesis.

In times of stress, protein synthesis takes a back seat to other events that are more important in terms of survival. The use of glutamine by the gut and immune system takes precedence over protein synthesis. When the body is subjected to stress, although glutamine is the most depleted amino acid as well as the last one to be replenished, little of this glutamine serves for the synthesis of structural or contractile protein. The increase in glutamine turnover rate seen in these various conditions likely represents an adaptive mechanism to the stressor for preservation of immune and visceral function.

Glutamine concentrations decrease and tissue glutamine metabolism increases markedly in many catabolic, stressful disease states, and whole body exchange rates of glutamine can exceed the body's total stores of glutamine by several-fold each day. Under stressful conditions, there is a constant requirement for de novo synthesis of glutamine to match the rate of utilization. In healthy skeletal muscle, intracellular glutamine concentrations can reach more than 33 times the extracellular concentrations.[144] The maximal synthetic rate of glutamine in human skeletal muscle (about 50 mmol/h) has been shown to be higher than that of any other amino acid.[145]

Thus although nonessential under normal conditions,[146] the demand for glutamine can exceed its supply during periods of stress (e.g., intense exercise, sepsis, and conditions generating an acid load), hence its classification as a conditionally essential amino acid.[147] This position has been supported by recent studies that have shown trophic effects of glutamine-supplemented diets on the growth of specific tissues and on total body nitrogen balance.[148]

In summary, the reduction of skeletal muscle protein synthesis is associated with a decrease of muscle-free glutamine proportional to the muscle protein catabolism. Protein catabolic states are accompanied by an increased rate of glycolysis and subsequently to an increased non-oxidative disposal of pyruvate, derived alanine. This process reduces the availability of intracellular nitrogen for glutamine synthesis, thereby causing a depletion of the intracellular glutamine pool which in turn suppresses protein synthesis.

Glutamine supplementation may offer athletes many advantages. Overall, the use of exogenous glutamine would spare intramuscular glutamine and result in decreased proteolysis and potentially increased levels of muscle protein. Gastrointestinal and immune functions would be maximized and the morbidity secondary to overtraining would be improved. Glutamine can efficiently release growth hormone and perhaps up-regulate other anabolic hormones. All of these factors strongly suggest that glutamine supplementation may play a major role in enhancing the effects of resistance training.

Glutamine and Overtraining — Besides being so versatile, or perhaps because of that, a new study suggests that glutamine can be used as a marker of overtraining.[149] Although none of the other parameters (including serum hormone and cortisol levels) measured showed any significant changes during the training season, glutamine levels correlated with the degree of successful training (measured by improvements in performance). The elevations in plasma glutamine concentration observed in response to long-term balanced training in this study may be distinguishable from previous reports of decreased glutamine concentrations in overtrained athletes,[150] making it a potentially valuable tool in the monitoring of overtraining in athletes.

The other side of the coin, of course, is to see if the use of supplemental glutamine has a positive effect on both preventing and alleviating the overtraining syndrome. It would because glutamine not only increases protein synthesis and decreases protein breakdown, but it also has positive effects on the immune system, which in turn can affect various parameters of the overtraining syndrome. Also, glutamine has recently been shown to act both as a substrate and as a regulator of gluconeogenesis (the production of glucose from other substrates such as amino acids, glycerol and lactic acid).[151] This is important because it provides a vital supply of fuel for both muscles and other tissues, including the brain, and thus may improve muscle and cognitive function during training and help attenuate some aspects of overtraining.

The bottom line is that supplemental glutamine can have significant effects on many aspects of athletic performance.

7.5.2.4 Amino Acid Metabolites — HMB and KIC

Alpha-Ketoisocaproic Acid (KIC) — Alpha-Ketoisocaproate (KIC), the keto-acid of leucine — is clearly the most important BCKA. KIC is anabolic and anticatabolic, particularly during catabolic states. Because any intensive, strenuous activity is also catabolic, there is every reason to believe that the BCKAs will prove to be of value to bodybuilders, power lifters, and aerobic athletes.

Both leucine and KIC are metabolized further to alpha-amino-n-butyrate and beta-hydroxy-beta-methylbutyrate. These compounds have not as yet been investigated in humans for their anabolic and protein sparing properties. However, they may have some anabolic and anticatabolic effects.

Although KIC is the transamination product of the BCAA leucine, and both tend to increase in parallel in the serum when exogenous leucine is used,[152] there is substantial evidence that it has anabolic- and protein-sparing properties separate from leucine.[153,154] On the other hand, leucine has properties apart from its transamination to KIC.

In one study, the effects of leucine, its metabolites, and the 2-oxo acids of valine and isoleucine on protein synthesis and degradation in incubated limb muscles of immature and adult rats were investigated.[155] The results seemed to point to an anabolic and anticatabolic effect of leucine that was found to stimulate protein synthesis and reduce protein catabolism. However, the anticatabolic effects of leucine, in contrast to its anabolic effects, required its transamination to the 2-oxo acid, 4-methyl-2-oxopentanoate or KIC. Although the oxo acid of leucine was found to have significant effects, the 2-oxo acids of valine and isoleucine did not affect protein synthesis or degradation.

Interestingly, the authors of this 1984 study said the effect of KIC in preventing muscle degradation was likely due to the accumulation within cells of a metabolite of KIC (such as HMB). They also said it is KIC rather than leucine that reduced the catabolic process. Supplements containing KIC in pharmacological doses have been shown to decrease the rate of 3-methylhistidine excretion by patients with Duchenne's muscular dystrophy.[156] 3-Methylhistidine, which occurs only in the myofibrillar proteins, is often used as an indicator of contractile protein degradation.[157]

The results of these studies confirmed the results obtained from an earlier study that concluded that KIC showed anticatabolic but not anabolic effects,[158] that KIC reduced muscle catabolism but did not stimulate protein synthesis. Leucine, on the other hand, seemed to affect protein synthesis. Interestingly enough, the authors concluded that neither of the other two BCAAs (isoleucine and valine) promoted protein synthesis.

Perhaps one of the more important actions of KIC (and also leucine) is its enhancement of the anabolic drive via stimulation of insulin secretion. Both leucine[159] and KIC[159] (and other amino acid compounds such as arginine, ornithine, and OKG) stimulate insulin secretion. Insulin increases the intercellular transport of amino acids and has both anabolic and anticatabolic effects.

Beta-Hydroxy-Beta-Methylbutyrate (HMB) — One of the newest anabolic/anticatabolic supplements to hit the market is beta-hydroxy-beta-methylbutyrate (HMB), a leucine catabolite. The classical pathway of leucine metabolism involves conversion to alpha-ketoisocaproate, transport into the mitochondria, and oxidation to HMG-CoA, which can then be converted to ketones. An alternative leucine metabolic pathway has been described. In this pathway, leucine is converted to KIC and KIC is oxidized to HMB by a cytosolic enzyme called KIC-dioxygenase.[160]

The HMB produced is further metabolized in at least three ways: The first fate is further metabolism to HMG-CoA. This cytosolic source of HMG-CoA plays at least some role in cholesterol synthesis. A second fate of HMB produced in the cell is loss in the urine. Previous feeding studies indicate that up to 40% of the HMB fed is lost in the urine and likely accounts for the relative short half-life of HMB of about one hour. The third fate of HMB appears to be further use by the cell.

HMB meets the criteria of a dietary supplement because it is found in some foods in small amounts (such as catfish and some citrus fruits), found in breast milk, and used and produced by body tissues. As yet, there has been no evidence that HMB is a necessary nutrient and that the body uses it preferentially for modulating protein synthesis. However, it seems to have effects on protein synthesis and may help maximize the anabolic effects of exercise.

HMB has been seriously studied in the past seven years and found to have an effect on protein synthesis and lean body mass. Animal studies have shown that HMB appears non-toxic and may counteract the effects of stress and increase growth and health of animals.[161–164]

One study looked at the effects of leucine and its catabolites on *in vitro*, mitogen-stimulated DNA synthesis by bovine lymphocytes.[165] The results suggest that leucine is necessary for mitogen-induced DNA synthesis by bovine lymphocytes and that this requirement for leucine can be partially met by KIC. When leucine was not limiting, KIC, HMB, and HMG at concentrations that might occur *in vivo* did not alter lymphocyte DNA synthesis *in vitro*. Thus it would appear that in some circumstances and in some tissues, HMB is lower down on the anabolic and anticatabolic scale than either leucine or KIC.

However, a few recent studies suggest that HMB has significant anticatabolic potential in skeletal muscle. Especially promising is a study in which supplementation with either 1.5 or 3 g of HMB per day was shown to partly prevent exercise-induced proteolysis/muscle damage and result in larger gains in muscle function associated with resistance training in humans.[166]

In this study, the effects of dietary supplementation of HMB were studied in two experiments. In Study 1, 41 untrained (no participation in a resistance training program for at least three months) subjects were randomized among three levels of HMB supplementation (0, 1.5, or 3.0 g HMB/day) and two protein levels and weight lifted (WL) 1.5 hours three days a week for three weeks. In Study 2, subjects were fed either 0 or 3.0 g HMB/day and WL for two to three hours six days a week for seven weeks.

In Study 1, HMB significantly decreased the exercise-induced rise in muscle proteolysis, as measured by urine 3-methylhistidine, during the first two weeks of exercise. Plasma creatine phosphokinase (CK), was also decreased with HMB supplementation. WL was increased by HMB supplementation when compared with the unsupplemented subjects during each week of the study.

After a one-week adaptation period, the three-week supplementation/exercise protocol was started. After only one week of training/supplementation, muscle protein breakdown in the group fed 3 g HMB was decreased 44% (compared with placebo). Muscle protein breakdown continued to be lower in the HMB group for the entire length of the study. A second indicator of muscle damage and muscle breakdown is the muscle-specific enzyme called creatine phosphokinase (CPK). This enzyme was also markedly decreased with HMB supplementation.

The biochemical indicators of muscle damage were also accompanied by demonstrable increases in muscle strength and muscle mass. Lean body mass increases for the 0, 1.5, and 3.0 g HMB/d were 0.4, 0.8, and 1.2 kg/3 weeks, respectively. Strength increases for the 0, 1.5, and 3 g HMB/d were 10%, 23%, and 29%, respectively.

In Study 2, in which the intensity of exercise was much higher, fat free mass was significantly increased in HMB supplemented subjects compared with the unsupplemented group at two, four, five, and six weeks of the study. This second part of the study may be of even more significance than the first part in that proteolysis would ordinarily be expected to be higher, with a danger of overtraining, and therefore the anticatabolic effects of HMB would be even more prominent.

Nissen et al. have subsequently carried out another study to see if HMB has similar effects in trained subjects. The results of this recent study were presented at the 1996 Experimental Biology Meeting on April 15, 1996. In this four-week, double-blind study, 3 g of HMB per day in capsules were given in three divided doses to trained and untrained subjects while they participated in an intense weight-training program.

HMB was equally effective for both the previously trained and untrained groups, so results were pooled for HMB supplementation. Overall, HMB increased lean body mass 4.44 lb or 3.1%, and decreased bodyfat by 2.17 lb, or 7.3% (both significantly better than control groups). The HMB-supplemented subjects also showed an increase in their bench-press strength of 22 lb, which represents a 37% absolute increase over that of controls, and similar results were found for other exercises.

In the past year or so, several studies have further shown the effectiveness of HMB in decreasing protein catabolism and increasing protein synthesis. Three studies on HMB's effects were presented at the Experimental Biology 98 meeting. The first study was set up to show the underlying mechanisms by which HMB enhances the gains in muscle strength and lean mass associated with resistance training.[167] The data from this study suggest that HMB exerts several effects on muscle cells. First it increases the muscle cell's oxidative capacity. This action apparently lasts beyond the exposure to HMB and might involve changes in oxidative enzymes. Increased fat oxidation by muscle may contribute to gains in lean body mass.[168] Second, HMB appears to exert a stabilizing effect on myotube membranes as evidenced by the decrease in LDH leak into the medium. This effect may be particularly beneficial during strength training because it would protect against some of the associated cellular injury. Finally, the effect of HMB on CK, an established differentiation marker, suggests that it might enhance expression of muscle-specific proteins.

The second study was set up to examine the effects of HMB supplementation on muscle damage following intense endurance exercise. Prior to and following four weeks of supplementation, CK and LDH were measured in 13 subjects. Subjects were paired according to their two-mile run times and past running experience. Treatments, either 3 g of HMB or 3 g of placebo, were randomly assigned in a double-blind fashion. The subjects ran a 20-K race following the fifth week of supplementation. CK and LDH were measured prior to the race, immediately post race, and one to four days after the race. Plasma CK and LDH levels were elevated in both the placebo- and HMB-treated subjects post race and for four days following the 20-K race. However, the placebo group had a higher CK and a trend to higher LDH levels when compared with the HMB-treated group. The HMB-treated group had lower CK levels two and three days after the race. The authors concluded that supplementation with HMB partially protects muscle from damage often associated with strenuous aerobic exercise.

The third study was set up to see if older adults participating in an exercise program five days a week responded by changes in body composition the same way as younger adults (as seen in a previous study[166]). Subjects (15 men and 16 women, mean age 70 ± 1 years) were randomly assigned in a double-blind fashion, receiving either 3 g/day of HMB or 3 g/day of a placebo (CON). Subjects participated in a walking program three days a week and strength training program two days a week for eight weeks. Skinfold (SF) measurements were obtained to estimate percent body fat at zero, four, and eight weeks of training. A single computerized tomography (CT) slice of the thigh and upper arm were also made at zero and eight weeks in 12 subjects from each group. The area of the fat and muscle regions were differentiated based on image density. Both groups significantly increased the area of muscle in the thigh as measured by CT during the eight weeks of training to the same extent. However, there was a significant reduction in the area of fat for the HMB group as compared with the CON group. After eight weeks, HMB-treated subjects gained significantly more FFM and lost more body fat than the CON-treated subjects as measured by SF. In summary,

HMB decreased whole body fat and increased lean content with regional changes in leg composition consisting primarily of decreased fat.

It has been shown that HMB significantly influences protein metabolism. It positively enhances the effects of exercise on body compositions in both older and younger adults.

HMB appears to regulate protein synthesis either through hormonal receptor effects (cortisol, testosterone, GH, IGF-I, insulin) or by modulating the enzymes responsible for muscle tissue breakdown. HMB may affect the metabolism of leucine and glutamine, and perhaps other anabolic and anticatabolic amino acids, or may decrease gluconeogenesis and the subsequent oxidation of amino acids in the intracellular amino acid pool and catabolism of skeletal muscle cellular protein.

HMB can enhance gains in lean body mass and strength in both trained and untrained subjects. HMB decreases muscle proteolysis, increases net protein synthesis, and speeds recovery from exercise-induced muscle damage and thus can significantly increase the anabolic effects of exercise. HMB can also speed the loss of body fat by increasing fat oxidation in muscle.

7.5.2.5 Amino Acid Derivatives — Creatine

There are several metabolically important compounds in the body that are derived from a small number of amino acids. One of the most important is creatine. Because creatine is covered in detail in Chapter 11 only some basic information is provided here.

Creatine is an amino acid derivative that is obtained from food (especially red meat — 2 lb of steak has about 4 g of creatine). It is also formed in the liver from the amino acids arginine, glycine, and methionine. Creatine is then taken up by skeletal muscle where it forms phosphocreatine, the high energy phosphate compound. In humans, over 95% of the total creatine content is located in skeletal muscle, of which approximately a third is in its free form. The remainder is present in a phosphorylated form.

Phosphocreatine serves as a backup source of energy for ATP, the immediate source of energy for muscular contraction. The amount of phosphocreatine in skeletal muscle partially determines the length of time that maximum muscle work can be done. Once the phosphocreatine is gone, ATP must be regenerated through the metabolism of substrates such as glycogen, glucose, fatty acids, ketones, and amino acids.

Although the building blocks of ATP can be recycled, creatine cannot due to the reactivity of the phosphoguanidine group in which the carboxyl group displaces the phosphate. The resultant cyclic compound is creatinine, which is excreted in the urine. A dramatic increase in muscle use, such as in high-intensity training for bodybuilding, results in an increase in creatine phosphate breakdown, an increase in creatinine excretion, and an increased synthesis of creatine from the amino acids arginine, glycine, and methionine.

There is reproducible and consistent data that CM supplementation increases lean body mass and strength. By increasing the PC in muscle, more energy is available for contraction decreasing the need for anaerobic and aerobic mechanisms (such as hepatic gluconeogenesis and oxidation of amino acids). And because under normal conditions muscle contraction places such a demand on ATP and PC that there is insufficient amounts available for active protein synthesis at the same time that muscle contractions are occurring, increasing the available intracellular energy may lead to an increase in protein synthesis and a decrease in protein catabolism.

7.6 RECOMMENDATIONS

Proteins and amino acids can affect muscle mass, strength, and athletic performance. Now learn how to use this information in the real world.

First, it is important to realize that increasing one's dietary protein intake and taking protein and amino acid supplements is only part of the story. Many other factors have to be considered before one realizes increases in muscle mass and strength and athletic performance. There is an ideal way to maximize your lean body mass and strength and enhance athletic performance. Below is a four-part plan.

7.6.1 Part One: Lifestyle Changes

First, athletes need to straighten out their lives. Too much stress, not enough sleep, and the use of drugs and alcohol are all counter productive. One cannot build a good body if the foundation is shaky.

For example, men studies have shown that sleep deprivation adversely affects testicular function, leading to lower serum levels of testosterone.[169] In both men and women, decreased testosterone levels and secretion rates are observed under stressful conditions (anesthesia, anxiety, hangover, exhaustion, undernutrition, overtraining) as well as with increased serum cortisol levels and ACTH stimulation. Drugs such as alcohol,[170–172] marijuana[173,174] and cocaine[175,176] also have adverse effects on serum testosterone levels.

To set up a foundation for the body one desires, one must optimize his or her lifestyle. That means keeping stress at bay as much as possible, getting proper sleep, and keeping away from excesses of alcohol and recreational drugs.

Although not too many of us abuse illicit drugs, alcohol may be another story.

7.6.1.1 Effects of Alcohol Intake on Protein Synthesis

It seems that everywhere you look there are articles on the positive effects of moderate alcohol intake on heart disease and longevity. Unfortunately, what many people consider moderate is often too much. That is especially true for those who want to maximize the anabolic effects of exercise.

Alcohol, either acutely or chronically, decreases protein synthesis and affects type 11 muscle fibers (the kind that hypertrophy best and give us that massively muscled look) more than type 1 fibers (the kind that give us that long-distance runner look). Excessive or binge use can decrease levels of testosterone and increase levels of cortisol and as well affect muscle cells that can result in significant muscle wasting, especially if protein intake is not adequate.

Several studies have shown the adverse effects of alcohol on protein synthesis. A study published in 1986 showed the effect of acute alcohol intake on protein synthesis in the whole body and in other tissues of the rat.[177] The study found that alcohol decreased whole-body protein synthesis by 41% as well as in individual tissues (liver: 60%; muscle: 75%; heart: 45%; kidney: 59%; spleen: 73%; plasma protein: 44%; lung: 64%). These data indicate a generalized effect of alcohol on protein synthesis.

Other earlier studies have also shown that alcohol or its metabolites, besides the effects on testosterone and cortisol, also has a direct inhibitory effect on protein synthesis.[178] Newer studies have also found both the indirect and direct effects of alcohol on protein synthesis and with chronic use, muscle wasting.[179]

One recent study looked at the effects of ethanol on skeletal muscle protein synthesis and protease activities in young male Wistar rats.[180] In this study, the alcohol-fed rats, compared with pair-fed controls, significant reductions in total protein, RNA, and DNA contents were seen only after 24 hours in all skeletal muscles studied: Changes were more marked in the muscles containing large proportions of type II fibers. The results suggest that the muscle compositional changes seen over acute periods of ethanol toxicity are predominantly associated with impaired synthesis of protein and that the contribution of cellular proteolytic systems may be minimal. The effects of ethanol on skeletal muscle protein metabolism are greater in muscles that contain a predominance of type II fibers than in those that contain mainly type I fibers. Ethanol's effects on muscle may be influenced by hormonal changes after 24 hours because protein synthesis is still compromised and free plasma T3 and corticosterone are altered at this time-point.

Alcohol, even in moderation can decrease serum testosterone levels and as such, can hamper the anabolic effects of exercise. Alcohol has also been shown to decrease protein synthesis up to 24 hours after use. It can also decrease fat oxidation.[181]

7.6.2   Part Two: Exercise

To be effective, exercise has to elicit an adequate adaptive response. If the work load is adequate, your body will respond to the stress of working out by increasing muscle mass and strength so that you can cope with further demands.

For example, if you are trying to increase muscle mass and strength, one of the ways to monitor whether or not you are doing enough to force increased muscle growth and fat burning is to listen to your body. If you have trained hard enough, your body will respond the next day with a certain amount of muscle soreness. This delayed onset muscle soreness (DOMS) is a signal to you that you have challenged your body with a workout that will force it to adapt. DOMS does not have to be the "I can't walk" type of soreness. It can just be a tightness and stiffness that lasts for several hours and is gone before you train again. And it does not have to happen after every workout. Once or twice a month you should go for that extra amount so that the next day it shows with some degree of DOMS.

To reach a new level of lean body mass, make one workout in four or five more strenuous than the rest so that the resulting DOMS lets you know that you are still making progress.

You can do this by increasing the weight and making sure that you go through the full range of movement for each repetition — a complete stretch and contraction in each rep is necessary to maximize the hormonal response to exercise. Increasing the number of reps you do (say, go from 8 reps to 20 reps for that one day), changing the way you do the exercise (for example, changing your hand spacing in any pressing movements), increasing the weight you use, going all out in your last set, doing some negative movements (eccentric) after your regular sets, and working a body part that you normally do not work are all ways of increasing the training load and forcing your body to adapt. This will usually result in some DOMS the day after training.

Before going further, eccentric, or negative, exercise should be defined. This is the concept of emphasizing the "negative," or "eccentric," component to exercising. Each exercise has a "positive," or "concentric," component and a "negative," or "eccentric," component. The positive component is moving the weight away from the earth (center) to some fixed position, and the negative component is that part from the fixed position back to the starting point or toward the earth (center). For example, with standing biceps curl, the positive component involves lifting the weight from the starting point where your arms are fully extended in front of you by contracting the biceps muscles to where your arms are fully flexed at the top. The negative component involves lowering the weight back to where the arms are again fully extended at rest, toward the earth.

An advanced training routine might consist of a workout in which you do your regular routine followed by two or three sets of one repetition of negative or eccentric exercise. The eccentric movements would result in some DOMS. You would do your next workout when most or all of the soreness is gone. This workout could be the same or different exercises done with a lighter weight just to stretch out and pump up the muscles. The next workout might be your regular workout with no eccentric movements, and the next after that would be a repeat of your regular routine, plus the eccentrics again. Thus every three or four workouts, you would give your body that extra push that would result in some DOMS the next day. That way, you know that your body is reacting to the workouts and that you are progressing.

7.6.3   Part Three: Diet.

Diets should be structured to suit the athletic activity. A diet high in complex carbohydrates may be necessary for endurance athletes but may be counterproductive for those who wish to maximize muscle mass and strength. The day of the high-complex carbohydrate, low-fat diet is long gone. First, although carbohydrates are important, their use keeps the metabolism in a carbo-hydrate-dependent mode and decreases the use of fat as a primary energy source.

As far as fats are concerned, they are not the villains they are made out to be. A moderate amount of fat in your diet can supply you with the essential fatty acids needed for optimum health and can increase serum testosterone and even maintain serum thyroid levels.

It is important to get a fair share of protein. Studies have shown that the anabolic effects of intense training are increased by a high-protein diet. And when you are trying to lose body-weight/body fat and maintain lean body mass, it is more important than ever to increase your daily protein intake. If you are trying to lose weight and/or body fat, it is important to keep your dietary protein levels high. That is because the body oxidizes more protein on a calorie-deficient diet than it would in a diet that has adequate calories. The larger the body's muscle mass, the more transamination of amino acids occurs to fulfill energy needs.

So how much protein should you take? On the average, a minimum of 1 g and a maximum of 1.6 g of high-quality protein per pound of bodyweight is recommended every day for any person who wants to maximize lean body mass while losing body fat.

Those who want to lose body fat will have to supplement their diet with extra protein because trying to get the protein needed from a diet is difficult to do without needlessly increasing the number of calories taken in.

Do not be overly worried about fat intake, but do not overdo it. First, if you are losing bodyweight/body fat, increasing fat intake will not impact your serum cholesterol levels unless you have a family predisposition. In many cases, serum cholesterol actually decreases with beneficial changes in the HDL/LDL ratio.

One more tip. Make sure you take some protein every three hours or so. Unlike what one might think, eating smaller amounts every three hours instead of larger amounts three times a day can result in a decrease in daily caloric intake, help keep you from being hungry, and increase the anabolic effects of exercise.

7.6.4 Part Four: Nutritional Supplements

Nutritional supplements are by far the most elusive, evasive, and difficult to figure out. The netherworld of nutritional supplements is a place where people fear to tread because they might lose their financial souls. And many of the ones who do are invariably lost to the gods of mumbo jumbo (better than steroids; you can eat all you want of whatever you want and lose weight; gain 40 lb. of muscle in one week).

But there is a light at the end of this dark nutritional tunnel. It is called research. This light can make us see what supplements work and which ones are just making the noise.

Again, it is not all that hard to do. It is easy to get lost when talking about the science of nutrition. All that talk about adrenergic receptors, uncoupling proteins, uncoupling oxidative phos-phorylation, lipolysis, lipogenesis, lipases, testosterone, growth hormone, IGF-1, insulin, thyroid hormone, cortisol, etc.

For now, look at what works and when to use it.

7.6.4.1 Some of the Most Useful Nutritional Supplements

Multiple vitamin. Take a good multiple vitamin and mineral pill every day. Taking one a day will assure you of getting certain amounts of the stress vitamins (Bs and vitamin C), vitamin A, vitamin D, vitamin E, calcium, chromium, magnesium, zinc, and the dozens more micronutrients that are necessary for optimal functioning.

Antioxidants. Taking an antioxidant supplement prior to training will help attenuate some of the free radical damage and cytokine response that increases with exercise and may also aid in preventing injuries.

Protein supplements. The best is a combination of soy and whey protein. Taking this combination of supplemental protein (one-to-one ratio) not only increases dietary protein, which should be even higher when trying to lose body weight and fat than at any other time, but it will also give your thyroid hormone and metabolic rate a boost. Make sure you take in at least 1 g of protein per pound of body weight every day, spread out in not more than three-hour intervals while you are awake. Take some before bed and as soon as you get up to decrease the catabolic effects of the eight- or so hour fast you go through while sleeping. If you wake up during the night, that is a good time to take some more protein and decrease even further the muscle catabolism.

As discussed above, taking some protein along with carbohydrates and even fats within an hour of training is good because this is one of the best ways to increase protein synthesis, maximize the anabolic effects of exercise, and speed recuperation.

Creatine Monohydrate. This supplement will increase lean body mass, increase strength and endurance, and help decrease body fat both directly and indirectly. Take a loading dose of 25 g per day for five days and then use 5 to 10 g per day as a maintenance dose. There is no need to take creatine either before or after training, although some athletes like to use it before training along with HMB.

Glutamine. This is anabolic in that it improves protein synthesis and decreases protein catabolism. It boosts the immune system, which is important when dieting and when regularly training. Glutamine also decreases hunger and cravings because the cells of the gastrointestinal tract use it extensively. Five grams of glutamine should be used both before and after training.

Branched chain amino acids. BCAAs not only improve protein metabolism but also help abolish visceral adipose tissue or VAT (the stuff most potbellies are made of). BCAAs also have been shown to increase energy levels for workouts and prolong exercise duration even when training under hot conditions. Interestingly enough, if you use the protein supplementation suggested above, you will get your daily quota of BCAAs because whey protein contains about 25% BCAAs.

HMB. Recent studies, some in publication, show that 3–5 g of HMB a day decreases protein catabolism and increases fat oxidation while dieting. HMB is best used spread out in three- or four-hour intervals and before training. In several studies, the use of HMB eliminated the loss of muscle mass while the participants lost substantial amounts of body fat.

7.7 SUMMARY

1. Athletes need significantly higher protein intakes than normal sedentary people. And depending on the sport, they may need specific protein and amino acid supplementation.
2. To keep the body in a positive anabolic state, protein must be consumed every two to three hours. Otherwise, catabolism of body protein occurs.
3. Certain amino acids have to be present in the dietary protein in specific amounts to have maximal protein synthesis and minimal protein catabolism.
4. The absence of adequate amounts of certain amino acids can result in decreased protein synthesis even in the presence of a high-protein diet.
5. Certain whole food protein supplements offer distinct advantages over high-protein foods.
6. Certain amino acids and their metabolites, either alone or in specific combinations, in pharmacological doses and at specific times (for example before and after exercise) regulate protein syntheses and protein catabolism (either by their direct effects or their effects on the anabolic and catabolic hormones) and can result in increased lean body mass that cannot be duplicated through the use of a high protein diet or specific foods.
7. The use of specific protein and amino acid supplements can have anabolic and anticatabolic effects (through their intrinsic activity and by stimulating anabolic and decreasing the effect of catabolic

hormones) similar to those obtained through the use of exogenous anabolic drugs including anabolic steroids and growth hormone.

8. The use of pharmacological doses of certain supplements, such as creatine monohydrate, that are derived from amino acids can result in an increased skeletal muscle hypertrophy that cannot be duplicated by the use of high-protein or specific foods.

9. The use of protein and amino acid supplements can have important effects on many other functions in the body, including the GI, antioxidant and immune systems that affect protein synthesis, lean body mass, and athletic performance.

10. Some amino acids trigger cellular reactions that initiate peptide formation and increase protein synthesis.

11. Oral ingestion of several amino acids in proper doses consistently and reproducibly elicit release of growth hormone and insulin in healthy athletes.

12. Ingestion of protein supplements or particular amino acids enhanced the results of resistance training by improving lean body mass (mostly muscle) and increasing strength, compared with control groups not using these supplements.

REFERENCES

1. Guyton and Hall, *Textbook of Medical Physiology*, Ninth Edition, W.B. Saunders Co., 1996, page 877.
2. Gerich, J. E., Control of Glycaemia, Baillieres *Clin. Endocrinol. Metab.* 1993; 7(3):551-86.
3. Nurjhan, N., Bucci, A., Perriello, G., et al., Glutamine: a major gluconeogenic precursor and vehicle for interorgan carbon transport in man, *J. Clin. Invest.,* 1995; 95(1):272-7.
4. Kaloyianni, M., Freedland, RA., Contribution of several amino acids and lactate to gluconeogenesis in hepatocytes isolated from rats fed various diets, *J. Nutr.,* 1990; 120(1):116-22.
5. Widhalm, K., Zwiauer, K., Hayde, M., Roth, E., Plasma concentrations of free amino acids during 3 weeks treatment of massively obese children with a very low calorie diet, *Euro. J. Pedia.,* 1989; 149(1):43-7.
6. Pozefsky, T., Tancredi, R. G., Moxley, R. T., Dupre, J., Tobin, J. D., Effects of brief starvation on muscle amino acid metabolism in nonobese man, *J. Clin. Invest.,* 1976; 57(2):444-9.
7. Fery, F., Bourdoux, P., Christophe, J., Balasse, E. O., Hormonal and metabolic changes induced by an isocaloric isoproteinic ketogenic diet in healthy subjects, *Diabete et Metabolisme* 1982; 8(4):299-305.
8. Cynober, L., Amino acid metabolism in thermal burns. Jpen: *J. Parenteral & Enteral Nutri.,* 1989; 13(2):196-205.
9. Lemon, P. W., Nagle, F. J., Effects of exercise on protein and amino acid metabolism, *Medicine & Science in Sports & Exercise,* 1981; 13(3):141-9.
10. Rothman, D. L., Magnusson, I., Katz, L. D., Shulman, R. G., Shulman, G. I., Quantitation of hepatic glycogenolysis and gluconeogenesis in fasting humans with (sup 13)C NMR, *Science,* 1991; 254:573-6.
11. Boirie, Y., Dangin, M., Gachon, P., et al., Slow and fast dietary proteins differently modulate post-prandial protein accretion, *Proc. Natl. Acad. Sci.,* USA Vol. 94, pp. 14930-14935, December 1997.
12. National Research Council: Recommended Dietary Allowances, 10th ed. Washington, D.C., National Academy of Sciences, 1989.
13. von Liebig, J., *Animal Chemistry or Organic Chemistry and Its Application to Physiology and Pathology* (translated by W Gregory), London, Taylor, and Walton 1842; p 144.
14. Fick, A. and Wislicenus, J., On the origin of muscular power. *Phil. Mag. J. Sci.,* 1866; 41:485-503.
15. Cathcart, E. P., Influence of muscle work on protein metabolism, *Physiol. Rev.,* 1925; 5: 225-243.
16. Astrand, P. O. and Rodahl, K., *Textbook of Work Physiology,* 3rd ed. McGraw-Hill Book Co., New York, 1986.
17. Lemon, P. W. R., Do athletes need more dietary protein and amino acids? *Int. J. Sport. Nutr.,* 1995; 5:S39-S61.
18. Kleiner, S. M., Bazzarre, T. L., and Ainsworth, B. E., Nutritional status of nationally ranked elite bodybuilders, *Int. J. Sport Nutr.,* 1994; 4(1):54-69.
19. Darden, E., Protein. *Nautilus,* 1981; 3(1):12-17.
20. Dohm, G. L., Protein nutrition for the athlete. *Clin. Sports Med.,* 1984; 3(3):595-604.

21. Lemon, P. W., Maximizing performance with nutrition: protein and exercise: update 1987, Medicine and science in sports and exercise 1987; 19(5):S179-S190.
22. Burke, L. M. and Read, R. S., Sports nutrition. Approaching the nineties, *Sports Med.,* 1989; 8(2): 80-100.
23. Lemon, P. W. and Proctor, D. N., Protein intake and athletic performance, *Sports Med.,* 1991; 12(5): 313-325.
24. Lemon, P. W., Protein requirements of soccer, *J. Sports Sci.,* 1994; 12:S17-22.
25. Lemon, P. W., Do athletes need more dietary protein and amino acids? *Int. J. Sport Med.,* 1995; 5:S39-S61.
26. Phillips, S. M., Atkinson, S. A., Tarnopolsky, M. A., et al., Gender differences in leucine kinetics and nitrogen balance in endurance athletes, *J. Appl. Physiol.,* 1993; 75:2134-2141.
27. Butterfield, G. E., Whole body protein utilization in humans, *Med. Sci. Sports Exerc.,* 1987; 19:S157-S165.
28. Piatti, P. M., Monti, L. D., Magni, F., et al., Hypocaloric high-protein diet improves glucose oxidation and spares lean body mass: comparison to hypocaloric high-carbohydrate diet, *Metabolism,* 1994; 43:1481-1487.
29. Fern, E. B., Bielinski, R. N., Schutz, Y., Effects of exaggerated amino acid and protein supply in man, *Experientia,* 1991; 47(2):168-72.
30. Bigard, A. X., Satabin, P., Lavier, P., et al., Effects of protein supplementation during prolonged exercise at moderate altitude on performance and plasma amino acid pattern, *Euro. J. Appl. Physiol. & Occup. Physiol.,* 1993; 66(1):5-10.
31. Dohm, G. L., Tapscott, E. B., Kasperek, G. J., Protein degradation during endurance exercise and recovery, *Med. Sci. Sports Exerc.,* 1987; 19(5):S166-S171.
32. Henriksson, J., Effect of exercise on amino acid concentrations in skeletal muscle and plasma, *J. Exp. Biol.,* 1991; 160:149-65.
33. Millward, D. J., Bates, P. C., Brown, J. G., et al., Role of thyroid, insulin and corticosteroid hormones in the physiological regulation of proteolysis in muscle, *Progress in Clinical & Biological Research,* 1985; 180:531-42.
34. Lemon, P. W., Protein requirements of soccer, *J. Sports Sci.,* 1994; 12:S17-22.
35. Manz, F., Remer, T., Decher-Spliethoff, E., et al., Effects of a high protein intake on renal acid excretion in bodybuilders, *Zeitschrift fur Ernahrungswissenschaft,* 1995; 34(1):10-5.
36. Sterck, J. G., Ritskes-Hoitinga, J., Beynen, A. C., Inhibitory effect of high protein intake on nephro-calcinogenesis in female rats, *Brit. J. Nutr.,* 1992; 67(2):223-33.
37. Wolfe, B. M., Giovannetti, P. M., Short-term effects of substituting protein for carbohydrate in the diets of moderately hypercholesterolemic human subjects, *Metabolism: Clinical & Experimental,* 1991; 40(4):338-43.
38. Hunnisett, A. G., Kars, A., Howard, J. M. H., Davies, S., Changes in plasma amino acids during conditioning therapy prior to bone marrow transplantation: Their relevance to antioxidant status, *Amino Acids,* 1993; 4(1-2):177-185.
39. Soon Cho, E., Krause, G. F., Anderson, H. L., Effects of dietary histidine and arginine on plasma amino acid and urea concentrations of men fed a low nitrogen diet, *J. Nutr.,* 1977; 107(11):2078-89.
40. Laidlaw, S. A., Kopple, J. D., Newer concepts of the indispensable amino acids, *Am. J. Clin. Nutr.,* 1987; 46(4):593-605.
41. Harper, A. E. and Yoshimura, N. N., Protein quality, amino acid balance, utilization, and evaluation of diets containing amino acids as therapeutic agents, *Nutrition,* 1993; 9(5):460-9.
42. Kihlberg, R., Bark, S., Hallberg, D., An oral amino acid loading test before and after intestinal bypass operation for morbid obesity, *Acta Chirurgica Scandinavica,* 1982; 148(1):73-86.
43. Rennie, M. J., Edwards, R. H., Krywawych, S., et al., Effect of exercise on protein turnover in man, *Clin. Sci.,* 1981; 61(5):627-39.
44. Lowell, B. B., Ruderman, N. B., Goodman, M. N., Regulation of myofibrillar protein degradation in rat skeletal muscle during brief and prolonged starvation, *Metabolism,* 1986; 35:1121-1127.
45. Li, J.B. and Goldberg, A. L., Effects of food deprivation on protein synthesis and degradation in rat skeletal muscle, *Am. J. Physiol.,* 1984; 246:E32-E37.
46. Dohm, G. L., Tapscott, E. B., Barakat, H. A., et al., Measurement of *in vivo* protein synthesis in rats during an exercise bout, *Biochem. Med.,* 1982; 27:367-372.

47. Dohm, G. L., Williams, R. T., Kasperek, G. J., Increased excretion of urea and N tau-methylhistidine by rats and humans after a bout of exercise, *J. Appl. Physiol.: Respir. Envir. Exer. Physiol.*, 1982; 52(1):27-33.

48. Millward, D. J., Davies, C. T., Halliday, D., Wolman, S. L., Matthews, D., Rennie, M., Effect of exercise on protein metabolism in humans as explored with stable isotopes. Federation Proceedings 1982; 41(10):2686-91.

49. Wolfe, R. R., Wolfe, M. H., Nadel, E. R., Shaw, J. H. F., Isotopic determinations of amino acid-urea interactions in exercise, *J. Appl. Physiol.*, 1984; 56:221-229.

50. Wolfe, R. R., Goodenough, R. D., Wolfe, M. H., Royle, G. T., Nadel, E. R., Isotopic analysis of leucine and urea metabolism in exercising humans, *J. Appl. Physiol.*, 1982; 52:458-466.

51. Devlin, J. T., Brodsky, I., Scrimgeour, A., Fuller, S., Bier, D. M., Amino acid metabolism after intense exercise, *Am. J. Physiol.*, 1990; 258(2 Pt 1):E249-55.

52. *Nutrition in Exercise and Sport,* edited by Ira Wolinsky and James F. Hickson, Jr., 1994 CRC Press, Boca Raton, FL, Page 127.

53. Morgan, H. E., Earl, D. C. N., Broadus, A., Wolpert, E. B., Giger, K. E., Jefferson, L. S., Regulation of protein synthesis in heart muscle. I. Effect of amino acid levels on protein synthesis, *J. Biol. Chem.*, 1971; 246:2152-2162.

54. Zawadzki, K. M., Yaspelkis, B. B. 3d, Ivy, J. L., Carbohydrate-protein complex increases the rate of muscle glycogen storage after exercise, *J. Appl. Physiol.*, 1992; 72(5):1854-9.

55. Okamura, K., Doi, T., Hamada, K., et al., Effect of amino acid and glucose administration during postexercise recovery on protein kinetics in dogs, *Am. J. Physiol.*, 1997 Jun;272(6 Pt 1):E1023-E1030.

56. Biolo, G., Tipton, K. D., Klein, S., Wolfe, R. R., An abundant supply of amino acids enhances the metabolic effect of exercise on muscle protein, *Am. J. Physiol.*, 1997 Jul;273(1 Pt 1):E122-E129.

57. Roy, B. D., Tarnopolsky, M. A., MacDougall, J. D., Fowles, J., Yarasheski, K. E., Effect of glucose supplement timing on protein metabolism after resistance training, *J. Appl. Physiol.*, 1997 June; 82(6):1882-1888.

58. Tarnopolsky, M. A., Bosman, M., Macdonald, J. R., Vandeputte, D., Martin, J., Roy, B. D., Postexercise protein-carbohydrate and carbohydrate supplements increase muscle glycogen in men and women, *J. Appl. Physiol.*, 1997 Dec 1;83(6):1877-1883.

59. Gautsch, T. A., Anthony, J. C., Kimball, S. R., Paul, G. L., Layman, D. K., Jefferson, L. S., Availability of eIF4E regulates skeletal muscle protein synthesis during recovery from exercise, *Am. J. Physiol.*, 1998 Feb;274(2 Pt 1):C406-C414.

60. Dragan, G. I., Wagner, W., Ploesteanu, E., Studies concerning the ergogenic value of protein supply and l-carnitine in elite junior cyclists, *Physiologie*, 1988; 25(3):129-132.

61. Dragan, G. I., Vasiliu, A., Georgescu, E., Research concerning the effects of Refit on elite weightlifters, *J. Sports Med. Physical Fitness*, 1985; 25(4):246-250.

62. Dragan, G. I., Vasiliu, A., Georgescu, E., Effects of Refit on Olimpic (sic) athletes, Sportorvosi Szemle/*Hungarian Review of Sports Medicine*, 1985; 26(2):107-113.

63. Dragan, I., Stroescu, V., Stoian, I., Georgescu, E., Baloescu, R., Studies regarding the efficiency of Supro isolated soy protein in Olympic athletes, *Rev. Roum. Physiol.*, 1992; 29(3-4):63-70.

64. Dragan, G. I., Ploesteanu, E., Selejan, V., Studies concerning the ergogenic value of Cantamega-2000 supply in top junior cyclists, *Rev. Roum. Physiol.*, 1991; 28(1-2):13-6.

65. Kreider, R. B., Klesges, K. H., Grindstaff, P., et al., Effects of ingesting supplements designed to promote lean tissue accretion on body composition during resistance training, *Int. J. Sports Nutr.*, 1996; 6:234-246.

66. Charlton, M. R., Adey, D. B., Nair, K. S., Evidence for a catabolic role of glucagon during an amino acid load, *J. Clin. Invest.*, 1996; 98(1):90-9.

67. May, M. E. and Buse, M. G., Effects of branched-chain amino acids on protein turnover, *Diabetes Metab. Rev.*; 1989; 5(3):227-245.

68. Herrling, P. L., Synaptic physiology of excitatory amino acids, *Arzneimittel-Forschung,* 1992; 42(2A):202-8.

69. Watkins, J. C., Some chemical highlights in the development of excitatory amino acid pharmacology, *Can. J. Physiol. Pharmacol.*, 1991; 69(7):1064-75.

70. Tsumoto, T., Excitatory amino acid transmitters and their receptors in neural circuits of the cerebral neocortex, *Neuroscience Research*, 1990; 9(2):79-102.

71. Nieoullon, A., [Excitatory amino acids, central nervous system neurotransmitters], *Therapie,* 1990; 45(3):281-5.

72. McEntee, W. J. and Crook, T. H., Glutamate: its role in learning, memory, and the aging brain, *Psychopharmacology,* 1993; 111(4):391-401.

73. Danbolt, N. C., The high affinity uptake system for excitatory amino acids in the brain, *Progress in Neurobiology,* 44(4):377-96, 1994 Nov.

74. Headley, P. M. and Grillner, S., Excitatory amino acids and synaptic transmission: the evidence for a physiological function, *Trends Pharmacol. Sci.,* 11(5):205-11, 1990 May.

75. Shinozaki, H. and Ishida, M., Excitatory amino acids: physiological and pharmacological probes for neuroscience research, *Acta Neurobiologiae Experimentalis,* 53(1):43-51, 1993.

76. Krebs, M. O., [Excitatory amino-acids, a new class of neurotransmitters. Pharmacology and functional properties], *Encephale,* 18(3):271-9, 1992 May-June.

77. D'Angelo, E. and Rossi, P., Excitatory amino acid regulation of neuronal functions, *Functional Neurology,* 7(2):145-61, 1992 Mar-Apr.

78. Farooqui, A. A. and Horrocks, L. A., Excitatory amino acid receptors, neural membrane phospholipid metabolism and neurological disorders. Brain Research - Brain Research Reviews, 16(2):171-91, 1991 May-Aug.

79. Rothstein, J. D., Kuncl, R., Chaudhry, V., et al., Excitatory amino acids in amyotrophic lateral sclerosis: an update, *Ann. Neurol.,* 1991;30:224-5.

80. Fonnum, F., Glutamate: a neurotransmitter in mammalian brain, *J. Neurochem.,* 1984;42:1-11.

81. Nicholls, D. and Attwell, D., The release and uptake of excitatory amino acids, *Trends Pharmacol. Sci.,* 1990;11:462-8.

82. Haber, S. N., Neurotransmitters in the human and nonhuman primate basal ganglia, *Human Neurobiology,* 5(3):159-68, 1986.

83. D'Souza, S. W. and Slater, P., Excitatory amino acids in neonatal brain: contributions to pathology and therapeutic strategies. Archives of Disease in Childhood Fetal & Neonatal Edition, 72(3):F147-50, 1995 May.

84. Singewald, N., Zhou, G. Y., Schneider, C., Release of excitatory and inhibitory amino acids from the locus coeruleus of conscious rats by cardiovascular stimuli and various forms of acute stress, *Brain Research,* 704(1):42-50, 1995 Dec 15.

85. Gietzen, D. W., Dixon, K. D., Truong, B. G., Jones, A. C., Barrett, J. A., Washburn, D. S., Indispensable amino acid deficiency and increased seizure susceptibility in rats, *Am. J. Physiol.,* 271(1 Pt 2):R18-24, 1996 Jul.

86. Ostroverkhov, G. E., Khokhlov, A. P., Maliugin, E. F., Terent'eva, V. B., Rykov, V. I., [Hepatoprotective effect of glutamine], *Ter Arkh,* 1974; 46 (1):89-96.

87. Kendler, B. S., Taurine: an overview of its role in preventive medicine, *Prev. Med.,* 1989; 18 (1):79-100.

88. Johnson, P. and Hammer, J. L., Histidine dipeptide levels in ageing and hypertensive rat skeletal and cardiac muscles, *Comp. Biochem. Physiol. B. Comp. Biochem.,* 1992; 103/4:981-984.

89. Brooks, G. A., Amino acid and protein metabolism during exercise and recovery, *Med. Sci. Sports Exerc.,* 1987; 19(5):S150-S156.

90. Algert, S. J., Stubblefield, N. E., Grasse, B. J., Shragg, G. P., Connor, J. D., Assessment of dietary intake of lysine and arginine in patients with herpes simplex, *J. Am. Diet Assoc.,* 1987; 87(11):1560-1561.

91. Mgbodile, M. U. K., Holscher, M., Neal, R. A., Possible protective role for reduced glutathione in aflatoxin B1 toxicity: effect of pretreatment of rats with phenobarbital and 3-methylcholanthrene on aflatoxin toxicity, *Toxicol. Appl. Pharmacol.,* 1975; 34:128-142.

92. Ryle, P. R., Chakraborty, J., Thomson, A. D., Effects of cysteine and antioxidants on the hepatic redox-state, acetaldehyde and triglyceride levels after acute ethanol dosing, *Alcohol,* 1987, Suppl 1:289-293.

93. Buse, M. G. and Reid, S. S., Leucine: a possible regulator of protein turnover in muscle, *J. Clin. Invest.,* 1975; 56:1250.

94. Rogers, P. J. and Blundell, J.E., Reanalysis of the effects of phenylalanine, alanine, and aspartame on food intake in human subjects [comment], *Physiol. Behav.,* 1994; 56(2):247-50.

95. Cooke, J. P., Singer, A. H., Tsao, P., Zera, P., Rowan, R. A., Billingham, M. E., Antiatherogenic effects of L-arginine in the hypercholesterolemic rabbit, *J. Clin. Invest.,* 1992; 90:1168-72.

96. Pitkow, H. S., Rainieri, J. J., Dwyer, P., Hormone potentiating capability of amino acids on lactational performance in rats injected with 7,12-dimethylbenzanthracene (DMBA) during gestation, *Drug Chem. Toxicol.*, 1986; 9:15-23.

97. Cynober, L., [Role of new nitrogen substrates during peri-operative artificial nutrition in adults]. [French] Annales Francaises d Anesthesie et de Reanimation 1995; 14(Suppl 2):102-6.

98. Castellino, P., Levin, R., Shohat, J., DeFronzo, R. A., Effect of specific amino acid groups on renal hemodynamics in humans, *Am. J. Physiol. Renal Fluid Electrolyte Physiol.*, 1990; 258(4):F992-F997.

99. Svanberg, E., Moller-Loswick, A. C., Matthews, D. E., et al., Effects of amino acids on synthesis and degradation of skeletal muscle proteins in humans, *Am. J. Physiol.*, 1996; 271(4 Pt 1):E718-E724.

100. Parry-Billings, M., Blomstrand, E., McAndrew, N., Newsholme, E. A., A communicational link between skeletal muscle, brain, and cells of the immune system, *Int. J. Sports Med.*, 1990; 11(Suppl 2):S122-8.

101. Fernstrom, J. D., Dietary amino acids and brain function, *J. Am. Dietetic Assoc.*, 1994; 94(1):71-7.

102. May, M. E. and Buse, M. G., Effects of branched-chain amino acids on protein turnover, *Diabetes Metab. Rev.*, 1989; 5(3):227-245.

103. Nair, K. S., Schwartz, R. G., Welle, S., Leucine as a regulator of whole body and skeletal muscle protein metabolism in humans, *Am. J. Physiol.*, 1992; 263(5 Pt 1):E928-34.

104. Shinnick, F. L. and Harper, A. E., Effects of branched-chain amino acid antagonism in the rat on tissue amino acid and keto acid concentrations, *J. Nutr.*, 1977; 107(5):887-95.

105. Boirie, Y., Gachon, P., Corny, S., et al., Acute postprandial changes in leucine metabolism as assessed with an intrinsically labeled milk protein, *Am. J. Physiol.*, 1996; 271(6 Pt 1):E1083-91.

106. Louard, R. J., Barrett, E. J., Gelfand, R. A., Effect of infused branched-chain amino acids on muscle and whole-body amino acid metabolism in man, *Clin. Sci.*, 1990; 79:457-466.

107. Candeloro, N., Bertini, I., Melchiorri, G., De Lorenzo, A., [Effects of prolonged administration of branched-chain amino acids on body composition and physical fitness], [Italian] *Minerva Endocrinologica*, 1995; 20(4):217-23.

108. Palmer, T. N., Gossain, S., Sugden, M. C., Partial oxidation of leucine in skeletal muscle, *Biochemistry & Molecular Biology International*, 1993; 29(2):255-62.

109. Sherwin, R. S., Hendler, R. G., Felig, P., Effect of ketone infusions on amino acids and nitrogen metabolism in man, *J. Clin. Invest.*, 1975; 55:1382-1390.

110. Pawan, G. L. and Semple, S. J., Effect of 3-Hydroxybutyrate in obese subjects on very-low-energy diets, *Lancet*, 1983; 1(8):15-18.

111. Thompson, J. R. and Wu, G., The effect of ketone bodies on nitrogen metabolism in skeletal muscle, *Comp. Biochem. Physiol.*, 1991; 100(2):209-16.

112. Alvestrand, A., Hagenfeldt, L., Merli, M., Oureshi, A., Eriksson, L. S., Influence of leucine infusion on intracellular amino acids in humans, *Euro. J. Clin. Invest.*, 1990; 20(3):293-8.

113. Blomstrand, E. and Newsholme, E. A., Effect of branched-chain amino acid supplementation on the exercise-induced change in aromatic amino acid concentration in human muscle, *Acta. Physiol. Scand.*, 1992; 146:293-298.

114. Montoya, A., Gomez-Lechon, M. J., Castell, J. V., Influence of branched-chain amino acid composition of culture media on the synthesis of plasma proteins by serum-free cultured rat hepatocytes, *In Vitro Cell Dev. Biol.*, 1989; 25(4):358-364.

115. Hunter, D. C., Weintraub, M., Blackburn, G. L., Bistrian, B. R., Branched chain amino acids as the protein component of parenteral nutrition in cancer cachexia, *Br. J. Surg.*, 1989; 76(2):149-153.

116. Schott, K. J., Gehrmann, J., Potter, U., Neuhoff, V., On the role of branched-chain amino acids in protein turnover of skeletal muscle, Studies *in vivo* with L-norleucine, *Z Naturforsch,* [C] 1985; 40(5-6):427-437.

117. Dohm, G. L., Beecher, G. R., Warren, R. Q., Williams, R. T., Influence of exercise on free amino acid concentrations in rat tissues, *J. Appl. Physiol.,: Resp. Envir. Exercise Physiol.*, 1981; 50(1):41-4.

118. Askanazi, J. Y. A., Carpentier, C. B., et al., Muscle and Plasma Amino Acids Following Injury: Influence of Intercurrent Infection, *Ann. Surg.*, 1980: 192:78-85.

119. Henriksson, J., Effect of exercise on amino acid concentrations in skeletal muscle and plasma, *J. Exp. Biol.*, 1991; 160:149-165.

120. Adibi, S. A., Metabolism of branched-chain amino acids in altered nutrition, *Metabolism: Clinical & Experimental*, 1976; 25(11):1287-302.

121. Carli, G., Bonifazi, M., Lodi, L., et al., Changes in the exercise-induced hormone response to branched chain amino acid administration, *Eur. J. Appl. Physiol.*, 1992; 64:272-277.

122. Carli, G., Bonifazi, M., Lodi, L., et al., Changes in the exercise-induced hormone response to branched chain amino acid administration, *Eur. J. Appl. Physiol.*, 1992; 64:272-277.

123. Buse, M. G., *In vivo* effects of branched chain amino acids on muscle protein synthesis in fasted rats, *Horm. Metab. Res.*, 1981; 13:502-505.

124. Kraemer, W. J., Endocrine response to resistance exercise, *Med. Sci. Sports Exer.*, 1988; 20:S152-S157.

125. Essen, P., Heys, S. D., Garlick, P., Wernerman, J., The separate and combined effect of leucine and insulin on muscle free amino acids, *Clin. Physiol.*, 1994; 14(5):513-25.

126. Torres, N., Tovar, A. R., Harper, A. E., Leucine affects the metabolism of valine by isolated perfused rat hearts: relation to branched-chain amino acid antagonism, *J. Nutr.*, 1995; 125(7):1884-93.

127. Blomstrand, E. and Newsholme, E. A., Effect of branched-chain amino acid supplementation on the exercise-induced change in aromatic amino acid concentration in human muscle, *Acta. Physiol. Scand.*, 1992; 146:293-298.

128. Blomstrand, E., Celsing, F., Newsholme, E. A., Changes in plasma concentrations of aromatic and branched-chain amino acids during sustained exercise in man and their possible role in fatigue, *Acta. Physiol. Scand.*, 1988; 133:115-122.

129. Ji, L. L., Miller, R. H., Nagle, F. J., Lardy, H. A., Stratman, F. W., Amino acid metabolism during exercise in trained rats: the potential role of carnitine in the metabolic fate of branched-chain amino acids, *Metabolism*, 1987; 36(8):748-52.

130. Fukagawa, N. K., Minaker, K. L., Young, V. R., Rowe, J. W., Insulin dose-dependent reductions in plasma amino acids in man, *Am. J. Physiol.*, 1986; 250(1 Pt 1):E13-7.

131. Calders, P., Pannier, J. L., Matthys, D. M., Lacroix, E. M., Pre-exercise branched-chain amino acid administration increases endurance performance in rats, *Med. Sci. Sports Exerc.*, 1997; 29(9):1182-1186.

132. Mittleman, K. D., Ricci, M. R., Bailey, S. P., Branched-chain amino acids prolong exercise during heat stress in men and women, *Med. Sci. Sports Exerc.*, 1998; 30(1):83-91.

133. Kapadia, C. R., Colpoys, M. F., Jiang, Z. M., et al., Maintenance of skeletal muscle intracellular glutamine during standard surgical trauma, *J. Parenter. Enteral. Nutr.*, 1985; 9:583-589.

134. Wasa, M., Bode, B. P., Abcouwer, S. F., Collins, C. L., Tanabe, K. K., Souba, W. W., Glutamine as a regulator of DNA and protein biosynthesis in human solid tumor cell lines, *Ann. Surg.*, 1996; 224(2):189-97.

135. Hall, J. C., Heel, K., McCauley, R., Glutamine, *Br. J. Surg.*, 1996; 83(3):305-12.

136. Neu, J., Shenoy, V., Chakrabarti, R., Glutamine nutrition and metabolism: where do we go from here?, *FASEB J.*, 1996; 10(8):829-37.

137. Rennie, M. J., Ahmed, A., Khogali, S. E., Low, S. Y., Hundal, H. S., Taylor, P. M., Glutamine metabolism and transport in skeletal muscle and heart and their clinical relevance, *J. Nutr.*, 1996; 126(4 Suppl):1142S-9S.

138. Anderson, K. E., *Hormones and Liver Function: Peptide Hormones and Catecholamines*, Schiff, Leon, Ed.; Schiff, Eugene R., Ed., Diseases of the Liver, Philadelphia: Lippincott, 1982. 6B. pp 199-211.

139. Newsholme, E. A., Newsholme, P., Curi, R., Challoner, E., Ardawi, S.. A role for muscle in the immune system and its importance in surgery, trauma, sepsis and burns, *Nutrition*, 1988;4:261-8.

140. Wernerman, J. and Vinnars, E., The effect of trauma and surgery on inter-organ fluxes of amino acids in man, *Clin. Sci.*, 1987; 73:129-133.

141. Rennie, M. J., Muscle protein turnover and the wasting due to injury and disease, *Br. Med. Bul.*, 1985; 41(3):257-64.

142. Bulus, N., Cersosimo, E., Ghishan, F., Abumrad, N. N., Physiologic importance of glutamine, *Metabolism: Clinical & Experimental*, 1989; 38(8 Suppl 1):1-5.

143. Furst, P., Albers, S., Stehle, P., Evidence for a nutritional need for glutamine in catabolic patients, Kidney International - Supplement 1989; 27:S287-92.

144. Rennie, M. J., Hundal, H., Babij, P., et al., Characteristics of a glutamine carrier in skeletal muscle have important consequences for nitrogen loss in injury, infection and chronic disease, *Lancet*, 1986; 2:1008-1012.

145. Golden, M. N., Jahoor, P., Jackson, A. A., Glutamine production rate and its contribution to urinary ammonia in normal man, *Clin. Sci.*, 1982; 62:299-305.

146. Rose, W. C., Amino Acid Requirements of Man, *Fed. Proc.*, 1949; 8:546-52.

147. Lacey, J. M. and Wilmore, D. W., Is glutamine a conditionally essential amino acid?, *Nutrition Reviews*, 1990; 48(8):297-309.

148. Smith, R. J., Glutamine metabolism and its physiologic importance, *J. Parenter. Enteral. Nutr.*, 1990; 14(4 Suppl):40S-44S.

149. Rowbottom, D. G., Keast, D., Garcia-Webb, P., Morton, A. R., Training adaptation and biological changes among well-trained male triathletes, *Med. Sci. Sports Exerc.*, 1997; 29 (9):1233-1239.

150. Rowbottom, D. G., Keast, D., Morton, A. R., The emerging role of glutamine as an indicator of exercise stress and overtraining, *Sports Med.*, 1996; 21(2):80-97.

151. Perriello, G., Nurjhan, N., Stumvoll, M., Bucci, A., Welle, S., Dailey, G., Bier, D. M., Toft, I., Jenssen, T. G., Gerich, J. E., Regulation of gluconeogenesis by glutamine in normal postabsorptive humans, *Am. J. Physiol.*, 1997; 272(3 Pt 1): E437-E445.

152. Alvestrand, A., Hagenfeldt, L., Merli, M., Oureshi, A., Eriksson, L. S., Influence of leucine infusion on intracellular amino acids in humans, *Euro. J. Clin. Invest.*, 1990; 20(3):293-8.

153. Flakoll, P. J., VandeHaar, M. J., Kuhlman, G., Nissen, S., Influence of alpha-ketoisocaproate on lamb growth, feed conversion, and carcass composition, *J. Anim. Sci.*, 1991; 69(4):1461-7.

154. Riedel, E., Hampl, H., Nundel, M., Farshidfar, G., Essential branched-chain amino acids and alpha-ketoanalogues in haemodialysis patients. Nephrology, Dialysis, Transplantation 1992; 7(2):117-20.

155. Mitch, W. E. and Clark, A. S., Specificity of the effects of leucine and its metabolites on protein degradation in skeletal muscle, *Biochem. J.*, 1984; 222:579-586.

156. Stewart, P. M., Walser, M., Drachman, D. B., Muscle Nerve, 1982; 5:197-201.

157. Young, V. R. and Munro, H. N., N-Methylhistidine (3-methylhistidine) and muscle protein turnover: an overview, *Fed. Proc.*, 1978; 37:2291-2300.

158. Tischler, M. E., Desautels, M., Goldberg, A. L., Does leucine, leucyl-tRNA, or some metabolite of leucine regulate protein synthesis and degradation in skeletal and cardiac muscle?, *J. Biol. Chem.*, 1982; 257:1613-1621.

159. Brouwer, A. E., Carroll, P. B., Atwater, I. J., Effects of leucine on insulin secretion and beta cell membrane potential in mouse islets of Langerhans, *Pancreas*, 1991; 6(2):221-8.

160. Van Koevering, M. and Nissen, S., Oxidation of leucine and alpha-ketoisocaproate to beta-hydroxy-beta-methylbutyrate *in vivo*, *Am. J. Physiol.*, 1992; 262(1 Pt 1):E27-31.

161. Nissen, S., Fuller, J. C. Jr., Sell, J., Ferket, P. R., Rives, D. V., The effect of beta-hydroxy-beta-methylbutyrate on growth, mortality, and carcass qualities of broiler chickens, *Poultry Sci.*, 1994; 73(1):137-55.

162. Gatnau, R., Zimmerman, D. R., Nissen, S. L., Wannemuehler, M., Ewan, R. C., Effects of excess dietary leucine and leucine catabolites on growth and immune responses in weanling pigs, *J. Anim. Sci.*, 1995; 73(1):159-65.

163. Nissen, S., Faidley, T. D., Zimmerman, D. R., Izard, R., Fisher, C. T., Colostral milk fat percentage and pig performance are enhanced by feeding the leucine metabolite beta-hydroxy-beta-methyl butyrate to sows, *J. Anim. Sci.*, 1994; 72(9):2331-7.

164. Van Koevering, M. T., Dolezal, H. G., Gill, D. R., Owens, F. N., Strasia, C. A., Buchanan, D. S., Lake, R., Nissen, S., Effects of beta-hydroxy-beta-methyl butyrate on performance and carcass quality of feedlot steers, *J. Anim. Sci.*, 1994; 72(8):1927-35.

165. Nonnecke, B. J., Franklin, S. T., Nissen, S. L., Leucine and its catabolites alter mitogen-stimulated DNA synthesis by bovine lymphocytes, *J. Nutr.*, 1991; 121(10):1665-72.

166. Nissen, S., Sharp, R., Ray, M., Rathmacher, J. A., Rice, D., Fuller, J. C. Jr., Connelly, A. S., Abumrad N., Effect of leucine metabolite beta-hydroxy-beta-methylbutyrate on muscle metabolism during resistance-exercise training, *J. Appl. Physiol.*, 1996;81(5):2095-2104.

167. Cheng, W., Phillips, B., and Abumrad, N., Effect of HMB on Fuel Utilization, Membrane Stability and Creatine Kinase Content of Cultured Muscle Cells, *FASEB J.*, 1998; 12:A950.

168. Cheng, W., Beta-hydroxy-beta-methylbutyrate increases fatty acid oxidation by muscle cells, *FASEB J.*, 1997; 11(3):A381.

169. Opstad, P. K. and Aakvaag, A., The effect of sleep deprivation on the plasma levels of hormones during prolonged physical strain and calorie deficiency, *Euro. J. Appl. Physiol. Occup. Physiol.*, 1983; 51(1):97-107.

170. Noth, R. H. and Walter, R. M. Jr., The effects of alcohol on the endocrine system, *Med. Clin. North Am.*, 1984; 68(1):133-146.

171. Babichev, V. N., Peryshkova, T. A., Aivazashvili, N. I., Shishkina, I. V., [Effect of alcohol on the content of sex steroid receptors in the hypothalamus and hypophysis of male rats], *Biull Eksp Biol. Med.*, 1989, 107 (2) p204-7.

172. Chung, K. W., Effect of ethanol on androgen receptors in the anterior pituitary, hypothalamus and brain cortex in rats, *Life Sci.*, 1989, 44 (4) p273-80.

173. Diamond, F. Jr., Ringenberg, L., MacDonald, D., et al., Effects of drug and alcohol abuse upon pituitary-testicular function in adolescent males, *Adolesc. Health Care*, 1986; 7(1):28-33.

174. Barnett, G., Chiang, C.W., Licko, V. J., Effects of marijuana on testosterone in male subjects, *Theor. Biol.*, 1983, 104 (4) p685-92.

175. Mendelson, J. H., Mello, N. K., Teoh, S. K., Ellingboe, J., Cochin, J., Cocaine effects on pulsatile secretion of anterior pituitary, gonadal, and adrenal hormones, *J. Clin. Endocrinol. Metab.*, 1989; 69(6):1256-1260.

176. Berul, C. I. and Harclerode, J. E., Effects of cocaine hydrochloride on the male reproductive system, *Life Sci.*, 1989; 45(1):91-5.

177. Tiernan, J. M. and Ward, L. C., Acute effects of ethanol on protein synthesis in the rat, *Alcohol*, 1986;21(2):171-179.

178. Preedy, V. R., Duane, P., Peters, T. J., Comparison of the acute effects of ethanol on liver and skeletal muscle protein synthesis in the rat, *Alcohol*, 1988; 23(2):155-62.

179. Preedy, V. R., Salisbury, J. R., Peters, T. J., Alcoholic muscle disease: features and mechanisms, *J. Pathol.*, 1994; 173(4):309-315.

180. Reilly, M. E., Mantle, D., Richardson, P. J., Salisbury, J., Jones, J., Peters, T. J., Preedy, V. R., Studies on the time-course of ethanol's acute effects on skeletal muscle protein synthesis: comparison with acute changes in proteolytic activity, *Alcohol Clin. Exp. Res.*, 1997; 21(5):792-798.

181. Doucet, E. and Tremblay, A., Food intake, energy balance and body weight control, *Eur. J. Clin. Nutr.*, 1997;51(12):846-855.

Supplements Containing Macronutrient Derivatives

CHAPTER 8

Carbohydrate Supplements in Exercise and Sport

Satya S. Jonnalagadda

CONTENTS

8.1 INTRODUCTION

An ergogenic aid is an agent or procedure that enhances energy production, energy control, or energy efficiency during exercise and/or sport performance, thereby providing the athlete with a competitive edge that cannot be obtained through normal training procedures.[1] Several types of ergogenic aids are available to athletes and sports enthusiasts, namely, nutritional, biomechanical, mechanical, physical, physiological, psychological or pharmacological substances or treatments.[1] These ergogenic aids can be used during training, competition, or during both training and competition. For instance, carbohydrate (CHO) supplementation can be used during both training and competition to enhance performance. The ultimate ergogenic agent selected by an athlete to aid performance should be safe, legal, and effective.

This chapter discusses the use of CHO as an ergogenic aid to enhance performance. Briefly, the type of CHO supplements, their usage, and their effectiveness in improving performance will be reviewed. Areas for future research will also be identified based on a review of the current literature.

8.2 DIETARY RECOMMENDATIONS

Diet has been shown to play a critical role in health and disease. Of the three macronutrients, CHO is the most important source of energy to a vast majority of the population because of its relatively low cost and widespread availability in all food sources. The current dietary recommendation for all individuals is that CHOs provide 55% of the daily energy intake, fat should provide no more than 30% of daily energy intake, and proteins should provide at least 15% of daily energy intake.[2] Dietary CHO and fat are the main energy substrates in healthy individuals, both during the fasting state and during prolonged exercise. Based on the 1994 Continuing Survey of Food Intakes by Individuals, the average daily CHO intake in the United States for adult males and females was 299 g/day (48% energy) and 209 g/day (51% energy), respectively.[3] Similarly, NHANES III observed a daily CHO intake of 280 g/day (47% energy) and 206 g/day (50% energy) by adult males and females in the United States, respectively.[4] The main contributors to the dietary CHO intake in the United States are grain products, fruits, and vegetables. Athletes participating in long-duration sports on average have been reported to consume 56.7% of energy as CHO.[5] On the other hand, athletes participating in short-duration sports have been observed to consume approximately 46.6% of total energy as CHO.[5] In the above instances, these intakes may not be sufficient to meet the demands of the sport.

Foods that contain CHO provide the major source of energy in the form of glucose, which is the main energy substrate for the central nervous system and the skeletal muscle. For the active individual, CHOs provide a ready source of energy for muscular activity. To meet the nutrient needs of physical activity and health, an athlete's training diet should provide 50% to 55% of the total energy as CHO, 12% to 15% from protein and 25% to 30% from fat.[6] At the present time, however, the actual CHO intake appropriate to meet the training and competition needs of athletes is under debate because their total dietary intake is influenced by their activity level, quality and quantity of training. A CHO intake of greater than 70% of daily energy intake has been proposed for athletes in training. However, such a blanket recommendation for all athletes is not appropriate because the daily energy intake varies between individual athletes and from one sport to another, depending on the type and intensity of activity.

Additionally, the form of CHO consumed and the timing of consumption has been shown to influence energy levels and physical performance capacity. Because dietary CHO intake significantly affects the body's CHO reserves and thereby energy stores, athletes and active individuals practice considerable dietary manipulations to optimize their CHO reserves and improve training and performance capacity. Although athletes have been advised to consume greater than 70% of energy as CHO,[7] many athletes consume less than the recommended amount mainly because of the bulk of high CHO diets, potentially jeopardizing their training and performance capacity. Optimizing blood glucose and muscle glycogen levels is important for athletic performance. Hypoglycemia and/or depleted muscle glycogen stores are associated with declining ability to exercise at a required intensity during prolonged activity. Therefore, consumption of CHO prior to exercise has been suggested as a means to increase muscle glycogen and maintain blood glucose levels during exercise.

Glycemic Index (GI) provides a way to compare blood glucose response of CHO foods.[8] It is a percentage value based on the area under the blood glucose response curve of a food containing 50 g of available CHO, divided by the area of the blood glucose response of 50 g of CHO in a reference food (white bread), multiplied by 100. The GI helps to standardize response areas of each individual's response to a standard food. It allows foods to be categorized as low, medium, or high GI, with low glycemic foods causing the least glycemic response and the high glycemic foods producing the greatest response. Therefore, knowing the GI of foods can be a useful guide to athletes and can lead to enhanced performance. Consuming low GI foods 30 to 60 minutes prior to exercise may lower the chance of rebound of blood glucose to hypoglycemic levels at onset of exercise and may provide essential substrates to the exercising muscle late in exercise. The slow rate of digestion and absorption of these foods will therefore result in the availability of glucose toward the end of the exercise and potentially increase and/or prolong performance. On the other hand, consuming high GI foods during exercise and after exercise will ensure that blood glucose levels are maintained throughout exercise and will increase the rate of muscle glycogen resynthesis by either increasing substrate availability (glucose) or increasing levels of glucose transporter and activating glycogen synthetase activity in muscle.[8] Therefore, fatigue during prolonged exercise (more than two hours) is associated with reduced body CHO reserves (blood glucose and muscle glycogen levels) and reduction in CHO oxidation.

CHO supplementation at the rate of 40–75 g CHO/h during exercise has been observed to improve performance by maintaining euglycemia and rate of CHO oxidation during the later stages of exercise. The optimal rate of supplementation varies depending on the intensity and duration of exercise and environmental conditions.[9] Resistance training and other forms of high-intensity, intermittent activities do not encounter reductions in blood glucose levels but can elicit glycogenolytic effects. The rate of glycogenolysis is greater during high-intensity anaerobic exercise than during aerobic endurance activity.[10] Therefore, the ingestion of CHO during intermittent exercise may reduce muscle glycogen degradation by increasing glycogen synthesis.

In the event that these CHO recommendations cannot be met by diet alone, supplementation may be an option to meet the energy needs of the active individual. This chapter examines the various CHO supplements available to athletes and their impact on physical performance. An overview of the influence of dietary CHO manipulation on physical performance is given elsewhere in this volume.

8.3 WHY USE CARBOHYDRATE SUPPLEMENTS?

Supplement usage among athletes is widespread. However, the rate of usage varies because of subtle differences in the definition of "supplements" in studies that have tried to document supplement usage. The type of supplements used can vary from vitamin and mineral supplements to CHO-electrolyte sports drinks to that of bran supplements. Also, the use of these supplements varies depending on the sport. In spite of variations in the type of supplement, it is the general consensus that athletes as a group use supplements more often (40–67%) than the general public.[11] In general, athletes tend to use supplements to 1) enhance performance (ergogenic aids), 2) compensate inadequate or poor dietary intakes, and 3) meet higher nutrient needs induced by heavy exercise. Therefore, several forms and type of supplements are available based on the needs of the athletes.

Daily CHO intake and pre-exercise CHO feeding affect skeletal muscle glycogen stores. With reduction in muscle glycogen stores, blood glucose utilization becomes increasingly important and is a function of both intensity and duration of exercise. CHO ingestion during low-intensity (30% $\dot{V}O_{2\,max}$) exercise increases blood glucose and insulin concentrations, resulting in a twofold increase in glucose uptake by the skeletal muscle. This, in turn, leads to elevations in blood glucose and reduction in the use of plasma free fatty acids during exercise. This increase in blood glucose has been associated with increased exercise performance. During moderate-intensity exercise (50–75% $\dot{V}O_{2\,max}$), CHO ingestion results in smaller changes in blood glucose and insulin compared with that observed during low-intensity exercise, probably due to greater glucose utilization by muscle and inhibition of pancreatic insulin secretion.

Two methods of CHO supplementation have commonly been used to increase exercise performance: 1) Increasing glycogen storage via CHO loading and 2) Consuming CHO during exercise. CHO loading, i.e., glycogen supercompensation, produces supranormal levels of muscle glycogen, which can result in improved performance. Glycogen supercompensation is designed for single endurance event performances and for any event lasting more than 90 minutes and resulting in exhaustion. However, it is not advisable to try glycogen supercompensation more than two or three times per month. Exogenous CHO supplement ingestion during exercise is also common among athletes. CHO ingestion during exercise can improve long-term endurance performance (lasting more than 90 minutes) and delay fatigue by 30 to 60 minutes. For individuals engaging in highly strenuous activities on successive days, rapid replenishment of CHO stores via CHO supplementation may be more advisable since CHO loading is not feasible.

A suggested mechanism for the ergogenic effect of a high-CHO training diet is an increase in storage of muscle glycogen prior to the start of the competition, resulting in a longer exercise time before fuel is depleted. However, this glycogen-loading procedure may benefit only individuals competing in events lasting 90 minutes or longer or those who start with compromised glycogen stores. On the other hand, consumption of CHO as a liquid or solid supplement during exercise has been observed to enhance aerobic endurance performance.[12] The amount of CHO consumed during exercise depends on the length of the performance, and the benefits of the supplement may be realized only when the CHO stores are dramatically reduced and may also depend on initial stores of muscle glycogen. CHO supplements during exercise potentially increase glucose availability in the blood and replace the utilization of muscle glycogen stores during exercise. Athletes competing in several events on a single day or on consecutive days need to prevent muscle glycogen depletion that occurs with prolonged activity. Therefore, the goal of the dietary regimen is to provide an adequate substrate, namely glucose, to stimulate muscle glycogen synthesis activity. Consumption of liquid CHO immediately after exercise has also been shown to increase muscle glycogen synthesis.[5]

8.3.1   Carbohydrate Supplements

Athletes participating in prolonged exercise are generally limited by their muscle glycogen stores. Insufficient CHO intake has been shown to result in chronic muscle glycogen depletion and fatigue, especially in endurance athletes who undertake strenuous training on a daily basis and in athletes involved in prolonged strenuous competition over successive days, such as bicycle tours. It has been suggested that these athletes consume 9–10 g of CHO/kg bodyweight/day, which is approximately 65–70% of total energy intake.[7] Although this high CHO intake is achievable through diet, the bulkiness and volume of the complex CHO foods make this recommendation impractical and uncomfortable for the athlete. Therefore, athletes more commonly use CHO supplements that provide low-bulk and a concentrated source of energy to achieve the recommended intake levels.

The CHO intake of athletes is achieved at meal times, and an equal amount of CHO is consumed in the form of snacks between meals, which is an important strategy for athletes because it allows them to achieve high CHO intake without the discomfort associated with consumption of large meals. Despite the recommendations to increase CHO intake to increase energy reserves, most athletes consume less than the recommended levels of CHO. For instance, U.S. Olympic marathon athletes consumed only 49–54% CHO,[13] thus potentially jeopardizing their training capacity and competition ability. The stored CHO, in the form of glycogen, is present in the muscle (79% of total), in the liver (14% of total) and in the form of glucose in the blood (7% of total). These CHO stores can meet the energy needs of moderate-intensity exercise for approximately two hours. Therefore, because of the limited body stores and the preference for CHO during exercise, it is important that body CHO stores are maintained with adequate amounts of carbohydrate before, during, and after exercise. The suggested mechanism for the ergogenic effect of a high-CHO training diet is an increase in muscle glycogen storage prior to competition, thereby resulting in a longer exercise time before the fuel is depleted.[14] Therefore, athletes must be taught to make wise food choices to optimize dietary CHO intake as well as to examine the potential use of CHO supplements to boost their total CHO intake and thereby their body stores.

The important characteristics of CHO supplements used by athletes are: readily digested, absorbed, and increase and/or maintain blood glucose levels during prolonged exercise.[15] These supplements are available in various forms, most commonly being liquid, semisolid (gels), or solid (Table 8.1).

Table 8.1 Carbohydrate Supplements*

	Size/Calories	CHO (g)	Protein (g)	Fat (g)
Solid Supplements				
Power Bar	65 g / 230 cals	45 g (14 g sugar)	10 g	2 g
Power Bar Harvest	65 g / 240 cals	45 g (16 g sugar)	7 g	4 g
Balance	50 g / 190 cals	22 g (18 g sugar)	14 g	6 g
PR*Bar	45 g / 190 cals	19 g (17 g sugar)	14 g	6 g
Clif	68 g / 250 cals	51 g (15 g sugar)	4 g	3 g
Exceed	280 cals	53 g	12 g	2 g
Gatorbar	220 cals	49 g	3 g	2 g
Semi-Solid Supplements				
Cril Shot	1.12 oz (31 g) / 100 cals	23 g	—	—
Squeezy	1 oz (28 g) / 80 cals	20 g	—	—
Gu	1.1 oz (31 g) / 100 cals	24 g	—	—
Hammer Gel	1.1 oz (31 g) / 100 cals	25 g	—	—
Pocket Rocket	1.3 oz (36 g) / 100 cals	25 g	—	—
Power Gel	1.4 oz (39 g) / 110 cals	28 g	—	—
ReLode	0.75 oz (21 g) / 80 cals	20 g	—	—
Ultra Gel	1.3 oz (36 g) / 133 cals	24 g	—	4 g
Liquid Supplements				
All Sport	8 oz (240 ml) / 70 cals	19 g	—	—
Gatorade	8 oz (240 ml) / 50 cals	14 g	—	—
Endura	8 oz (240 ml) / 62 cals	16 g	—	—
PowerAde	8 oz (240 ml) / 70 cals	19 g	—	—
Sports Toddy	8 oz (240 ml) / 46 cals	9 g	—	—
10-K	8 oz (240 ml) / 60 cals	15 g	—	—
XLR8	8 oz (240 ml) / 62 cals	15 g	—	—
Hydra Fuel	8 oz (240 ml) / 70 cals	17 g	—	—

*   This is not an inclusive list of all available CHO supplements

Solid and semisolid CHO supplements in the form of sports bars and gels (Table 7.1) are high-calorie, high-CHO snacks. They are typically easy to digest and provide an energy boost. However, both have an acquired taste because they typically tend to be mealy, gooey, and sometimes too sweet. The best sports bar is one that provides a similar proportion of CHO, fat, and protein typical of a healthy diet. Solid supplements typically, in addition to CHO, also contain extra nutrients such as protein, fat, vitamins, minerals, and fiber.[11] Additionally, some solid supplements may contain herbs and other stimulants, some of which are banned substances. Most solid CHO supplements typically provide 200–300 kcal. Gels, on the other hand, provide 75–100 kcal, with the predominant source of energy contributed by CHO. However, some may contain extra amino acids and caffeine. Solid CHO supplements that provide low-bulk and concentrated source of CHO are currently available to meet the CHO recommendations to enhance exercise. At rest, the gastric emptying rate of solid foods is significantly slower than liquid foods. Therefore, solid CHO supplements may provide a slow and sustained release of glucose and may be a better pre-exercise food choice than liquid CHO supplements, which empty rapidly and raise blood glucose levels more quickly and to a greater extent. Because of that, liquid CHO supplements may be a better choice during and after exercise to enhance endurance and promote glycogen repletion.[14] When consuming these solid and semi-solid supplements, it is important that athletes consume adequate amounts of fluids.

Liquid CHO supplements (Table 8.1), typically in the form of CHO-electrolyte sports drinks, provide CHO to replace glycogen stores expended during exercise. However, the CHO content of these drinks should be of the appropriate concentration to prevent gastrointestinal disturbances.[16] Typically, at about a concentration of 6–8%, CHO in these drinks has been observed to be absorbed 30% faster than water. Additionally, these sports drinks also contain sodium, potassium, and other common electrolytes that are lost through sweat. Therefore, important qualities of CHO drinks are 1) allow rapid delivery of fluids to tissues; 2) provide adequate CHO source for use during endurance exercise; 3) provide low level of electrolytes; 4) are palatable and refreshing during exercise; and 5) do not cause gastrointestinal disturbances. Currently available commercial CHO-electrolyte beverages appear to meet this profile, and their effectiveness in increasing exercise performance will depend on their appropriate use during exercise. Taking liquid CHO immediately after exercise can potentially increase muscle glycogen resynthesis. Because post-exercise anorexia is quite common and most athletes cannot consume solid foods, liquid CHO drinks can, therefore, be used to provide adequate amounts of CHO to increase muscle glycogen stores.

The main CHO component in most supplements is glucose, which serves as the energy substrate for the exercising skeletal muscle. Glucose is the only form of CHO that the skeletal muscle can easily mobilize for energy and store as glycogen. However, other CHO components, namely sucrose and maltodextrose (multiple glucose units), have also been used in developing liquid CHO supplements. These solutions are presumed to empty rapidly from the stomach and thereby supply glucose at a higher rate. On the other hand, ingestion of fructose during prolonged exercise has not been shown to improve performance, probably because of the slower rate of fructose absorption and the need for hepatic conversion of fructose to glucose prior to its availability to the exercising skeletal muscle.[16] Additionally, consuming large quantities of fructose can cause gastrointestinal distress such as diarrhea and vomiting. Therefore, athletes opting to use CHO supplements should be aware of the composition of the supplement and make a selection based on their reason for supplementation.

Research dealing with CHO supplements in athletes has dealt with three areas of concern: 1) The effect of CHO feedings on muscle and liver glycogen before an event; 2) Performance enhancement during exercise; and 3) Muscle and liver glycogen replenishment after exercise.

8.3.2   Role of Carbohydrate Supplements

During times of increased CHO needs, such as heavy training, intense competition, and multiday endurance events, athletes need to rely on CHO-dense liquids and foods, which contain predominantly simple CHOs, to meet their energy needs. Depending on the type of CHO food ingested, the metabolic responses, i.e., blood glucose and insulin response, vary depending on the rate of digestion and absorption of the ingested food. The Glycemic Index of foods varies depending on the CHO composition, and it is possible that some simple and complex CHOs are easily absorbed and therefore have high Glycemic Indexes, whereas other simple CHOs such as fructose have low Glycemic Indices.[8] Therefore, the type of carbohydrate ingested is important, suggesting that during times of increased requirements athletes should ingest CHOs that are easily absorbed and have high Glycemic indexes.

Ingested CHO enters the blood stream as glucose, and in the resting state, it is stored in the liver and muscle as glycogen (Figure 8.1). Muscle glycogen stores are affected by exercise, dietary carbohydrate intake, and training status. Liver glycogen is used to maintain blood glucose levels between meals, providing adequate energy supply to the central nervous system, erythrocytes, and kidneys. During exercise, muscle glycogen is broken down and is the major source of energy (Figure 8.1). The primary cause of fatigue during exercise is CHO availability to the exercising muscle. It has been demonstrated that increasing dietary CHO intake can improve high-intensity exercise performance, while inadequate CHO intake impairs performance.[14] During the early part of exercise, most of the CHO energy is derived from muscle glycogen (Figure 8.1). As exercise progresses, muscle glycogen is reduced and contributes less to CHO requirements of exercise, and there is an increased reliance on blood glucose to meet the energy needs (Figure 8.1). After three hours of exercise while drinking only water, i.e., fasting, the majority of the carbohydrate energy is derived from glucose metabolism, which is taken from the blood to the exercising muscle. However, when CHO is ingested throughout exercise and glucose remains high in the blood, fatigue can be delayed because blood glucose serves as the predominant CHO fuel during the latter stages of exercise. Fatigue during exercise is often associated with the depletion of glycogen in the contracting muscle, and the pattern of muscle glycogen depletion is influenced by the mode of exercise. Therefore, consumption of CHO during prolonged continuous exercise will ensure that sufficient CHO will be available during the later stages of exercise and it is essential that these individuals ingest CHO well in advance of fatigue. The type and amount of CHO ingested and the timing of CHO ingestion not only influences blood glucose levels but also influences exercise capacity. However, the extent to which CHO feedings improve performance in events less than two hours long and not limited by CHO availability is less clear.

Ingestion of large amounts of CHO (120–300 g) during continuous cycling at approximately 70% $\dot{V}O_{2\,max}$ produced a modest increase in blood glucose levels and delayed onset of fatigue by an hour. Muscle glycogen utilization also was not altered in spite of the increased duration,

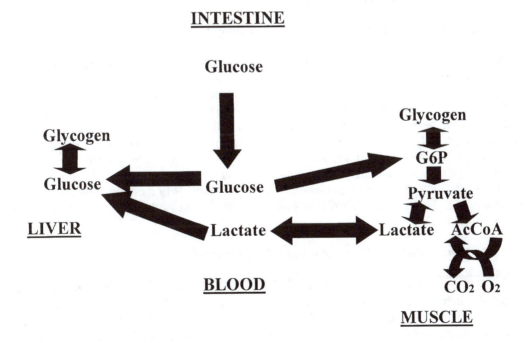

Figure 8.1 Carbohydrate interactions during exercise.

suggesting that a sparing effect of muscle glycogen occurs with CHO ingestion.[15] Similarly, during prolonged running, CHO ingestion increased blood glucose level, which was associated with improved endurance capacity and performance and muscle glycogen sparing was observed. This response to CHO ingestion during exercise is influenced by the intensity of the exercise protocol. Using blood glucose as an energy source increases as muscle glycogen levels decrease, which usually occurs late in the exercise period and during increased exercise intensity. However, in the later stages of exercise, blood glucose levels can decrease, which limits its availability as an energy source. Therefore, ingestion of CHO during exercise can prevent this reduction in blood glucose and increase availability of an energy substrate.

During exercise, blood insulin levels decrease, which increases the release of free fatty acids and the release of glucose from liver to provide adequate energy substrates to the exercising muscle. However, with reduced insulin levels, muscle uptake of glucose is also reduced, which could influence performance. Therefore, increasing insulin levels during or after exercise with carbohydrate feeding can increase rates of glycogen re-synthesis and increase recovery.

8.3.3   Composition of Carbohydrate Supplements

Glucose, sucrose and maltodextrins (multiple glucose units) appear to be equally effective in maintaining blood glucose concentration and CHO oxidation and in improving performance. Glucose is the energy substrate the exercising muscle uses and is the optimal CHO supplement. Sucrose has also been shown to be effective in maintaining plasma glucose concentrations and in enhancing exercise performance. Maltodextrins are also commonly used because they are presumed to empty rapidly from the stomach and thereby supply glucose at a higher rate. Additionally, these maltodextrin solutions are not very sweet and are thought to be more palatable. On the other hand, ingesting fructose during prolonged exercise has not been shown to improve performance, probably because of the slower rate of fructose absorption and the need for hepatic conversion of fructose into glucose prior to its availability to the skeletal muscle. Additionally, eating large amounts of fructose may cause some gastrointestinal distress.[16]

8.3.4   Carbohydrate Supplements and Performance

CHO loading, i.e., increased CHO intake in association with reduced exercise, results in elevated and/or supercompensated glycogen content in muscles that are frequently used. This CHO-loading regimen is associated with increased endurance time, especially in exercises of greater than 65% $\dot{V}O_{2\,max}$ and a duration of greater than 90 minutes.[17] Additionally, ingesting CHO immediately before or during intense exercise has also been shown to improve performance. Ingesting glucose polymer solutions (10%) resulted in a significantly smaller reduction in total power output during high-intensity cycle ergometer endurance performance for one hour with the effect most demonstrable after 40 minutes of exercise. Ingestion of CHO prior to exercise (30 g) and during exercise (120 g) was equally effective in maintaining total power output.[18] In these situations, the type of CHO ingested plays an important role in influencing blood glucose levels and restoring muscle energy stores.

8.3.4.1   Liquid and Solid Carbohydrate Supplements

Table 8.2 summarizes the studies examining the effect of CHO supplementation on various factors that influence exercise performance.[16–45] As can be seen, not all studies have reported positive effects of CHO supplements on exercise performance. The major limiting factors for prolonged heavy exercise are dehydration and CHO depletion. Replenishment of body fluids with CHO-containing beverages should benefit prolonged exercise. Fluid ingestion during exercise can minimize dehydration and help maintain performance. Liquid CHO ingestion during exercise not only

Table 8.2 Summary of Selected Research on the Response to Carbohydrate Ingestion During Exercise

Reference	Subjects	Type and duration of exercise	Exercise intensity % $\dot{V}O_2$ max	Type and amount of CHO	Blood glucose response	Blood insulin response	Muscle glycogen	Other effects
Jeukendrup et al.[19]	Well-trained cyclists	Constant intensity cycling, 2 hours (n=7)	60%	10% LG, 10% LG +5% MCT	↑	N/A	N/A	↑ plasma fatty acids
Roy et al.[20]	Resistance trained	Knee extensor, 4 sets, 10 reps (n=8)	85% of 1 max rep	1 g/kg LG	↑	↑	N/A	↓ protein breakdown, ↑ protein balance
Robergs et al.[21]	Well-trained cyclists	Cycle ergometer, 2 hours (n=8)	65%	L CHO (Exceed), S CHO 75 g (0.6g/kg/h)	↑ / →	→ / →	N/A	↑ glycerol, ↑ lactate
Hawley et al.[22]	Well-trained cyclists	Cycle ergometer, 1-hour time-trial (n=6)	N/A	S CHO (4–5 g/kg)	↔	N/A	↔	No improvement in 1-hour cycle time-trial
Fallowfield and Williams[23]	Well-trained runners	Constant pace treadmill running, 90 min (n=17)	70%	GP (6.9, 19.3%)	↑	↑	N/A	↑ plasma free fatty acids, ↑ plasma gycerol
Nicholas et al.[24]	Game players (soccer, rugby, hockey, or basketball)	Intermittent, high-intensity, shuttle runs (n=6)	> 55%	S CHO (10g/kg)	↔	N/A	N/A	↑ running time and distance, ↑ lactate
Davis et al.[25]	Physically active, untrained	Intermittent, high-intensity, cycle ergometry (n=16)	1-minute bouts at 120–130%, 3-minute rests	L CHO (18%)	↑	↑	N/A	↑ time to fatigue, ↑ number of exercise bouts, ↑ lactate, ↓ free fatty acids
Ferrauti et al.[26]	Tennis players	Interrupted tennis match, 4 hour (n=16)	N/A	CHO polymer (7.6%)	↑	→	N/A	↓ free fatty acids and glycerol, ↑ lactate
Taintzas et al.[27]	Recreational runners	Run to exhaustion (n=11)	70%	L CHO (5.5% and 6.9%)	↑ @ 20 minutes	N/A	N/A	↑ time to exhaustion, ↑ free fatty acids and glycerol

continued

Table 8.2 (continued) Summary of Selected Research on the Response to Carbohydrate Ingestion During Exercise

Reference	Subjects	Type and duration of exercise	Exercise intensity % VO_{2max}	Type and amount of CHO	Blood glucose response	Blood insulin response	Muscle glycogen	Other effects
Jeukendrup et al.[28]	Trained triathletes	Cycling, 3 hours (n=9)	57%	L CHO (15%)	↔	N/A	↓	↑ free fatty acids and glycerol
Anantaraman et al.[18]	Healthy individuals	Cycle ergometer, 1 hour (n=5)	90%	GP (10%)	↑	N/A	N/A	↑ total work
Rauch et al.[17]	Endurance cyclists	Cycling (2 hours) with sprints (1 hour) (n=8)	75%	S CHO (6.15 g/kg)	↔	N/A	↑	↑ power output ↑ speed and distance
Ball et al.[29]	Trained cyclists	Cycle ergometer, 50 minutes (n=8)	80%	L CHO (7%)	N/A	N/A	N/A	↑ peak power → RPE
Swensen et al.[30]	Trained cyclists	Cycle ergometer, to exhaustion (n=5)	70%	GP (7%) GP/PL (6.25/0.75%)	↔	↔	N/A	
Jenkins et al.[31]	Moderately trained	Five, 60s of all-out periods of cycling (n=14)	56.6%	S CHO (83%)	↔	N/A	N/A	↑ work output
Cole et al.[32]	Trained cyclists	Cycle ergometer, 105 minutes (n=10)	70%	G-S CHO (6%) HF (8.3%) HGP (8%)	↑	N/A	N/A	
Mason et al.[33]	Trained	Cycling, 2 hours (n=6)	65%	L CHO (5%) S (CHO)	↑	N/A	N/A	
Wagenmakers et al.[34]	Trained cyclists	Cycle ergometer, 2 hours (n=8)	70–75%	L CHO (166 g/L)	↑	N/A	↓	↑ lactate
Leatt and Jacobs[35]	Soccer players	Soccer game, 90 minutes (n=10)		GP (7%)	↑	N/A	↓	Utilized 39% less glycogen
Reed et al.[36]	Healthy, untrained	Cycle ergometer, 2 hours (n=8)	60–65% and 70–75%	GP (3 g/kg) S CHO (3 g/kg)	→	→	↔	
Mitchell et al.[37]	Trained cyclists	Cycle ergometer, 2 hours (n=10)	70%	L CHO (6–18%)	↑	N/A	↔	↑ work out

Study	Subjects	Protocol	Intensity	Supplement				Results
Flynn et al.[38]	Trained cyclists	Cycle ergometer, 105 minutes (n=7)	65%	Pre-exercise S CHO	↑	↑	N/A	↓ glycerol; ↑ performance
Murray et al.[16]	Healthy, untrained	Cycle ergometer, 115 minutes (n=12)	65–80%	L CHO (6%); G; F; Suc	↑	↑ ↔ ↑	N/A	↑ performance time; → performance time; →↓ free fatty acids; ↑ performance time
Brewer et al.[39]	Recreational runners	Treadmill, run to exhaustion (n=30)	70%	Complex S CHO (70%); Simple S CHO (70%)	↔	N/A	N/A	
Ivy et al.[40]	Trained cyclists	Cycle ergometer, 70 minutes (n=12)	68–88%	L CHO (25%), post-exercise	↑	↑	↑	↑ performance time; → free fatty acids
Hargreaves and Briggs[41]	Trained cyclists	Cycle ergometer, 2 hours (n=5)	70%	L GP (30 g)	↑	↔	↔	↑ performance time
Flynn et al.[42]	Trained cyclists	Cycle ergometer, 2 hours (n=8)	70%	L CHO (G, F, M) (2–7.7%)	↑	N/A	↔	↑ performance time
Coyle et al.[43]	Trained cyclists	Cycle ergometer, 4 hours (n=7)	70%	L GP (2 g/kg)	↑	↑	↔	↑ performance time; → free fatty acids
Fielding et al.[44]	Healthy, untrained	Cycle ergometer, 4 hours (n=9)	50%	S CHO (86 g)	↑	N/A	↔	↑ time to exhaustion
Hargreaves et al.[45]	Healthy, untrained	Cycle ergometer, 4 hours (n=10)	50%	S CHO (43 g)	↑	N/A	→	↑ performance time

G = glucose; F = fructose; S = sucrose; M = maltodextrose; GP = glucose polymer; L CHO = liquid carbohydrate; S CHO = solid carbohydrate; MCT = medium-chain triglyceride; PL = polylactate; RPE = rate of perceived exertion; ↑ = increase; ↓ = decrease; ↔ = no change; N/A = not available; n = number of subjects.

helps prevent hypoglycemia but can also serve as a fuel source to the working muscle that can be immediately utilized, thereby delaying onset of fatigue. Additionally, ingesting CHO and electrolytes in liquid form helps offset body fluid losses from sweating and lower vascular stress and hyperthermia associated with exercise induced dehydration. Therefore, the American College of Sports Medicine[46] recommends that runners drink 100–200 ml of fluid every 2–3 km, but this depends on the pace of the exercise/run, rate of dehydration due to sweating, environmental conditions and gastrointestinal comfort. The fluids consumed by these athletes are typically liquid CHO solutions. Coyle and Montain[47] recommend that exercising individuals consume solutions that provide 4–8% CHO.

Rate of gastric emptying is influenced by the volume of fluid consumed and CHO concentration of the solution. As the volume of fluid intake increases, the rate of gastric emptying increases. The rate of CHO delivery into the intestines increases as CHO concentration of the drink increases to about 5–8%.[47] Neufer et al[48] observed an increase in gastric emptying after ingestion of a solution containing maltodextrin and glucose (5% and 7.1%) followed by 15 minutes of running at 50–70% $\dot{V}O_{2\,max}$, which was approximately 38% greater during the running trials, with an overall average increase of 22% in CHO delivery. This could probably be due to an increase in mechanical movement of fluid within the stomach or may involve an exercise-induced hormonal control. Flynn et al[42] observed higher blood glucose concentrations after 60 minutes of exercise with consumption of CHO drinks containing maltodextrin plus glucose, maltodextrin plus fructose, or maltodextrin plus high-fructose corn syrup, all containing approximately 10% CHO, compared to water, in well-trained cyclists working at 70% $\dot{V}O_{2\,max}$. In spite of these differences in blood glucose levels, no significant improvement in performance was observed nor did it lower glycogen utilization. This suggests that the intensity of performance may influence the utilization of CHO supplements and their glycogen sparing effects. The optimal formulation of sports drinks and/or liquid CHO supplements is not clearly defined. It is commonly believed that maltodextrin solutions may offer an advantage because they can deliver more CHO without compromising fluid replenishment, thereby decreasing the risk of dehydration, heat illness, and stomach upset due to the lower osmolality and slower stomach emptying rate of these solutions.

Davis et al[49] using deuterium-labeled beverages, observed blood glucose concentrations to peak within 20 minutes after ingestion of 8% glucose-fructose mix and 30 minutes after ingestion of 6% glucose-fructose mix, 6% maltodextrin and 10% glucose-fructose mix. The plasma glucose concentrations after ingestion of these CHO electrolyte drinks was higher than after drinking water at 20 and 30 minutes ($p < 0.05$). Similarly, insulin concentrations increased rapidly 20 to 30 minutes after ingesting a CHO drink. The gastric emptying rate is also influenced by a variety of factors, such as fluid temperature, osmolality, sodium content, pH, calorie content, and electrolyte content. Therefore, the primary determinant of gastric-emptying is the calorie content of the ingested fluid, whereas its composition (simple vs. maltodextrins) may have little effect, suggesting that CHO beverages with >2.5% and ≤ 10% CHO may offer the advantage of delivering more CHO during prolonged intense exercise.

Reed et al[36] examined the effect of liquid and solid CHO supplements on the rate of gastric emptying and their effect on muscle glycogen storage post-exercise in healthy college-age men. The liquid CHO supplement provided 5% CHO (glucose polymers 70%, glucose 15%, sucrose 15%), and the solid CHO consisted of rice/banana cake supplemented with glucose with similar CHO content and calorie density. After two hours of cycling, subjects received 3 g CHO/kg bodyweight of liquid or solid CHO or intravenous glucose infusion. Although the blood glucose response after exercise after the intravenous glucose infusion was three times that after the liquid or solid supplement no differences were observed in the muscle glycogen storage rate during the first two-hour post-exercise (liquid 6.1, solid 6.3, intravenous 7.0 µmol/g wet weight/h) or second two hours of recovery (liquid 4.2, solid 4.7, and intravenous 4.3 µmol/g wet weight/h), suggesting that the rate of muscle glycogen storage after exercise is similar when 3 g CHO/kg body weight is administered in liquid or solid form and the rate of storage is not limited by the gastric emptying rate of the supplement.

Similarly, Flynn et al[38] examined the influence of CHO feeding (as meal) prior to exercise and CHO feeding (as liquid) during exercise on substrate utilization in highly trained cyclist and triathletes cycling at 65% of $\dot{V}O_{2\,max}$. Interestingly, although no significant differences were observed in the response to sub-maximal exercise or performance when a high CHO meal was ingested four or eight hours before exercise, CHO feeding in form of 7.7% glucose polymer/fructose solution improved performance, blood glucose levels were significantly greater ($p < 0.05$) throughout the exercise compared to placebo trials, while fat mobilization, i.e., blood glycerol levels, were significantly lower ($p < 0.05$) with the CHO feeding. Additionally, pre-exercise meals ingested four to eight hours before exercise did not significantly differ in their effects on substrate use and performance.

Rauch et al[17] supplemented the normal diets of endurance-trained cyclists with additional CHO in the form of potato starch (10.52 g/kg body mass/d) for three days prior to exercise. Subjects cycled for two hours at 75% of $\dot{V}O_{2\,max}$ with five 60-second sprints at 100% $\dot{V}O_{2\,max}$ at 20 minute intervals followed by a 60-minute performance ride. Increasing CHO intake by 72% for three days prior to exercise trial elevated muscle glycogen, improved power output, and extended distance covered in one hour. Additionally, muscle glycogen utilization was increased after CHO loading compared with after the normal diet.

Endurance exercise lasting 90 minutes or more is typically limited by dehydration and depletion of CHO stores. The efficacy of CHO feedings during intense exercise lasting less than 60 minutes or for intermittent, high-intensity exercise that imitates the demands of many competitive and recreational sports has not been well studied. Davis et al.[25] examined the effects of CHO feedings on fatigue during repeated, high-intensity cycling bouts lasting approximately 60 minutes in untrained men and women. Subjects consumed 6% CHO beverage (Gatorade, 4 ml/kg bodyweight) every 20 minutes during exercise. The average time to fatigue increased after the CHO trial, approximately 27 minutes delay in fatigue, compared with the placebo trial. Plasma glucose and insulin concentrations increased with CHO feeding. Ingestion of CHO beverages immediately before and during intermittent, high-intensity cycling delayed fatigue in these individuals, which could potentially improve performance during the last minutes of any event. This can have implications for sports such as soccer, hockey, basketball, and football, which have varying durations and intensity of actions and activity. However, the influence of CHO feeding during these types of sports has not been studied extensively.

Similarly, Tsintzas et al.[27] examined the effect of ingestion of 5.5% CHO electrolyte solution during the first hour of treadmill running on the onset of fatigue in male recreational runners who ran to exhaustion at 70% $\dot{V}O_{2\,max}$. The time to exhaustion was significantly longer (124.5 minutes) compared with just drinking water (109.6 minutes) ($p < 0.05$). Blood glucose concentrations at 20 minutes were significantly higher with CHO supplement, but no differences were observed at any other time compared with the water trial. On the other hand, plasma free fatty acids and glycerol concentrations were higher ($p < 0.05$) at 60 minutes in the water trial compared with the CHO trial, suggesting that ingestion of a 5.5% CHO solution during the first hour of prolonged running exercise improves endurance capacity by approximately 14%. Additional benefits could have potentially been gained if the CHO solution was ingested throughout exercise.

Ball et al.[29] examined the effect of CHO electrolyte replacement drink (2 ml/kg bodyweight), ingested just after the onset of and throughout a high-intensity cycle ergometer exercise bout, on sprint capacity, i.e., peak, minimum, and maximum power, which was significantly higher after the CHO-electrolyte trial ($p < 0.05$) potentially by sparing muscle glycogen during the high-intensity cycling. The rate of perceived exertion was lower during the CHO-electrolyte trial than during the placebo trial.

One of the most important criteria for CHO supplement taken during exercise is that it is readily digested and absorbed and increases and/or maintains blood glucose levels during prolonged exercises. Therefore, the supplement form is important. Mason et al.[33] compared the metabolic effects of liquid and solid CHO supplements during prolonged exercise in subjects working at 65% $\dot{V}O_{2\,max}$. Subjects consumed either 500 ml of rice-based liquid (5% CHO) or a food bar (25 g

CHO) taken with 500 ml water during the exercise. Both types of supplements significantly increased blood glucose levels (p < 0.05); however, no significant differences were observed between the two supplements. No differences in O_2 uptake, respiratory exchange ratios, or heart rate were observed between trials, suggesting that supplements with similar CHO concentrations are effective in a similar fashion irrespective of the physical form (liquid or solid). Additionally, consuming water with the solid supplement could have assisted in increased gastric emptying and thereby increased glycemic response, explaining the similar blood glucose concentration with the liquid and solid supplements.

Resistance training has become a popular mode of exercise among athletes and the general population. Although a lowering in blood glucose typically is not observed during resistance training, glycogenolytic effects have been observed with such training. Therefore, CHO ingestion could potentially increase performance by maintaining muscle glycogen stores in repeated sessions of resistance training and could enhance protein synthesis and hypertrophy associated with resistance training. Glycogen depletion could potentially occur if high-intensity bouts are repeated, resulting in fatigue and reduced force production. Therefore, CHO ingestion could potentially increase endurance capacity by decreasing muscle glycogen degradation due to the increase in glycogen synthesis occurring in periods between the high-intensity activities.[10] Additionally, CHO ingestion could lower hepatic glycogenolysis and gluconeogenesis because it replaces the hepatic glycogen stores that serve as the source of blood glucose. Lambert et al.[50] examined the effects of a CHO beverage (10% glucose polymer) ingestion on multiple bouts of leg extensions either before exercise or after the 5th, 10th, and 15th sets. The number of sets and repetitions performed were higher after ingestion of glucose polymer solution compared with the placebo. On the other hand, Conley et al.[51] observed higher blood glucose levels before exercise, immediately after exercise, and one and two hours after exercise when CHO was consumed 15 minutes before and during sets of 10 repetitions of squats at 65% of 1 RM with three minutes of rest between sets. The increase in blood glucose could be responsible for increased insulin levels and glycogen synthesis rates after exercise when CHO was consumed. However, no increase in exercise performance was observed as a result of CHO ingestion. Similarly, Vincent et al.[52] did not observe an increase in isokinetic resistance exercise performance following a free weight workout consisting of eight exercises when CHO was consumed immediately before the exercise session. Although the reasons for these differences are unclear, the definition of muscle failure and the type of resistance exercise in these studies could contribute to the variations in results, suggesting that the type of resistance exercise influences the utility of the ingested CHO.

In addition to glucose, lactate is an important gluconeogenic precursor during exercise and is rapidly oxidized by the skeletal muscle. Lactate serves as a CHO substrate for exercising muscle and potentially as a performance-enhancing agent via the "lactate shuttle," whereby CHO from the inactive muscles is redistributed as lactate to the active muscle, thus providing another source of energy to the exercising muscle (Figure 8.1). A lactate supplement (Poly L-Lactate) was developed as an additive to existing sports drinks and contains molecules of lactate that are ionically bound to amino acid.[53] The ingestion of this polymer form of lactate during moderate-intensity exercise has been observed to maintain plasma glucose concentrations similar to that of maltodextrin;[53] however, its exact mechanism of action is unclear. Fahey et al.[53] found that Poly L-Lactate helped sustain blood glucose levels during three hours of cycling at 50% of $\dot{V}O_{2\,max}$, suggesting that it may improve endurance. However, Swensen et al.[30] did not observe any significant effects on time to exhaustion of cyclists exercising at 70% $\dot{V}O_{2\,max}$ with the consumption of 5% Poly L-Lactate compared with a glucose polymer solution.

Fluid ingestion during exercise can minimize dehydration, and consumption of CHO solutions during exercise can improve performance. The ideal fluid consumed during exercise is one that maximizes the delivery of CHO without slowing the rate of emptying from the stomach. Although fructose has a higher rate of gastric emptying compared with the other sugars, when consumed alone, fructose is absorbed more slowly from the intestine and lowers exercise capacity compared with glucose and sucrose. However, when consumed in combination with glucose, these potential problems with fructose can be avoided. Therefore, high fructose corn syrup (HFCS) (50% fructose and 50% glucose) could potentially assist in endurance exercise. Cole et al.[32] examined the effect of 6% glucose-sucrose, 8.3% HFCS, 6.3% HFCS, plus 2% glucose polymer solutions consumed during exercise on performance capacity of highly trained cyclists exercising at 70% $\dot{V}O_{2\,max}$. Although blood glucose concentrations were higher with all three CHO supplements compared with a placebo, no significant differences were observed in total work performance. This could potentially be a result of similar initial muscle glycogen stores, which has been demonstrated to influence the ergogenic benefits of CHO ingestion. Additionally, the dietary CHO intake can also influence the muscle glycogen stores and thereby the ergogenic effect of the supplemental CHO.

Based on CHO supplementation during cycling studies, it has been suggested that CHO ingestion during exercise delays the onset of fatigue by maintaining euglycemia and oxidation of blood glucose at high rates late in exercise rather than reducing the rate of muscle glycogen utilization. In most studies on running, CHO ingestion results in elevated blood glucose levels compared with controlled conditions and has been shown to improve endurance capacity and performance in most, but not all, studies in the absence of declining blood glucose and CHO oxidation rates.[27,54-56] Therefore, CHO ingestion during running could potentially improve running capacity by delaying the development of glycogen depletion in the exercising muscle fibers.[15]

In addition to the type of CHO supplement, the amount and timing of CHO ingestion plays an important role in determining the effect of CHO ingestion on muscle glycogen utilization. Rate of gastric emptying can be increased by ingesting a large bolus (5–8 ml/kg bodyweight) of a CHO solution immediately before exercise and a subsequent ingestion of smaller volumes (2 ml/kg bodyweight) every 15–20 minutes thereafter. This pattern increases blood glucose and insulin levels during the first hour of exercise and muscle glycogen utilization is lowered.[27] CHO ingestion at a rate of 45 g/hour may therefore be required to produce changes in muscle glycogen utilization during constant intensity and intermittent exercise. The optimal rate of supplement will vary, however, depending on the type of exercise, intensity, duration and environmental conditions. A dose-response relationship between CHO supplement intake and improvement in exercise capacity does not seem to exist, and the relationship between the amount of CHO supplement intake, percent improvement in exercise capacity and extent of muscle glycogen utilization requires further study.

8.4 SUMMARY AND RESEARCH NEEDS

Glycogen is an important source of energy for exercises of various durations and intensities, but it is stored in limited amounts in the body. Depletion of muscle glycogen stores results in fatigue and reduces performance capacity. Therefore, CHO ingestion is critical in maintaining glycogen stores in the liver and muscle. During exercise, CHO supplements may improve performance capacity and training volume. A 5–10% CHO beverage consumed during exercise at a rate adequate to supply 30–70 g CHO/hour is recommended. For prolonged competitive events, it can prevent a decline in blood glucose and potentially conserve muscle glycogen.[5] Glycogen stores can be replenished most readily when CHO is consumed soon after the activity at the rate of at least 40–60 g/hour.

For resistance exercises, the ergogenic effects of CHO are less clear. Experimental evidence suggests two potential metabolic mechanisms that may explain the ergogenic effects of CHO ingestion during exercise: 1) During prolonged exercise, at a time when muscle glycogen contribution to energy metabolism is diminished, restoration of euglycemia and increased oxidation of blood glucose; and 2) Delay in muscle glycogen depletion and onset of fatigue by decreasing the rate of muscle glycogen utilization. Both mechanisms are influenced by the type and intensity of the exercise, amount, type and timing of CHO ingestion, pre-exercise nutrition, and training status of the individual. Table 8.3 summarizes the CHO recommendations for active individuals.[57] Based

Table 8.3   Summary of Recommendations on Carbohydrate Supplement Use By Athletes

For Recreational Athletes:

Consume a healthy diet (<30% fat, 10–12% protein and remainder from CHO)
During exercise, avoid dehydration consume fluids that may contain CHO

For Endurance Athletes:

For optimal training and enhanced performance, consume 500–600 g CHO (7–10 g CHO/kg
  bodyweight) of moderate to high glycemic foods or supplement foods with CHO beverages
During hours before endurance exercise, consume 4–5 g CHO/kg body weight three to four hours
  before exercise or consume up to 2 g CHO/kg body weight one to two hours before exercise
During endurance exercise, consume 0.1–0.2 g CHO/kg body weight per 15–20 min interval of a
  solution containing 5–10% CHO
During hours after endurance exercise, consume CHO immediately and at two hour intervals after
  exercise or consume as much as 1.2 g CHO/kg bodyweight every 15 minutes for four hours

For Sprint Athletes:

Consume 5–8 g CHO/kg body weight to maintain at least normal body CHO reserves
Ingest CHO-containing beverages during intermittent exercise such as soccer and ice hockey

Adapted from: Sherman, W.M., Carbohydrate supplements as potential modifiers of physical activity,
Abstract from NIH Workshop: The role of dietary supplements for physically active people
http://www.healthy.net/library/books/nihdietarysupplements/sherman.htm, Accessed 1/9/98.[57]

on the review of the available evidence and knowledge, the following recommendations are made
for future investigations:

1. Determine the ideal CHO consumption for endurance sports.
2. Develop a better understanding of the mechanism of the benefit of CHO consumption during exercise
    to make appropriate dietary recommendations.
3. Examine the effect of CHO beverages ingested just prior to performance on high-power exercise
    performance.
4. Determine the influence of CHO supplementation on resistance exercise performance and its mech-
    anism of action.
5. Examine the relationship between the amount of CHO consumed, percent improvement in exercise
    capacity, and extent of muscle glycogen utilization.
6. Examine the combined effects of liquid vs. solid CHO supplements on serum glucose and perfor-
    mance to maximize their beneficial effects.
7. Examine the synergistic effects of consumption of other ergogenic aids, such as MCT, amino acids,
    vitamins and minerals, in conjunction with CHO supplements on exercise performance.

ACKNOWLEDGMENT

The author would like to thank Dr. Christine Rosenbloom for reviewing the chapter and
providing useful feedback.

REFERENCES

1. Williams, M.H., Beyond Training. How Athletes Enhance Performance Legally and Illegally, Cham-
    paign, IL, *Human Kinetics*, 1989.
2. *Food and Nutrition Board, Commission of Life Sciences*, Recommended Dietary Allowances, 10th
    edition. National Research Council, Washington, D.C., 1989.

3. Wilson, J.W., Enns, C.W., Goldman, J.D., Tippett, K.S., Mickle, S.J., Cleveland, L.E., and Chahil, P.S., Data tables: Combined results from USDA's 1994 and 1995 Continuing Survey of Food Intake by Individuals and 1994 Diet and Health Knowledge Survey [Online]. ARS Food Surveys Research Group. Available (under "Releases"): <http://www/barc.usda.gov/bhnrc/foodsurvey/home.htm> Accessed 8/28/97.

4. McDowell, M.A., Briefel, R.R., Alaimo, K., Bischof, A.M., Caughman, C.R., Carroll, M.D., Loria, C.M., Johnson, C.L., Energy and macronutrient intakes of persons ages 2 months and over in the United States: Third National Health and Nutrition Examination Survey, Phase I, 1988-91, *Advance Data from Vital and Health Statistics*, No:255, National Center for Health Statistics, Hyattisville, MD, 1994.

5. Walberg-Rankin, J., Dietary carbohydrate as an ergogenic aid for prolonged and brief competitions in sport, *Intl. J. Sport Nutr.*, 5, S13, 1995.

6. American Dietetic Association. Timely statement of the American Dietetic Association: Nutrition guidance for adolescent athletes in organized sports, *J. Am. Diet. Assoc.*, 96, 611, 1996.

7. Costill, D. L., Carbohydrates for exercise: dietary demands for optimal performance, *Intl. J. Sports Med.*, 9, 1, 1988.

8. Walton, P. and Rhodes, E.C., Glycemic index and optimal performance, *Sports Med.*, 23, 164, 1997.

9. Coggan, A. R. and Swanson, S. C., Nutritional manipulation before and during endurance exercise: effects on performance, *Med. Sci. Sports Exerc.*, 24, S331, 1992.

10. Conley, M. S. and Stone, M. H., Carbohydrate ingestion/supplementation for resistance exercise and training, *Sports Med.*, 21, 7, 1996.

11. Burke, L. M. and Read, R. S. D., Dietary supplements in sport, *Sports Med.*, 15, 43, 1993.

12. Coggan, A. R. and Coyle, E. F., Effect of carbohydrate feedings during high-intensity exercise, *J. Appl. Physiol.*, 65, 1703, 1988.

13. Deuster, P.A., Kyle, S.B., Mosee, P.B., Vigersky, R.A., Singh, A., and Schoomaler, E.B., Nutritional intakes and status of highly trained amenorrheic and eumenorrheic female runners, *Fertil. Steril.*, 46, 636, 1986.

14. Maughan, R., Effects of diet composition on the performance of high intensity exercises, in *Nutrition and Sport* (Ed., Monod, H.), Masson, Paris, 200, 1990.

15. Tsintzas, K. and Williams, C., Human muscle glycogen metabolism during exercise: effect of carbohydrate supplementation, *Sports Med.*, 15, 7, 1998.

16. Murray, R., Paul, G.L., Seifert, J.G., Eddy, D.E., and Halaby, G.A., The effect of glucose, fructose and sucrose ingestion during exercise, *Med. Sci. Sports Exerc.*, 21, 275, 1989.

17. Rauch, H.G.L., Rodger, I., Wilson, G.R., Belonji, J.D., Dennis, S.C., Noakes, T.D., and Hawley, J.A., The effects of carbohydrate loading on muscle glycogen content and cycling performance, *Intl. J. Sport Nutr.*, 5, 25, 1995.

18. Anantaraman, R., Carmines, A. A., Gaesser, G. A., and Weltman, A., Effects of carbohydrate supplementation on performance during 1 hour of high-intensity exercise, *Intl. J. Sports Med.*, 16, 461, 1995.

19. Jeukendrup, A. E., Thielen, J. H. C., Wagenmakers, A. J. M., Brouns, F., and Saris, W. H. M., Effect of medium-chain triacylglycerol and carbohydrate ingestion during exercise on substrate utilization and subsequent cycling performance, *Am. J. Clin. Nutr.*, 67, 397, 1998.

20. Roy, B. D., Tarnopolsky, M. A., MacDougall, J. D., Fowles, J., and Yarasheski, K. E., Effect of glucose supplement timing on protein metabolism after resistance training, *J. Appl. Physiol.*, 82, 1882, 1997.

21. Robergs, R.A., McMinn, S.B., Mermier, C., Leadbetter III, G., Ruby, B., and Quinn, C., Blood glucose and glucoregulatory hormone responses to solid and liquid carbohydrate ingestion during exercise, *Intl. J. Sport Nutr.*, 8, 70, 1998.

22. Hawley, J. A., Palmer, G. S., and Noakes, T. D., Effects of 3 days of carbohydrate supplementation on muscle glycogen content and utilization during a 1-h cycling performance, *Eur. J. Appl. Physiol.*, 75, 407, 1997.

23. Fallowfield, J. L., and Williams, C., The influence of a high carbohydrate intake during recovery from prolonged, constant-pace running, *Intl. J. Sport Nutr.*, 7, 10, 1997.

24. Nicholas, C. W., Green, P. A., Hawkins, R. D., and Williams, C., Carbohydrate intake and recovery of intermittent running capacity, *Intl. J. Sport Nutr*, 7, 251, 1997.

25. Davis, L. M., Jackson, D. A., Broadwell, M. S., Queary, J. L., and Lambert, C. L., Carbohydrate drinks delay fatigue during intermittent, high-intensity cycling in active men and women, *Intl. J. Sport Nutr.*, 7, 261, 1997.

26. Ferrauti, A., Weber, K., and Struder, H.K., Metabolic and ergogenic effects of carbohydrate and caffeine beverages in tennis, *J. Sports Med. Phys. Fitness*, 37, 258, 1997.

27. Tsintzas, O-K., Williams, C., Wilson, W., and Burrin, J., Influence of carbohydrate supplementation early in exercise on endurance running capacity, *Med. Sci. Sports Exerc.*, 28, 1373, 1996.

28. Jeukendrup, A. E., Saris, W. H. M., Brouns, F., Halliday, D., and Wagenmakers, A. J. M., Effects of carbohydrate (CHO) and fat supplementation on CHO metabolism during prolonged exercise, *Metabolism*, 45, 915, 1996.

29. Ball, T. C., Headley, S. A., Vanderburgh, P. M., and Smith, J.C., Periodic carbohydrate replacement during 50 min of high-intensity cycling improves subsequent sprint performance, *Intl. J. Sport Nutr.*, 5, 151, 1995.

30. Swensen, T., Crater, G., Bassett, D. R., and Howley, E. T., Adding polylactate to a glucose polymer solution does not improve endurance, *Intl. J. Sports Med.*, 15, 430, 1994.

31. Jenkins, D. G., Palmer, J., and Spillman, D., The influence of dietary carbohydrate on performance of supramaximal intermittent exercise, *Eur. J. Appl. Physiol.*, 67, 309, 1993.

32. Cole, K. J., Grandjean, P. W., Sobszak, R. J., and Mitchell, J. B., Effect of carbohydrate composition on fluid balance, gastric emptying, and exercise performance, *Intl. J. Sport Nutr.*, 3, 408, 1993.

33. Mason, W.L., McConnell, G., and Hargreaves, M., Carbohydrate ingestion during exercise: Liquid vs. solid feedings, *Med. Sci. Sports Exerc.*, 25, 966, 1993.

34. Wagenmakers, A. J. M., Becker, E. J., Brouns, F., Kuipers, H., Soeters, P.B., Van Der Visse, G. J., and Saris, W. H. M., Carbohydrate supplement, glycogen depletion and amino acid metabolism during exercise, *Am. J. Physiol.*, 260, E883, 1991.

35. Leatt, P. B.,and Jacobs, I., Effect of glucose polymer ingestion on glycogen depletion during a soccer match, *Can. J. Sport Sci.*, 14, 112, 1989.

36. Reed, M.J., Bronzinick, J.T., Lee, M.C., and Ivy, J.L., Muscle glycogen storage post-exercise: Effect of mode of carbohydrate administration, *J. Appl. Physiol.*, 66, 720, 1989.

37. Mitchell, J. B., Costill, D. L., Houmard, J. A., Fink, W. J., Pascoe, D. D., and Pearson, D. R., Influence of carbohydrate dosage on exercise performance and glycogen metabolism, *J. Appl. Physiol.*, 67,1843, 1989.

38. Flynn, M. G., Michaud, T. J., Rodriguez-Zayas, J., Lambert, C. P., Boone, J. B., and Moleski, R. W., Effects of 4- and 8-h pre-exercise feedings on substrate use and performance, *J. Appl. Physiol.*, 67, 2066, 1989.

39. Brewer, J., Williams, C., and Patton, A., The influence of high carbohydrate diets on endurance running performance, *Eur. J. Appl. Physiol.*, 57, 698, 1988.

40. Ivy, J. L., Katz, A. L., Cutler, C. L., Sherman, W. M., Coyle, E. F., Muscle glycogen synthesis after exercise: effect of time of carbohydrate ingestion, *J. Appl. Physiol.*, 64,1480, 1988.

41. Hargreaves, M. and Briggs, C. A., Effect of carbohydrate ingestion on exercise metabolism, *J. Appl. Physiol.*, 65,1553, 1988.

42. Flynn, M. G., Costill, D. L., Hawley, J. A., Fink, W. J., Neufer, P. D., Fielding, R. A., and Sleeper, M. D., Influence of selected carbohydrate drinks on cycling performance and glycogen use, *Med. Sci. Sports Exerc.*, 19, 37, 1987.

43. Coyle, E. F., Coogan, A. R., Hemmert, M. K., and Ivy, J. L., Muscle glycogen utilization during prolonged strenuous exercise when fed carbohydrate, *J. Appl. Physiol.*, 61,165, 1986.

44. Fielding, R. A., Costill, D. L., Fink, W. J., King, D. S., Hargreaves, M., and Kovaleski, J. E., Effect of carbohydrate feeding frequencies and dosage on muscle glycogen use during exercise, *Med. Sci. Sports Exerc.*, 17, 472, 1985.

45. Hargreaves, M., Costill, D. L., Coggan, A., Fink, W. J., and Nishibata, I., Effect of carbohydrate feedings on muscle glycogen utilization and exercise performance, *Med. Sci. Sports Exerc.*, 16, 219, 1984.

46. American College of Sports Medicine. Position Statement: Exercise and fluid replacement, *Med. Sci. Sports Exerc.*, 28, I, 1996.

47. Coyle, E. F. and Montain, S. J., Benefits of fluid replacement with carbohydrate during exercise, *Med. Sci. Sports Exerc.*, 24, S324, 1992.

48. Neufer, P. D., Costill, D. L., Fink, W. J., Kirwan, J. P., Fielding, R. A., and Flynn, M. G., Effects of exercise and carbohydrate composition on gastric emptying, *Med. Sci. Sports Exerc.*, 18, 658, 1986.

49. Davis, J. M., Burgess, W. A., Slentz, C. A., and Bartole, W. P., Fluid availability of sports drinks differing in carbohydrate type and concentration, *Am. J. Clin. Nutr.*, 51, 1054, 1990.

50. Lambert, C.P., Flynn, M.G., Boone, J.B., Michaud, T. J., and Rodriguez-Zaya, J., Effects of carbohydrate feeding on multiple-bout resistance exercise. *J. Appl. Sports Sci. Res.*, 5, 192, 1991.

51. Conley, M. S., Stone, M. H., Marsit, J. L., O'Bryant, H. S., Nieman, D. C., Johnson, R. L., Butterworth, D., and Keith, R., Effects of carbohydrate ingestion on resistance exercise, *J. Strength Condition. Res.*, 9, 201, 1995.

52. Vincent, K. R., Clarkson, P. M., Freedson, P. S., DeCheke, M., Effect of a pre-exercise liquid, high carbohydrate feeding on resistance exercise performance, *Med. Sci. Sports Exerc.*, 25, S194, 1993.

53. Fahey, T. D., Larsen, J. D., Brooks, G. A., Colvin, W., Henderson, S., and Lay, D., The effect of ingesting polylactate or glucose polymer drinks during prolonged exercise, *Intl. J. Sport Nutr.*, 1, 249, 1991.

54. Sasaki, H., Maeda, J., Usui, S., and Ishiko, T., Effect of sucrose and caffeine ingestion on performance of prolonged strenuous running, *Intl. J. Sport Med.*, 8, 261, 1987.

55. Riley, M. L., Israel, R. G., and Holbert, D., Effect of carbohydrate ingestion on exercise endurance and metabolism after 1-day fast, *Intl. J. Sport Med.*, 9, 320, 1988.

56. Wilber, R. L., and Moffat, R. J., Influence of carbohydrate ingestion on blood glucose and performance in runners, *Intl. J. Sports Nutr.*, 2, 317, 1992.

57. Sherman WM, Carbohydrate supplements as potential modifiers of physical activity, Abstract from NIH Workshop: The role of dietary supplements for physically active people <http://www.healthy.net/library/books/nihdietarysupplements/sherman.htm>, Accessed 1/9/98.

CHAPTER 9

Lipid Supplements in Exercise and Sports

Timothy P. Carr and Russell L. Cowles

CONTENTS

9.1 INTRODUCTION

Lipid supplementation as a means of enhancing exercise performance has received limited attention in the scientific community. Although much is known about the utilization of lipids as an energy source during exercise (as discussed in Chapter 6), information regarding the consumption of lipid supplements as an adjunct to diet is sparse and inconclusive. The majority of studies conducted focus on the use of the so-called medium-chain triglycerides (MCTs) as an ergogenic aid, although supplementation with omega-3 fatty acids and other long-chain fatty acids has also been reported. This chapter reviews the current scientific literature examining the effectiveness and safety of using lipid supplements to enhance exercise performance.

9.2 TYPES AND FUNCTION OF LIPID SUPPLEMENTS

MCTs are structurally similar to naturally-occurring triglycerides except that the esterified fatty acids are limited to those containing 6–12 carbons. MCTs are manufactured by a commercial process utilizing medium-chain fatty acids hydrolyzed and fractionated from kernel oils, such as coconut and palm kernel oil. The traditional fractionation process is based on distillation and isolates primarily caproic (C6:0), caprylic (C8:0), and capric acid (C10:0), although some "contamination" of lauric acid (C12:0) occurs.[1] The isolated medium-chain fatty acids are then randomly esterified to glycerol to form MCTs. Consequently, the approximate percentage of the fatty acids in MCT will reflect the quantity and distribution of medium-chain fatty acids fractionated from the original oil. When coconut oil is used, the typical fatty acid distribution in MCT is 1–2% caproic, 65–75% caprylic, 25–35% capric, and 1–2% lauric acid.[1] Alternatively, specific medium-chain fatty acids may be further purified and esterified to glycerol to produce MCTs containing a single fatty acid (e.g., tricaprylin).

Application of MCTs in human nutrition was first introduced in the 1950s for the treatment of disorders related to lipid absorption. Because of their increased solubility in biological fluids, MCTs facilitate the action of pancreatic lipase so that the fatty acids are hydrolyzed faster and more completely than triglycerides containing long-chain fatty acids.[2] Medium-chain fatty acids do not require bile salts for absorption, nor are they re-esterified to glycerol in the intestinal cell, as are long-chain fatty acids.[3] Consequently, most medium-chain fatty acids are absorbed directly into the hepatic circulation, making them a more immediate fuel source compared with long-chain fatty acids. The purported benefit of MCT supplementation in exercise performance is therefore based on the ability of medium-chain fatty acids to be absorbed directly to the liver for oxidation. It should be noted that if a benefit is to be realized, MCT must be ingested as a supplement to diet because medium-chain fatty acids do not exist in a concentrated form independent of long-chain fatty acids in the natural food supply.

In the liver, medium-chain fatty acids rapidly cross the mitochondrial membranes where they undergo β-oxidation to form acetyl-CoA. Some of the acetyl-CoA can be used to synthesize long-chain fatty acids, although most is converted to ketone bodies and delivered to peripheral tissues where they can serve as an immediate energy source.[2] Unlike long-chain fatty acids, medium-chain fatty acids can migrate into the mitochondrial matrix in the absence of carnitine.[4] MCT supplements also stimulate insulin release in a manner similar to glucose, although the specific mechanism of action on the pancreas is uncertain.[2] In this way, the metabolic function of ingested MCT is more reflective of dietary carbohydrate than native triglycerides.

Ingestion of omega-3 fatty acids has also been examined as an ergogenic aid. The rationale for omega-3 fatty acid supplementation is based on observations that the deformability of red blood cells decreases during exercise,[5,6] possibly impeding blood flow and delivery of oxygen to the muscles. Incorporation of omega-3 fatty acids into membranes is thought to increase deformability of red blood cells,[7,8] thereby enhancing oxygen transport and possibly improving exercise performance. Omega-3 fatty acid supplementation is generally achieved by ingesting fish oil capsules, as certain fish oils are rich sources of eicosapentaenoic acid (C20:5) and docosahexaenoic acid (C22:6). Increased intake of omega-3 fatty acids can also be achieved by eating more fish, although this type of dietary modification would not be considered lipid supplementation.

9.3 LIPID SUPPLEMENTS AND EXERCISE PERFORMANCE

Several laboratories have examined the usefulness of MCT in exercise performance. These studies are summarized in Table 9.1. Each laboratory used different methods to document performance outcomes and to administer MCT supplements. All of the studies were conducted in young males who were either trained or non-trained.

Jeukendrup and colleagues[9–12] recently published a series of studies in trained athletes given MCTs (as tricaprylin) in carbohydrate-based supplements before and during exercise. In three of their studies,[9–11] subjects received 29 g of MCT in a glucose polymer drink and exercised at 57–70% $\dot{V}O_{2\,max}$. A consistent finding in these experiments (conducted under similar conditions) was an increase in plasma β-hydroxybutyrate, indicating an increase in ketone body production. The authors concluded that although oral MCT could serve as an additional energy source during exercise, the contribution of MCT to total energy expenditure was small and MCT did not significantly influence carbohydrate utilization or glycogen breakdown.[9–11] In a fourth study, Jeukendrup et al.[12] showed that high MCT supplementation (85 g) also resulted in elevated plasma β-hydroxybutyrate. A time trial was included in this study to measure performance gains resulting from high MCT intake. The study demonstrated that large amounts of MCT ingested during prolonged exercise provoked gastrointestinal problems and lead to decreased exercise performance.[12]

Table 9.1 Summary of Research Articles Addressing MCT Supplementation and Exercise Performance

Reference	Date	Subjects	Number of Subjects	Age, Mean (range)	Type of MCT	Delivery of MCT	Total Supplement Consumed	Pattern of Intake	Type of Exercise	Major Outcomes
Jeukendrup et al.[9]	1995	Male, trained	8	28.8	Tricaprylin	Glucose polymer drink	1) 214 g CHO 2) 149 g CHO, plus 29 g MCT 3) 214 g CHO, plus 29 g MCT	Given before exercise and every 20 minutes	Cycling at 57% $\dot{V}O_{2\,max}$ for three hours	MCTs increase β-hydroxybutyrate MCT 3–7% total energy expenditure
Jeukendrup et al.[10]	1996	Male, trained	8	28.9	Tricaprylin	Glucose polymer drink	Same as above	Same as above	Cycling at 70% $\dot{V}O_{2\,max}$ for three hours	MCTs increase β-hydroxybutyrate Low CHO intake does not increase MCT oxidation
Jeukendrup et al.[11]	1996	Male, trained	9	26	Tricaprylin	Glucose polymer drink	1) 214 g CHO 2) 149 g CHO, plus 29 g MCT	Same as above	Cycling at 65% $\dot{V}O_{2\,max}$ for three hours	MCTs increase β-hydroxybutyrate MCTs do not affect CHO utilization or glycogen breakdown
Jeukendrup et al.[12]	1998	Male, trained	7	Not reported	Tricaprylin	Glucose polymer drink	1) 170 g CHO 2) 170 g CHO, plus 85 g MCT 3) 85 g MCT	Given before exercise and every 15 minutes	Cycling at 60% $\dot{V}O_{2\,max}$ for two hours, plus time trial	MCTs increase β-hydroxybutyrate High MCT supplements cause GI distress and decrease exercise performance
Massicotte et al.[13]	1992	Male, non-trained	6	22.8	Tricaprylin	Hot drink, undefined	1) Water 2) 25 g MCT 3) 57 g CHO	Single dose before exercise	Cycling at 61% $\dot{V}O_{2\,max}$ for two hours	MCTs increase epinephrine release similarly to CHO MCTs do not affect CHO utilization

continued

Table 9.1 (continued) Summary of Research Articles Addressing MCT Supplementation and Exercise Performance

Reference	Date	Subjects	Number of Subjects	Age, Mean (range)	Type of MCT	Delivery of MCT	Total Supplement Consumed	Pattern of Intake	Type of Exercise	Major Outcomes
Decombaz et al.[14]	1983	Male, non-trained	12	(17–19)	Undefined	Instant coffee drink, decaffeinated	1) 25 g MCT 2) 50 g CHO	Single dose before exercise	Cycling at 60% $VO_{2\,max}$ for one hour	MCTs increase ketone bodies CHO incresases insulin and lactate
Ivy et al.[15]	1980	Male, trained	10	22.8	Undefined	Mixed with cereal and skim milk	1) 30 g MCT 2) 30 g LCT	Single dose before exercise	Cycling or treadmill at 70% $VO_{2\,max}$ for one hour	MCTs increase β-hydroxybutyrate LCTs increase triglycerides
Van Zyl et al.[16]	1996	Male, trained	6	20	Undefined	Glucose polymer drink	1) 200 g CHO 2) 86 g MCT 3) 200g CHO, plus 86 g MCT	Given after warm-up and every ten minutes	Cycling at 60% $VO_{2\,max}$ for two hours, plus time trial	MCTs increase β-hydroxybutyrate MCTs only decrease performance MCT/CHO combination increases performance

The four studies of Jeukendrup and colleagues[9–12] provide important information regarding the metabolism of MCT in the body under exercise conditions. In exercise bouts lasting three hours, it was demonstrated that MCT utilization was not dependent on muscle glycogen stores,[11] suggesting MCT metabolism was independent of carbohydrate usage. The data also indicate that MCT supplementation in excess of 29 g may be detrimental to exercise performance.

Massicotte et al.[13] tested the effect of MCT supplementation in non-trained males, in contrast to the previous studies. The research protocol also differed from the studies of Jeukendrup and colleagues because the subjects were given 25 g of MCT or 57 g carbohydrate as single doses one hour prior to exercise. The rationale for providing the nutrients prior to exercise was to allow adequate time for the lipid to be fully absorbed and available for use as energy. The study was designed to examine the change in oxidation of exogenous macronutrients and to measure hormonal changes. Results from the study verified Jeukendrup's observation that MCT ingestion increases plasma β-hydroxybutyrate. In addition, both carbohydrate and MCT ingestion slowed the usual decrease in insulin, reduced the rise of glucagon, and inhibited epinephrine release normally seen during prolonged exercise.[13]

Decombaz et al.[14] administered MCT and carbohydrate (maltodextrin) in separate trials to non-trained males one hour prior to exercise. Consistent with other reports, these investigators documented an increase in plasma β-hydroxybutyrate with MCT supplementation. Carbohydrate supplementation resulted in insulin release and elevated lactate in muscle. Neither the MCT nor carbohydrate supplement altered the utilization of glycogen stores during exercise. In both treatment groups, glycogen stores were utilized at a similar rate. Consistent with other research,[11] the data of Decombaz et al.[14] suggest that MCT supplementation does not necessarily spare glycogen during exercise.

Ivy et al.[15] reported a study using well-trained male athletes who ingested MCT and long-chain triglycerides (LCT) mixed with cereal and skim milk. The subjects received supplements prior to exercise and were required to cycle or run on a treadmill at 70% $\dot{V}O_{2\,max}$ for one hour. In a preliminary experiment, the subjects ate various amounts of MCT to select a level that would be easily tolerated and absorbed. Subjects who consumed 50–60 g of MCT suffered abdominal cramping and diarrhea. Therefore, the investigators selected a 30 g dose for the primary study. MCT supplementation resulted in higher serum ketone levels, while LCT ingestion caused a predictable increase in serum triglycerides. In both cases, the respiratory exchange ratio ($VCO_2/\dot{V}O_2$) was similar during exercise. When given in combination with carbohydrate (i.e., cereal meal), the authors concluded that neither MCT nor LCT was a significant energy source during prolonged exercise.[15]

In contrast to the previously discussed research regarding MCT supplementation, Van Zyl et al.[16] reported that ingestion of MCT before and during exercise reduced oxidation of muscle glycogen. The study involved six endurance-trained cyclists who received MCT alone (86 g) or with carbohydrate. The subjects were required to cycle for two hours and then were asked to complete a 40-km time trial. Similar to the work of Jeukendrup and co-workers,[12] Van Zyl et al.[16] noted that MCT-only supplementation resulted in a marked reduction in performance, possibly due to gastrointestinal problems. In contrast, subjects who consumed MCT supplements with carbohydrate completed the 40-km time test with faster times. Muscle lactate levels were decreased when subjects ingested the MCT/carbohydrate mixture. Therefore, it was concluded that a glycogen-sparing effect could be achieved when the subject took high amounts of MCT supplements with carbohydrate during exercise.[16]

Supplementation with omega-3 fatty acids has also been examined, although much less extensively than MCT. Leaf and Rauch[17] reported in 1988 that supplementation with 6 g of fish oil per day increased $\dot{V}O_{2\,max}$ based on treadmill performance, although increasing supplementation to 12 g per day did not further improve performance. In contrast, more-recent studies have been unable to document enhanced performance with fish oil supplementation. Oostenbrug et al.[18] gave 6 g fish oil daily for three weeks to eight well-trained male cyclists, while eight other cyclists received a placebo supplement. Exercise performance was monitored using an endurance test on a cycle ergometer. No difference in exercise performance was observed between the groups.[18] In another recent study, Raastad et al.[19] provided 5.2 g fish oil per day to 15 male soccer players for ten weeks, while 13 soccer players received 5.2 g corn oil per day. These investigators were also unable to detect an effect of fish oil supplementation on exercise performance despite significant increases in plasma concentration of eicosapentaenoic and docosahexaenoic acid. Because of the lack of research examining supplemental omega-3 fatty acids, it is still uncertain how these acids affect exercise performance.

9.4 SUMMARY AND RECOMMENDATIONS

The search for ergogenic aids to enhance exercise performance has led investigators to examine lipid supplements, particularly MCTs. Due to their solubility in biological fluids, the digestion, absorption, and oxidation of MCT is more reflective of carbohydrates than naturally occurring triglycerides. The major rationale for focusing on MCTs in prolonged exercise is the hope that MCTs might act to spare muscle glycogen more efficiently than supplemental carbohydrate. MCT supplements have been shown to decrease muscle lactate acumulaton during exercise, to decrease catecholamine secretion, and to promote ketogenesis. Each metabolic response could conceivably enhance exercise performance. However, the bulk of the evidence suggests that MCTs are at best equal to dietary carbohydrate in their ability to be used as an energy source. In general, exogenous carbohydrate and MCT supplements produced similar results with regard to their oxidizability; both fuel sources are about 50% oxidized during exercise and appear to contribute up to 10% of total energy used. Whether MCTs spare muscle glycogen during prolonged exercise is still uncertain and appears to depend on the amount of MCT ingested. A major disadvantage of MCT supplementation is that high amounts exceeding about 30 g during an exercise bout can provoke gastrointestinal problems, thus decreasing exercise performance.

The ability of omega-3 fatty acids to enhance exercise performance has also been examined, although their purported mechanism of action is quite different than that for MCTs. Omega-3 and other long-chain fatty acids are much more lipophilic and are absorbed via the lymph chylomicron system. Long-term supplementation of omega-3 fatty acids is thought to increase the deformability of red blood cells and, therefore, their oxygen-carrying capacity. Although supplementation with omega-3 fatty acids produces elevated plasma omega-3 fatty acids, enhanced exercise performance has not been clearly demonstrated. A disadvantage of omega-3 fatty acid supplementation is that, unlike MCTs, they require several weeks of ingestion to elicit metabolic changes that could possibly increase the oxygen-carrying capacity of red blood cells.

Based on the available research, it is questionable how effective lipid supplementation in the form of MCTs or omega-3 fatty acids is on exercise performance. Omega-3 fatty acid supplementation does not appear to be harmful at moderate doses, but supplemental MCT can cause abdominal cramping and diarrhea. More research is needed before MCT use can be declared a safe and effective means of enhancing exercise performance.

REFERENCES

1. Babayan, V.K., Medium-chain triglycerides – their composition, preparation, and application, *J. Am. Oil Chem. Soc.*, 45, 23, 1968.
2. Bach, A.C. and Babayan, V.K., Medium-chain triglycerides: an update, *Am. J. Clin. Nutr.*, 36, 950, 1982.
3. Bell, S.J., Bradley, D., Forse, R.A., and Bistrian, B.R., The new dietary fats in health and disease, *J. Am. Diet. Assoc.*, 97, 280, 1997.
4. Bremer, J., Carnitine and its role in fatty acid metabolism, *Trends Biochem. Sci.*, 2, 207, 1980.

5. Galea, G. and Davidson, R.J.L., Hemorrheology of marathon running, *Int. J. Sports Med.*, 6, 136, 1985.
6. Van der Brug, G.E., Peters, H.P.F., Hardeman, M.R., Schep, G., and Mosterd, W.L., Hemorheological response to prolonged exercise; no effects of different kinds of feedings, *Int. J. Sports Med.*, 16, 231, 1995.
7. Terano, T., Hirai, A., Hamazaki, T., Kobayashi, S., Fujita, T., Tamura, Y., and Kumagai, A., Effect of oral administration of highly purified eicosapentaenoic acid on platelet function, blood viscosity and red cell deformability in healthy human subjects, *Atherosclerosis*, 46, 321, 1983.
8. Cartwright, I.J., Pockley, A.G., Galloway, J.H., Greaves, M., and Preston, F.E., The effects of dietary ω-3 polyunsaturated fatty acids on erythrocyte membrane phospholipids, erythrocytes deformability and blood viscosity in healthy volunteers, *Atherosclerosis*, 55, 267, 1985.
9. Jeukendrup, A.E., Saris, W.H.M., Schrauwen, P., Brouns, F., and Wagenmakers, A.J.M., Metabolic availability of medium-chain triglycerides coingested with carbohydrates during prolonged exercise, *J. Appl. Physiol.*, 79, 756, 1995.
10. Jeukendrup, A.E., Saris, W.H.M., Van Diesen, R., Brouns, F., and Wagenmakers, A.J.M., Effect of endogenous carbohydrate availability on oral medium-chain triglyceride oxidation during prolonged exercise, *J. Appl. Physiol.*, 80, 949, 1996.
11. Jeukendrup, A.E., Saris, W.H.M., Brouns, F., Halliday, D., and Wagenmakers, A.J.M., Effect of carbohydrate (CHO) and fat supplementation on CHO metabolism during prolonged exercise, *Metabolism*, 45, 915, 1996.
12. Jeukendrup, A.E., Thielen, J.J.H.C., Wagenmakers, A.J.M., Brouns, F., and Saris, W.H.M., Effect of medium-chain triacylglycerol and carbohydrate ingestion during exercise on substrate utilization and subsequent cycling performance, *Am. J. Clin. Nutr.*, 67, 397, 1998.
13. Massicotte, D., Peronnet, F., Brisson, G.R., and Hillaire-Marcel, C., Oxidation of exogenous medium-chain free fatty acids during prolonged exercise: comparison with glucose, *J. Appl. Physiol.*, 73, 1334, 1992.
14. Decombaz, J., Arnaud, M.-J., Milon, H., Moesch, H., Philippossian, G., Thelin, A.-L., and Howald, H., Energy metabolism of medium-chain triglycerides versus carbohydrates during exercise, *Eur. J. Appl. Physiol.*, 52, 9, 1983.
15. Ivy, J.L., Costill, D.L., Fink, W.J., and Maglischo, E., Contribution of medium and long chain triglyceride intake to energy metabolism during prolonged exercise, *Int. J. Sports Med.*, 1, 15, 1980.
16. Van Zyl, C.G., Lambert, E.V., Hawley, J.A., Noakes, T.D., and Dennis, S.C., Effects of medium-chain triglyceride ingestion on fuel metabolism and cycling performance, *J. Appl. Physiol.*, 80, 2217, 1996.
17. Leaf, D.A. and Rauch, C.R., Omega-3 supplementation and estimated $\dot{V}O_{2\,max}$: a double blind randomized controlled trial in athletes, *Ann. Sport Med.*, 4, 37, 1988.
18. Oostenbrug, G.S., Mensink, R.P., Hardeman, M.R., De Vries, T., Brouns, F., and Hornstra, G., Exercise performance, red blood cell deformability, and lipid peroxidation: effects of fish oil and vitamin E, *J. Appl. Physiol.*, 83, 746, 1997.
19. Raastad, T., Hstmark, A.T., and Strmme, S.B., Omega-3 fatty acid supplementation does not improve maximal aerobic power, anaerobic threshold and running performance in well-trained soccer players, *Scand. J. Med. Sci. Sports*, 7, 25, 1997.

CHAPTER 10

Protein and Amino Acid Supplements in Exercise and Sport

Luke R. Bucci and Lisa Unlu

CONTENTS

10.1 INTRODUCTION

This chapter will familiarize readers with the predominant proteins that are utilized as dietary supplements for sports nutrition applications. Unlike other reviews on protein and exercise, this chapter will present practical information on characteristics of commercially available proteins, distinguishing why certain proteins are attractive to physically active consumers, and provide a cost analysis of commercially available protein sources and dietary supplements. Trends in the dietary supplement industry will also be illustrated. Effects of protein supplements in physically active individuals will be only briefly presented. Guidelines for reasonable use of protein supplements for physical activities will be listed. Fruitful areas for future research will also be pinpointed. Protein requirements and metabolism during exercise are covered in another chapter in this book[1] and several other recent reviews[2-6] and will not be discussed in this chapter.

Historically, strength athletes and weightlifters have always consumed a lot of protein.[3,7,8] A recent review of nutrient intakes of body builders found that typical protein intakes were almost 200 g for competitive male bodybuilders (three times the Recommended Daily Allowance [RDA] for protein) and 100 g for female bodybuilders (twice the RDA for protein).[3] A survey of supplement use in high school athletes in 1984 found that 22% consumed protein drinks, 9% consumed amino acid supplements, and 17% consumed either weight-gain or weight-loss products (which contain high levels of protein).[8] Thus, several (between 22 and 48%) high school athletes consume dietary supplements to increase protein intake. This and other findings reviewed in 1998 by Bazzarre[3] and Marquardt, et al.[8] indicate that protein supplementation has been, and is, widespread in athletes trying to increase muscular strength and body mass. Thus, protein supplements remain an area of interest for consumers and dietary supplement providers.

10.1.1 Rationale for Protein Supplements

Protein supplements have proliferated because they fill a need for consumers. The primary reasons why people use protein supplements instead of simply eating more protein-rich foods are most likely simplicity, convenience, and lack of concomitant fat intake. Protein supplements also make possible the manufacture of meal replacements with specific macronutrient and micronutrient compositions to facilitate muscle gain, muscle maintenance, and weight loss (body fat loss). The widespread availability of meal replacements as diet aids owes much to technologies fostered by the demand for protein supplements.

10.1.2 Increased Requirements for Dietary Protein Intake With Exercise

Recent reviews on protein requirements in exercising individuals have generally agreed upon an increased requirement over the RDA.[2-6] The current RDA of 0.8 g/kg/d was based on needs of sedentary subjects. However, much research has shown that to maintain nitrogen balance and prevent a predominance of amino acid oxidation, both endurance and strength exercise increase protein requirements past the current RDA.[2-6] Currently, endurance athletes require 1.0–1.4 g/kg/d, while strength athletes require 1.4–1.8 g/kg/d to achieve nitrogen balance. In extreme cases of exercise stress, short-term (lasting about one to two weeks) protein requirements may be between 2.0–3.0 g/kg/d.

10.1.3 Consumer Awareness of Increased Protein Needs

The increased need for protein intake for exercising individuals is well-known by both recreational and student athletes,[3,8] who usually show greater nutrition knowledge than sedentary subjects on surveys. Media (books and magazines) was a primary source of nutrition information for exercising individuals, indicating that exercising individuals keep abreast of the latest information concerning protein requirements as well as being exposed to advertisements for protein supplements. Thus, exercising individuals understand that they need more dietary protein and at the same time want to preserve leanness or reduce body fat. This drives individuals to seek low-fat sources of dietary protein. Protein supplements offer a convenient source of low-fat, high-quality protein, which is a major reason why protein supplements have become popular.

A survey of *Muscle & Fitness*, the leading (by paid circulation) popular magazine (January 1998 issue) devoted to exercise, found that 29 out of 54 (53.7%) advertisements for dietary supplements were devoted to protein supplements or weight gain/meal replacement products.[9] *Flex*, a leading magazine targeted at bodybuilders had 35 out of 65 (53.8%) dietary supplement advertisements with protein.[10] Survey of *Bicycling*, *Runner's World*, *Running Times*, and *Triathlete* showed a combined total of 18 advertisements for dietary supplements.[11] Only 4 out of 18 (22.2%) advertisements were for a protein product, but including meal replacements (bars) increased protein-containing supplement advertisements to 11 (61.1%). Thus, protein supplements are a major emphasis in dietary supplements targeted toward strength athletes, and a majority of the supplement advertisements found in endurance athlete magazines were for protein-containing products.

10.1.4 Protein Supplements — Advantages Over Foodstuffs

Protein supplements have advantages over foodstuffs for exercising individuals, as listed in Table 10.1. These claimed advantages seem to outweigh the perceived disadvantage of higher cost compared with foodstuffs for consumers of protein supplements.

Table 10.1 Advantages of Protein Supplements Over Foodstuffs

1. Convenient and flexible preparation (no cooking necessary)
2. No or very low-fat (replace fat-containing, high-protein foodstuffs)
3. Storage (no refrigeration needed)
4. Shelf life and stability (better transportability)
5. Simplicity: As a component of meal replacements/weight gain products, dietary manipulations of protein, carbohydrate, and fat caloric intakes are easier
6. Keeping track of caloric intake and calories from protein, carbohydrate, and fat is easier
7. Comparable or lower cost than many (but not all) high-protein foodstuffs
8. Placebo effect (knowledge that one is helping one's self and taking control may lead to stimulation of mental placebo effects)
9. Additional source of calories with poor potential for conversion to body fat if excess is consumed (compared to excess fat or carbohydrate calories)
10. Hormonal changes after ingestion of protein are anticatabolic and/or anabolic compared with carbohydrates or fat
11. Addition of other micronutrients (for meal replacements and weight gain products) enhances food value of protein supplements over foodstuffs
12. Taste may be more acceptable to some individuals, especially if other foodstuffs can be added to protein products (e.g., protein powder smoothies with fruit)
13. Much less chance of food-borne microbial contamination.

Upon closer examination, protein powders can be a similar or more cost-effective source of protein per dollar than vegetables, grains, nuts, cheeses, fish, and most beef when discounted protein powder products are purchased (Table 10.2).[12] Meal-replacement products, weight-gain products,

Table 10.2 Cost Comparisons of Protein Sources

Foodstuff[a]	Approx. \$/kg[b]	g protein/\$1.00
Beef, ground	4.38	46
Beef, round steak	7.25	42
Pork chops	6.59	32
Fresh fish filets	8.79	27
Tuna, canned	6.63	35
Chicken breasts (skinless, boneless)	7.69	30
Turkey breast	5.48	38
Nonfat milk	0.66	48
Nonfat powdered milk	6.87	51
Cheddar cheese	7.69	33
Whole eggs	1.58	76
Egg substitute	4.55	24
Tofu	3.25	34
Peanut butter	4.14	53
Pinto beans	1.64	119
Rice	3.18	26
Pasta (wheat flour)	2.94	43
Raisin Bran cereal	4.97	20
Meal replacement powders (n=10)[c]	21–34	17d (10–24)[e] (12–48)[f]
High protein bars (n=6)[g]	20–25	13 (8–17) (10–34)
Sports bars (n=6)[h]	18–22	8 (5.5–10) (7–20)
Weight gain products (n=16)[i]	10–17	16 (8–28) (10–56)
Milk/egg protein powders (n=4)[j]	25–29	22 (19–26) (24–52)
Whey protein powders (n=19)[k]	30–40	20 (9–45) (11–90)
Whey protein isolate powders, ion-exchange (IEW)sources (n=5)[m]	40–50	20 (14–24) (18–48)
Whey protein isolate powders, cross-flow microfiltered sources (n=5)[n]	40–55	19 (15–23) (19–46)
Soy protein powders (n=3)[o]	27	31 (29–33) (38–62)

a Foodstuffs were sampled from local grocery stores in Salt Lake City, UT in 1998.

b Prices/kg refer to retail pricing for foodstuffs and protein supplements. Foodstuff pricing was from local grocery stores in Salt Lake City, UT in 1998, and protein supplement prices (both suggested retail prices and discount prices) were obtained from Nutrition Express and Power System mail order catalogs from 1997/1998. These values are intended for comparative purposes only, and they will fluctuate continuously, depending upon purchase amount, crop conditions, market conditions, and availability.

c Meal replacement powders typically contain protein, carbohydrates, little or no fat, and vitamin/mineral mixtures, sometimes with additional nutrients such as amino acids or herbs. Meal replacement products typically contained proprietary blends of milk, whey, and egg protein blends.

d An average retail cost/kg from the indicated number of products.

e Values in the first set of parentheses refer to the range of suggested retail prices from the indicated number of products.

f Values in the second set of parentheses refer to the range of discounted prices from the indicated number of products (typically 20–50% of suggested retail prices) available from sales pricing, discount mass merchandisers, mail order catalogues and internet ordering sources.

g High-protein sports bars typically contain 20–30 g protein/bar from mixtures of soy, milk, whey, and egg sources, along with carbohydrates and other nutrients.

h Sports bars typically contain 5–20 g protein/bar from soy, milk, whey and egg sources, along with carbohydrates and other nutrients.

i Weight-gain products typically contain protein (20–200 g per serving) from mixtures of whey and/or milk sources, along with carbohydrates, vitamins, minerals and other nutrients. Some products contain less carbohydrate than protein calories, and some contain two to five times more carbohydrate calories than protein calories. These products contain little or no fat.

Table 10.2 (continued) Cost Comparisons of Protein Sources

j Milk and egg protein powders typically contain mixtures of various grades of milk, whey, casein, and egg protein sources (16–55 g per serving), along with little or no carbohydrates and fat. Additional nutrients, other than flavorings, are seldom added.

k Whey protein powders contain a wide variety of protein purities (34 to more than 93%) based on the raw material source, accounting for the large variation in pricing. Sources can range from whey powder (33% protein or less) to different grades of whey protein concentrates (34–85%) to whey protein isolates (more than 90%), and various mixtures of each of these sources. Typically, 15–55 g protein per serving is suggested, and additional nutrients (other than flavoroings) are seldom added.

l Ion-exchange whey protein isolates are generally acknowledged as the highest-quality protein sources. These products usually contain flavoring and few, if any, additional nutrients.

m Cross-flow microfiltered whey protein isolates are also acknowledged as the highest quality protein sources. These products usually contain flavoring and few, if any, additional nutrients.

n Soy protein isolate products typically contain flavoring and few, if any, additional nutrients.

sports bars, and protein powders purchased at suggested retail prices are less cost-effective than foodstuffs (Table 10.2). However, the higher cost of protein from meal-replacement products and sports bars reflects the additional carbohydrates and other nutrients in the product rather than a greater expense for protein. Except for nonfat powdered milk and some egg substitutes, the foods that cost less than protein powders contain considerable quantities of fat or carbohydrates, which contribute to undesirable intake of excess calories for athletes wishing to maintain or reduce body fat levels (such as body builders, cyclists, long-distance runners, triathletes, gymnasts, wrestlers, and most recreational athletes). Powdered milk contains considerable amounts of lactose, which may cause gastrointestinal disturbances in many individuals.

For the cost of one or two restaurant dinners or a week's supply of inexpensive meats ($20), an individual can consume approximately 50 g per day of supplemental protein for at least an entire month from protein powder.[12] The variation in cost of protein supplements is large and depends primarily on two factors: 1) protein source and 2) retail vs. discount pricing. Clearly, exercising individuals view protein powders as a cost-effective, convenient, and safe source of dietary protein. When protein powders are purchased at discount prices, they are frequently more cost-effective than foodstuffs as a dietary protein source, a distinct advantage over foodstuffs.

10.2 PROTEIN SUPPLEMENTS

Recent advancements in extraction and purification of proteins from various sources have made relatively pure proteins available at affordable prices. These advancements have removed most of the consumer objections to palatability and organoleptic properties that labeled early protein supplements as foul tasting and unfriendly to gastrointestinal tracts. As a result, competition in the market place has led to an enormous variety of protein supplements, exemplified by the supplement product types listed in Table 10.3. Three major protein sources are used in protein supplements: 1) milk, 2) egg, and 3) soy.

Most commercially available proteins are purified by similar means. Ultrafiltration of a solution containing protein, salts, carbohydrates, and fats (usually as micelles) through filter membranes with pore sizes larger than 0.1 μm retains fat micelles, leaving protein, carbohydrates and salts. Ultrafiltration through membranes with molecular weight cutoff of 5000 daltons retains proteins and removes salts, carbohydrates, and other small molecules. Diafiltration pumps distill water through the membrane to further remove small molecules, and increase protein concentration. Drying can be accomplished by a variety of methods, including evaporation and spray drying. Isolation of protein from food sources requires a large investment in large pieces of equipment.

Table 10.3 Protein Supplement Types

Protein powders (containing protein varying in purity from 34% to almost 100%)

Meal replacement powders, bars, or drinks (containing protein, carbohydrates, vitamins, minerals, and sometimes other nutrients or fats)

Weight gain powders (containing protein, carbohydrates, and sometimes fats, vitamins, minerals, and other nutrients)

Weight loss powders (containing protein, carbohydrates, and sometimes fats, vitamins, minerals, and other nutrients)

Bars (some bars contain 25 g or more of protein and are advertised as a dietary protein source)

Ready-to-drink liquids (may or may not contain carbohydrates and other nutrients)

Pills (tablets, capsules, or wafers containing protein and sometimes other nutrients)

Protein hydrolysates (in powder, beverage, bar, or pill forms)

Amino acids (in combinations of 18 or more that approximate protein or mixtures of a few amino acids or individually — these may be stand-alone products or added to other protein-containing supplements)

10.2.1   Milk Proteins

10.2.1.1 Characteristics of Commercially Available Milk Proteins

Milk proteins (almost always bovine source) are commercially available as whole milk proteins, caseinates, and whey proteins. Milk protein is approximately 80% caseins (α, β, γ, and κ subtypes) and 20% whey proteins (α-lactalbumin, β-lactoglobulin, bovine serum albumin, immunoglobulins, lactoferrin, lactoperoxidase). Each individual milk protein is available in purity exceeding 95%; however, milk protein isolates, caseinates, and whey proteins are most common in commercial use. Characteristics of commercially available milk protein fractions are listed in Table 10.4.

Milk protein isolates are produced from skim milk by two basic methods: 1) ultrafiltration, diafiltration (to concentrate protein) and drying, or 2) low or high heat pasteurization, precipitation, washing, and drying. Milk protein concentrates and isolates contain more than 90% protein (Table 10.4) and are commonly used in foods and dietary supplements.

Caseinates are produced from skim milk by heating or other coagulating techniques, removing liquid whey, washing and resolubilization with sodium, potassium or calcium hydroxides, and drying. Caseinates used for dietary supplements are generally produced by acid, as opposed to rennet casein production used for cheese making. Caseinates are commercially available as sodium, potassium, or calcium caseinates, each with different solubility and mixability characteristics. Protein purity is over 90% (Table 10.4).

Whey proteins are extracted from liquid whey produced as a byproduct of cheese or casein manufacturing.[13] Liquid whey is 0.6% protein and 93% water, with lactose, ash and milk fat. Liquid whey is perishable, similar to milk, and must be handled accordingly. Whey protein concentrates (about 80% protein) are produced from liquid whey by clarification, ultrafiltration, diafiltration, and drying. Whey protein isolates (>90% protein) are produced from liquid whey by a variety of techniques. Initial concentration of protein can be accomplished by mixing liquid whey with an ion-exchange resin to bind protein, followed by washing to remove non-protein solids, washing the protein off of the resin, and concentration by ultrafiltration and diafiltration, followed by drying. This process produces ion-exchange whey protein isolate (Table 10.4).

The other major type of whey protein isolate is called cross-flow microfiltered whey protein isolate. Production from liquid whey involves initial protein concentration by ultrafiltration with a two-way flow to remove lactose, salts and fat micelles, followed by ultrafiltration, diafiltration, and drying (Table 10.4).

Table 10.4 Comparison of Characteristics and Cost of Commercial Protein Sources

Ingredient*	Nonfat Dry Milk	Milk Protein Isolate	Whey Protein Concentrate (34)	Whey Protein Concentrate (75)	Whey Protein Concentrate (85)	Rennet Caseinate	Calcium Caseinate	Sodium Caseinate	Potassium Caseinate	Ion-Exchange Whey Protein Isolate (BiPro)
Supplier	Dairy America	New Zealand Milk Products	Avonmore	Calpro	Calpro	New Zealand Milk Products	New Zealand Milk Products	New Zealand Milk Products	Erie Foods Int'l	Davisco
Source	milk / dairy	milk / dairy	milk / dairy	milk / dairy	milk / dairy	milk / dairy	milk / dairy	milk / dairy	milk / dairy	milk / dairy
Proximate										
Protein (%) (dry basis)	33–34	93	35	79	86	89	93	93–95	91–93	90
Fat (%)	0.8–1.25	1.1	3–5	6–8	5	0.3–0.5	1.5	1.1	1.1	1
Cholesterol (mg/100g)	25	20	97	220–240	230	na	20	20	na	17
Carbohydrates (%)	54	< 1.0	51	8–10	4	about 1.6	0.1	0.1	0.2	1
Lactose (%)	51	0.2	50	8–10	4	0.05–0.1	0.1	0.1	0.2	1
Moisture (%)	4	4.3	3.5	4	4	11	4	4	9.3	5
Ash (%)	8.2	3.6	8	3	3	7.8	3.4	3.6	3.9	3
Minerals										
Sodium (mg/100g)	494	1200	550	150–300	100–200	5	10	1300	600	525
Potassium (mg/100g)	1674	< 20	1660	500–750	350–500	10	< 20	< 20	1350	na
Calcium (mg/100 g)	1250	50	550	300–500	300–500	2800	1400	< 100	55	142
Phosphorus (mg/100 g)	990	700	560	250–400	250–400	1600	800	800	720	52
Iron (mg/100 g)	0.4	na	0.6	na	na	na	na	na	0.5	1.5
Magnesium (mg/100 g)	110	< 30	100	40–60	35–50	80	< 40	< 30	4	18
Amino Acid Profile (mg/100 g protein)										
Alanine	3.28	3.50	4.94	4.82	4.82	3.00	3.00	3.00	3.22	5.60
Arginine	3.45	3.50	2.19	3.18	3.18	3.80	3.70	3.70	3.59	3.00

continued

Table 10.4 (continued) Comparison of Characteristics and Cost of Commercial Protein Sources

Ingredient*	Nonfat Dry Milk	Milk Protein Isolate	Whey Protein Concentrate (34)	Whey Protein Concentrate (75)	Whey Protein Concentrate (85)	Rennet Caseinate	Calcium Caseinate	Sodium Caseinate	Potassium Caseinate	Ion-Exchange Whey Protein Isolate (BiPro)
Amino Acid Profile (mg/100 g protein)										
Aspartic Acid	7.22	8.00	11.35	12.26	12.26	6.80	6.90	6.90	7.18	12.30
Cysteine/Cystine	0.88	0.60	2.35	2.28	2.28	0.40	0.40	0.40	0.37	1.90
Glutamic Acid	19.94	20.80	15.13	15.41	15.41	20.70	20.90	20.90	19.80	17.70
Glycine	2.02	1.90	2.06	2.00	2.00	1.90	1.80	1.80	1.73	1.90
Histidine	2.58	2.70	2.22	2.41	2.41	3.00	2.90	2.90	3.09	2.00
Isoleucine	5.76	4.40	6.00	6.41	6.41	4.10	4.60	4.60	4.95	5.40
Leucine	9.33	10.30	11.01	11.60	11.60	9.10	9.10	9.10	8.42	13.50
Lysine	7.55	8.10	9.13	9.83	9.83	7.70	7.70	7.70	7.30	10.90
Methionine	2.39	3.30	1.88	2.35	2.35	3.00	2.90	2.90	3.22	3.50
Phenylalanine	4.60	5.00	3.28	3.56	3.56	5.40	5.10	5.10	4.95	3.40
Proline	9.22	9.50	5.94	6.28	6.28	10.40	10.40	10.40	9.65	4.80
Serine	5.18	6.20	5.63	6.24	6.24	5.60	5.80	5.80	5.82	4.50
Threonine	4.30	4.50	7.44	8.44	8.44	3.80	4.30	4.30	4.58	5.30
Tryptophan	1.34	1.40	1.97	1.80	1.80	1.50	1.20	1.20	1.24	1.50
Tyrosine	4.60	5.20	1.97	3.26	3.26	5.80	5.50	5.50	4.70	3.90
Valine	6.37	5.70	5.50	6.09	6.09	5.40	5.70	5.70	6.19	5.40
Aromatic Amino Acids (phe & tyr)	9.19	10.20	5.25	6.82	6.82	11.20	10.60	10.60	9.65	7.30
Sulfur Amino Acids (met & cys)	3.27	3.90	4.22	4.63	4.63	3.40	3.30	3.30	3.59	5.40
Branched Chain Amino Acids (leu, iso, val)	21.46	20.40	22.51	24.10	24.10	18.60	19.40	19.40	19.55	24.30
Typical Raw Material Cost ($/kg)	2.50	6.00	1.50	6.00	7.00	—	6.00	6.00	5.00	10.00

Ingredient	Cross-Flow Microfiltration Whey Protein Isolate (Provon)	Whey Protein Hydrolysate	Casein Hydrolysate	Soy Protein Concentrate	Soy Protein Isolate	Soy Protein Isolage (w/ Ca)	Glutamine Peptide	Egg Albumen (dried)	Hydroglyzed Collagen
Supplier	Avonmore	New Zealand Milk Products	New Zealand Milk Products	ADM	Protein Tech. Int'l	Protein Tech. Int'l	CPC	Sonstegard Foods	Traco Labs
Source	milk / dairy	milk / dairy	milk / dairy	soybean	soybean	soybean	wheat	egg	bovine collagen
Proximate									
Protein (%) (dry basis)	92–95	90	90	70	90	84	81	87	97
Fat (%)	< 1	3.8	0.8	3	4	4.5	4.5	0.25	< 0.1
Cholesterol (mg/100g)	1.5	na	na	0	0	0	0	0	0
Carbohydrates (%)	1	about 2.2	3.1	16	< 1.0	< 1.0	9–12	16	< 0.1
Lactose (%)	< 1	0.3	0.1	0	0	0	0	0	0
Moisture (%)	5	4.3	4.5	8	5	5	4.5	5–8	4–8
Ash (%)	3	3.0–3.5	5.6	5	5	10	3.6	4.9	< 0.9
Minerals									
Sodium (mg/100g)	250	1400	2100	1200		800	350–660	1200	na
Potassium (mg/100g)	300	100	30	300		800	90–730	1100	na
Calcium (mg/100 g)	600	200	100	250		2900	35–750	50	na
Phosphorus (mg/100 g)	210	200	700	700		2000	150–500	100	na
Iron (mg/100 g)	9.3	na	na	9		14	3–4.5	0.3	na
Magnesium (mg/100 g)	90	30	20	100		na	20–40	80	na
Amino Acid Profile (mg/100 g protein)									
Alanine	5.60	5.20	3.00	4.60	4.30	4.30	2.60	5.77	10.50
Arginine	1.70	3.00	3.70	7.90	7.60	7.60	2.90	5.43	9.90
Aspartic Acid	12.70	12.30	6.90	11.90	11.60	11.60	3.00	10.18	6.70
Cysteine/Cystine	2.50	2.90	0.40	1.40	1.30	1.30	1.20	2.59	0.40
Glutamic Acid	19.70	18.30	20.90	19.00	19.10	19.10	37.90	13.29	11.70
Glycine	2.00	2.30	1.80	4.60	4.20	4.20	3.30	3.49	27.10

continued

Table 10.4 (continued) Comparison of Characteristics and Cost of Commercial Protein Sources

Ingredient	Cross-Flow Microfiltration Whey Protein Isolate (Provon)	Whey Protein Hydrolysate	Casein Hydrolysate	Soy Protein Concentrate	Soy Protein Isolate	Soy Protein Isolage (w/ Ca)	Glutamine Peptide	Egg Albumen (dried)	Hydroglyzed Collagen
Histidine	1.80	1.90	2.90	2.80	2.60	2.60	1.80	2.26	1.80
Isoleucine	6.80	5.50	4.80	5.20	4.90	4.90	4.00	5.66	1.70
Leucine	10.90	14.20	9.10	8.50	8.20	8.20	7.00	8.41	3.40
Lysine	9.50	10.20	7.70	6.90	6.30	6.30	1.40	6.80	4.10
Methionine	3.10	2.40	2.90	1.50	1.30	1.30	1.50	3.44	0.50
Phenylalanine	2.50	3.80	5.10	5.40	5.20	5.20	5.30	5.82	2.00
Proline	6.30	5.10	10.40	5.60	5.10	5.10	13.20	3.91	16.00
Serine	5.30	5.00	5.80	5.10	5.20	5.20	4.40	6.88	3.30
Threonine	8.30	5.50	4.30	4.20	3.80	3.80	2.20	4.55	2.10
Tryptophan	2.00	2.30	1.20	1.20	1.30	1.30	0.80	1.23	na
Tyrosine	3.10	3.90	5.50	4.00	3.80	3.80	3.40	3.91	0.40
Valine	6.40	5.90	5.70	5.40	5.00	5.00	4.00	6.37	3.00
Aromatic Amino Acids (phe & tyr)	5.60	7.70	10.60	9.40	9.00	9.00	8.70	9.73	2.40
Sulfur Amino Acids (met & cys)	5.60	5.30	3.30	2.90	2.60	2.60	2.70	6.03	0.90
Branched Chain Amino Acids (leu, iso, val)	24.10	25.60	19.60	19.10	18.10	18.10	15.00	20.45	8.10
Typical Raw Material Cost ($/kg)	10.00	9.00	22.00	3.50	3.50	3.00	13.00	6.50	12.00

10.2.1.2 Attributes of Milk Proteins

Table 10.5 lists some advantages and disadvantages from a consumer viewpoint for the major proteins used in dietary supplements. Because of the long-standing size of dairy and cheese industries, milk proteins remain the most common form of protein found in dietary supplements. Large-scale production yields comparatively low-cost proteins, making milk protein powders rival foods in cost-effectiveness. Consumers perceive, milk proteins as being the best protein in terms of quality (a topic to be discussed later). Milk proteins are acceptable for lacto-ovo vegetarians.

Table 10.5 Comparative Advantages and Disadvantages of Protein Sources in Protein Supplements

Protein Source	Advantages	Disadvantages
Whey proteins	Perceived as highest quality protein Taste and mixability Rapid digestion and uptake of amino acids Familiar source	Cost
Casein	Lower cost Perception as high quality Range of grades (mixability, taste) May provide delayed release of amino acid uptake compared with whey	Some grades do not mix well Perception as inferior to whey Taste
Egg protein	Perception as the highest quality protein Familiar source Ease of mixing	Taste Cost
Soy protein isolates	Lower cost Suitable for strict vegetarians Successful human research on athletes Taste Ease of mixing Isoflavone content Complete protein for humans	Incorrect perception as having a lower protein quality (from PER data) Taste Isoflavones perceived as estrogenic by some consumers
Whey protein hydrolysates	Perception as highest quality Fastest uptake of amino acids	High cost Taste Mixability Hypothetical advantages unproven in athletes
Free-form amino acid mixtures	Customized formula No other calories (highest purity) Non-protein amino acids	Tryptophan unavailable (any formula would be incomplete) High cost Taste Mixability Hypothetical advantages of mixtures unproven in athletes

Whey proteins in particular have been singled out as the ultimate form of protein based on essential amino acid composition, branched-chain amino acid (BCAA) content, sulfur amino acid content, taste acceptance, ease of mixing, stability in liquids, and rapidity of digestion (especially when compared with caseinates). Although whey protein isolates cost more than other proteins in dietary supplements, the perceived advantages and excellent organoleptic properties have made whey protein the protein of choice for weightlifters. This perception has been fueled by articles and advertisements in popular magazines. Many consumers know the difference between cross-flow microfiltered and ion-exchange whey proteins, as well as the theoretical advantages of one over the other. Attention to very small differences in lactose and fat content and preservation of glutamine residues are used as selling points to distinguish the two types of whey protein isolate. Whether these minor differences have any distinctions for producing muscular gains has not been studied in exercising humans.

10.2.1.3 Studies on Milk Protein Supplementation in Exercising Humans

Most of the human clinical trials of protein supplementation and exercise have used milk proteins. Incredibly, some studies did not specify the type of protein supplement used or referred to a commercial product as a protein source. In most cases, the commercial products used in those studies have contained milk proteins. All types of commercial milk proteins have been used in human clinical studies (milk protein isolates, caseinates, whey proteins). In addition, numerous studies of protein supplementation in post-surgical settings, diabetes, growth of children, and protein metabolism studies have used milk protein supplements. The sheer volume of human studies over the past 50 years that use milk proteins has solidified the perception of milk protein as a viable protein supplement in the minds of consumers and precludes an analysis in this chapter. Most of the results from studies on protein supplementation and exercise used milk proteins, and readers should look at the relevant chapter in this volume and reviews on protein metabolism.[1-6]

10.2.2   Egg Proteins

10.2.2.1 Characteristics and Attributes of Commercially Available Egg Proteins

Egg protein is produced commercially from chicken egg whites (ovalbumin) or whole eggs by typical procedures outlined above (Table 10.4). Egg protein has been a reference protein for determining human protein needs, and consumers generally perceived it as an excellent source of a complete protein, equal to whey proteins (Table 10.5). Like milk proteins, egg protein supplements are acceptable to lacto-ovo vegetarians. In the past, egg protein powders were regarded as the premier protein supplement. However, egg proteins cost more than other pure proteins, which has greatly reduced the number of egg protein products in the marketplace, especially because pure grades of whey proteins have appeared. Egg proteins are frequently added to protein powders, usually in small amounts (less than 5% of total protein), to gain consumer confidence and acceptance without increasing product cost.

10.2.3   Soy Proteins

10.2.3.1 Characteristics of Commercially Available Soy Proteins

Like whey proteins, soy proteins have been a subject for extensive industrial research to produce a virtually pure protein isolate in commercial quantities. Soy protein is produced from soybeans via water extraction, followed by precipitation, washing and drying procedures to yield either a soy protein concentrate (approximately 70% protein) or soy protein isolates (90% protein). Some extraction procedures use ethanol/water mixtures, which remove isoflavones. Various grades of soy proteins have varying organoleptic properties (ease of mixing, taste).

In the past, low protein purity of soy-derived protein sources led to consumer dissatisfaction due to gastrointestinal disturbances, poor taste, and poor mixability. Although these objections have been successfully eliminated, the image of poor tolerance of soy protein remains in the minds of many consumers. The significantly lower cost of soy protein isolates compared with egg, whey, and some milk proteins has made soy protein supplements more attractive.

10.2.3.2 Attributes of Soy Protein

Soy protein possesses some unique characteristics that separate it from animal-derived proteins (Table 10.5), and it appears to benefit exercising individuals. First, soy protein isolates contain isoflavone glucosides (mostly genistin and diadzin — 0.68–2.49 mg/g). The health-promoting benefits of soy isoflavones and soy products are a fertile field of research. Research suggests that isoflavones are mostly responsible for antioxidant actions, thyromimetic properties,[14] cancer prevention, reduction of cardiovascular disease risk factors, maintenance of bone mass, and amelioration of female gynecological complaints.[15–17] Many of these studies compared soy protein to casein, thus making soy protein appear to be more desirable than casein for humans.

Second, soy protein contains a higher percentage (35%) of five "critical cluster" amino acids, including glutamine, lysine, and the BCAAs than other proteins, such as whey, casein, egg, and beef (see Figure 10.1). In theory, these are the amino acids preferred for fortification of proteins by the dietary supplement industry, and they have hypothetical benefits for exercising individuals.

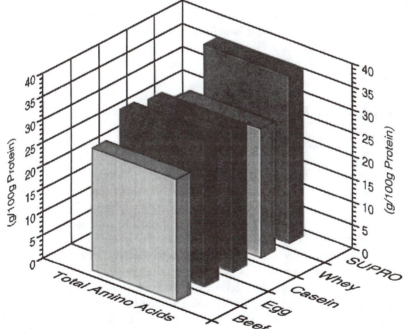

Figure 10.1 Diagram illustrating the amount of "critical cluster" amino acids (glutamine, leucine, isoleucine, valine, and lysine) in different protein sources. These amino acids are hypothesized to be of primary importance, among amino acids, for muscle metabolism. Supro refers to isolated soy protein.

Soy protein isolates are generally less expensive than whey and egg proteins (see Table 10.2), and possess favorable organoleptic properties such as mixability, taste, texture, and ease of flavoring. Recent data has confirmed that soy protein is complete for humans, and has similar biological value, as illustrated by PDCAAS scores (Table 10.6), in humans to milk, beef, and egg proteins.[18,19] This fact has been overlooked by many health care professionals, the public, and especially strength athletes because of reliance on animal studies of protein utilization and

Table 10.6 Comparison of Protein Quality

Protein	PDCAAS	PER
Egg	1.00	2.8
Milk protein	1.00	2.8
Casein	1.00	2.9
Whey	1.00	3.0
Soy	1.00	1.8
Beef protein	0.92	2.3
Wheat	0.43	1.5
Pork skin (collagen)	0.08	—

Abbreviations: Protein Digestability Corrected Amino Acid Score (PDCAAS) — scale used to assess protein quality for humans based on content of amino acids and corrected for digestion; Protein Efficiency Ratio (PER) — scale used to assess protein quality based on ability to support growth in young rats (not directly applicable to humans).

Values adapted from educational brochures from New Zealand Milk Products (North America) Inc., Santa Rosa, CA, and Brody, T. *Nutritional Biochemistry*, 2nd ed., Academic Press, 1998, 470.

promotional activities of other protein suppliers. This is in spite of the fact that soy protein-based formulas have been used successfully for many years in growth of infants as the sole source of protein. Infant growth has the highest protein requirements of sedentary humans, and thus represents a practical test for biological value of soy protein in humans. Nevertheless, the perception that soy protein is inferior in quality to animal proteins still exists, limiting marketability of soy protein to strength athletes.

10.2.3.3 Studies on Soy Protein Supplementation in Exercising Humans

Soy protein isolate supplementation has been studied repeatedly in practical settings with athletes.[20–26] Four double-blind, placebo-controlled studies on elite Romanian athletes administered 1.5 g/kg/d additional protein from isolated soy protein for 8 to 16 weeks during stressful training periods.[20–23] Athletes ranged from endurance sports to swimmers to gymnasts. In general, lean body mass was preserved or increased, muscular strength was maintained or increased, and urinary mucoproteins (an indicator of exercise stress) were decreased in soy protein-supplemented subjects, while adverse changes were noticed in placebo subjects. The study on female gymnasts[23] found increased serum thyroxine and prolactin levels compared to decreases in the placebo group. These results fit a thyromimetic mechanism[14] as one of soy protein's properties in athletes. A double-blind study by Husaini on young, elite, Indonesian badminton players found improvements in $\dot{V}O_{2\,max}$ and iron status.[24] An open trial of individualized dietary changes, including supplementation with a soy protein beverage, was performed on five professional baseball players by Shilstone.[25] All five subjects noticed large decreases in weight (3–12.5 lb) and body fat mass (–2.6 to –6.3%), but the results were not statistically significant because the sample size was small. An unpublished abstract by Min from the Training Center of the National Sports Commission for China reported improvements in blood rheology, body fat, strength diathesis, and "sports ability," although no details were given, after administration of a soy protein beverage.[26] A soy-based candy bar to increase dietary intake of protein in sportsmen was described by Wittig de Pena in Chile, although no studies on effects were performed.[27] University of Nebraska sports teams use soy protein beverages as part of their training (Ellis, D., personal communication, 1998).

In summary, supplementation trials with soy protein in human athletes have been associated with improvements in training and recovery. The results certainly fit the proposed advantages of soy proteins. It must be noted that so far, no study on soy protein supplementation and exercise has been published in easily accessible or major sports-related journals, compared with the wealth of peer-reviewed, published studies on soy protein supplementation for other health issues. Nevertheless, soy protein is an under-recognized means of providing high-quality protein for exercising individuals and perhaps may possess other benefits due to isoflavone content and actions.

10.2.4 Other Proteins

Although a wide variety of semi-purified or purified proteins from other animal or vegetable sources are commercially available, high costs and perceived advantages of milk, egg, or soy proteins prevent other protein sources from being commercially important as protein supplements. Vegetable protein sources are usually mixed with amino acids or protein hydrolysates to improve their biological value, which drives prices higher. Protein supplements using rice, pea, beet, wheat gluten, and, occasionally, other grain proteins have appeared on the marketplace, but they have been unsuccessful with consumers compared with milk, egg, and soy products.

Likewise, fish proteins, bovine blood proteins, feather/hair (keratin) proteins, and muscle proteins have been commercially available and have appeared as protein supplements, but have also been unsuccessful with consumers.

10.2.4.1 Gelatin (Collagen)

One protein that remains in commerce as a dietary supplement is collagen (gelatin). Because of its low price and widespread availability, collagen protein has been used in liquid protein-sparing, low-calorie diets, mostly in the 1970s, with harmful consequences.[28] Because deaths were associated with ingestion of collagen products as a sole source of protein intake for weight loss, collagen protein has a negative image with consumers and regulatory agencies, and it is seldom found in protein supplements. Use of gelatin in other foodstuffs that are not protein supplements (such as Jello® brand desserts) and as food additives continues unabated, because these foods are not perceived as protein sources. Collagen is also a protein of very poor quality, a fact readily noticed by nutrition-savvy consumers. These facts have relegated collagen to a few remaining liquid protein supplements. Some products have additional amino acids or additional proteins added to improve biological value. Identity of collagen protein in a product can be confirmed by the presence of hydroxyproline in an amino acid analysis when such information is present on the label.

Interestingly, in the 1930s and 1940s, when gelatin was first available commercially in large quantities, gelatin was briefly, but intensely, studied as an ergogenic aid for athletes.[29] Research interest was spurred by the fact that gelatin was rich in glycine, a precursor for creatine, which was being studied for relief of muscular fatigue in muscular dystrophy and other medical conditions.[29–31] Although three initial studies of gelatin supplementation to exercising individuals found large increases in work capacity, these experiments were not properly controlled and measured training effects.[32–34] Other reports, most of which had acceptable experimental control, found no performance benefits for delayed muscle soreness, race times from 500 to 1500 m, walking, cycle ergometry, swim times for 60 to 100 y races, weight lifting or arm ergometer work.[35–41] Doses of gelatin ranged from 30 to 60 g daily for long time periods, providing an additional 7.5 to 14 g of glycine to the diet. The poor uptake of glycine-containing hydroxyproline peptides[42] and the presence of other amino acids (preventing glycine from exerting any specific effects) may have accounted for lack of results. Thus, gelatin is not an ergogenic aid for athletes. Gelatin cannot be relied upon for a sole source of dietary protein intake, but it still could be a low-cost source of supplemental protein, albeit with less efficiency than other sources of protein.

10.3 PROTEIN HYDROLYSATES

10.3.1 Milk Protein Hydrolysates

Protein hydrolysates are produced from purified protein sources by heating with acid or preferably, addition of proteolytic enzymes, followed by purification procedures as outlined for proteins, with lower molecular weight cutoff for membrane filtration steps. Enzyme hydrolysis is greatly preferred because acid hydrolysis oxidizes cysteine and methionine, destroys some serine and threonine, and converts glutamine and asparagine to glutamate and aspartate, respectively, lowering protein quality and biological value. Table 10.4 lists some characteristics of milk protein hydrolysates, and Table 10.5 lists comparative advantages and disadvantages.

Both casein hydrolysates and whey protein hydrolysates have been used extensively in human clinical studies for elaborating protein digestion, protein metabolism, post-surgical healing, and many other uses. In general, protein hydrolysates have been documented to cause faster and more even uptake of amino acids when compared with isonitrogenous amounts of whole proteins or free-form amino acid mixtures.[43-45] This is a desirable trait for athletes who wish to maximize amino acid delivery to muscles. As a result, several dietary supplements that claim to contain protein hydrolysates (especially whey protein hydrolysates) have been marketed. However, definitive research on whether such products enhance recovery from exercise compared with whole protein supplementation has not been reported. Nevertheless, consumers perceive whey protein hydrolysate products as the ultimate type of protein supplement.

10.3.2 Collagen Hydrolysates

Enzymatic hydrolysates of collagen (gelatin) are being studied in Europe as a treatment for chondropathia patellae and osteoarthritis (Beuker, F., 1996, unpublished data on file).[46-51] Open and double-blind clinical trials have all shown slow but significant amelioration of symptoms and reduction in analgesic dosages after four weeks of administration of 7–10 g/d of collagen hydrolysate. Furthermore, administration of 10 g of collagen hydrolysate to athletes resulted in higher concentrations of plasma amino acids, which in theory may facilitate recovery from strenuous exercise (Beuker, F., unpublished data, 1996). For specific uses (joint injuries), collagen hydrolysates with hydroxyproline-containing peptides may represent a unique form of protein supplementation compared with other protein supplements.

10.3.3 Glutamine Peptides

The recent surge in popularity of glutamine as an ergogenic aid for recovery,[52-54] the knowledge that protein hydrolysates may enhance absorption of an amino acid over that of an equivalent amount in protein or in free-form,[43-45] and the fact that glutamine is converted to glutamate by cooking and normal processing has led to a commercial source for a protein hydrolysate rich in glutamine (38%) (Table 10.4). Wheat is the starting material for glutamine peptides. However, the relatively high cost and poor taste of glutamine peptides have limited widescale use in protein powders.

10.3.4 Peptide FM

Also known as Borep™, Peptide-FM is a mixture of protein hydrolysates from bovine and wheat sources. Studies from Japan have found that Peptide-FM decreases fat uptake from a meal and leads to reduced body weight in humans after daily supplementation (unpublished data on file, 1996). Animal studies indicated that Peptide-FM may have metabolic effects on the liver to increase oxidation of fats (unpublished data on file, 1996). Peptide-FM has appeared in some sports nutrition products as an aid for lowering body fat. No studies in athletes have been performed to measure body composition changes.

10.3.5. Other Sources (Fish, Soy, Egg, Vegetable)

Although other proteins have been used to prepare hydrolysates commercially, there is virtually no presence of these hydrolysates in dietary supplements targeted at exercising individuals.

10.4 AMINO ACIDS

Since the 1989 ban on tryptophan for supplements (but not for infant formulas, parenteral or enteral feeding products) in the United States, the number of amino acid mixtures as dietary supplements has dropped. Less than 10% of advertised protein supplement products were claimed to be predominantly free-form amino acids.[9,10] Because a mixture of 100% free-form amino acids cannot contain tryptophan, it would by definition be an incomplete protein source and unacceptable to consumers of protein supplements. The comparative higher cost and poorer organoleptic properties of free-form amino acid mixtures relative to high-quality grades of protein and protein hydrolysates have also contributed to their decline in popularity. Rather, specific amino acids are frequently used to fortify protein supplements or are combined with other nutrients.

Amino acids most commonly used to fortify protein supplements are glutamine, BCAAs, taurine, methionine (soy proteins), arginine, and ornithine. Although a prodigious amount of research on the effects of glutamine and BCAA supplementation to exercising individuals is accumulating, the effects of glutamine or BCAA enrichment in protein supplements is not defined. Effects from other additional amino acids is relatively unknown. The doses of added amino acids in protein supplements frequently does not reach the doses used in human clinical studies.

One study by Kreider et al. compared a protein-rich (67 g per day of protein with 64 g per day carbohydrate) weight gain formula (Phosphagain™) containing 7.2 g of additional L-glutamine, 6.2 g of additional taurine and 20 g of creatine to another weight gain product (Gainers Fuel® 1000) containing 60 g per day of protein and 290 g of carbohydrates.[55] A maltodextrin placebo (190 g per day) group was also included. Thirty resistance-trained male subjects in three different groups were studied for 28 days. Both protein powder groups showed significantly greater gains in body mass, but the amino acid-supplemented group (Phosphagain™) showed greater increases in lean muscle mass, whereas the Gainers Fuel® 1000 group showed significantly increased body fat mass and percentage with no increase in lean body mass (compared with maltodextrin placebo). The mixture of protein, creatine, glutamine, and taurine led to significant increases in lean body mass, but the relative contributions of each major ingredient cannot be pinpointed.

In summary, free-form amino acids as a sole protein source have fallen out of favor. Free-form amino acids are still frequently used as value-added components of protein supplements, meal replacements, and weight gain products.

10.5 SUMMARY AND CONCLUSIONS

10.5.1 Industry Trends

As stated previously, strength athletes and weightlifters have traditionally focused on high dietary intakes of protein, including protein supplements.[4,7,8] The availability, forms, purity, and sophistication of protein supplements have reached overwhelming proportions in the 1990s, especially because increased protein requirements have been documented.[1-6] Consumers seek the highest biological value, nitrogen retention, digestibility, ease of mixing, and taste from protein supplements. Currently, whey protein hydrolysate is the *most desired* protein supplement. The *most popular* is whey protein. The best value is soy protein isolate. Protein supplements have evolved from inexpensive, lower potency, milk proteins to pure milk protein fractions with predigested peptides. Competitive pressures have spawned several protein supplements with value-added ingredients (such as creatine or free-form amino acids) to convince consumers that they are getting a better product.

So far, there have not been any head-to-head comparisons in exercising individuals of the effects of different proteins on nitrogen balance, muscle mass or strength. Thus, consumers are assailed with hypothetical advantages or disadvantages of different proteins extrapolated from animal studies or enteral/parenteral clinical nutrition fields. Even so, these hypothetical arguments are convincing and attractive to consumers, as evidenced by the popularity of whey protein and whey protein hydrolysates.

Trends in the dietary supplement sports nutrition industry include marketing protein powders with value-added ingredients (such as protein hydrolysates, creatine, or free-form amino acids), removal of even tiny amounts of fats and carbohydrates from protein sources (higher purity), passing on decreased price of raw materials to consumers, greater reliance on scientific literature or published research studies to promote advantages, and a return to unembellished protein powders.

Another recent trend is to advertise a large amount of protein per serving (up to 60 g at one time), a manifestation of the "horsepower" race of dose escalation common to dietary supplements. In contrast, another trend is to mix proteins with rapid uptake (such as whey protein or whey protein hydrolysates) with a slower-digesting protein (caseinates) and/or soluble fibers to prevent the adaptive response by the body of increasing amino acid oxidation (catabolism) when increased levels of amino acids are present. This concept is based on a report by Biorie and others comparing whole body leucine kinetics in healthy adults after ingestion of identical amounts of leucine from either whey or casein proteins.[56] Net leucine balance over the seven-hour after a meal was more positive with casein than with whey, which was partly explainable by a greater oxidation of leucine after whey protein ingestion.

Whey protein is the preferred protein for strength athletes, and it forms the majority of protein powder products. In fact, the market has become so sophisticated that certain types of whey protein are preferred. Either Cross-Flow Microfiltered (CFM) whey protein isolate or Ion-Exchange whey protein isolate (IEW), which represent different methods of extraction and purification, are recognized as superior forms of whey proteins. Work is in progress to provide whey protein fractions (lactalbumin and lactoglobulin) in bulk. For weightlifters, a goal of reproducing the whey protein makeup of human milk is desired, as this mimics human protein requirements during time of greatest need (infant growth). Preservation of glutamine residues is also preferred in whey proteins. Frequently, advertisements and product label copy for whey protein products explain the advantages of each type of whey protein compared with other forms.

Analysis of whey protein products by amino acid analysis and size exclusion chromatography finds that some products do not provide whey protein hydrolysates as stated on their labels (Feliciano, J., unpublished data, 1997), although whey protein is present. Marketing or quality control of these products may be regarded as questionable, but consumers still get benefits from a pure protein.

10.5.2 Guidelines for Use of Protein Supplements

Are protein supplements necessary? Who would benefit from protein supplements? How much is effective? Are protein supplements safe? While protein intake from foodstuffs alone can be increased to any level of protein intake desired, many persons do not want the preparation time, do not want a concomitant fat or carbohydrate intake, or are vegetarian. Also, most persons do not have sufficient skills to gauge their protein intake from foods. Protein supplements allow one to know exactly how much protein is being consumed, taking the guesswork out of eating enough protein from foods. Protein powders can be mixed into shakes or smoothies, and other foods or calories can be added. Furthermore, protein supplements are easily transportable and last longer before spoilage than high-protein foodstuffs. Control over dietary protein intake and convenience are major reasons why protein supplements are popular.

There is even some evidence to suggest that protein from supplements is handled differently than protein from foodstuffs. Studies investigating intestinal protein uptake from the 1970s and 1980s found that protein hydrolysates are absorbed into the bloodstream faster with a less biased amino acid composition than whole proteins or foodstuffs.[43-45] However, whether this apparent advantage over ingestion of foodstuffs has a practical effect of faster muscle mass accretion or improved recovery from exercise has not been adequately tested in exercising individuals. Nevertheless, documented advantages of protein supplements over foodstuffs (faster uptake of amino acids, higher biological value) remain attractive to consumers.

Table 10.7 lists guidelines for using protein supplements.[1-6,12,55] If supplemental protein intake is desired, it is important for each person to try various protein supplement sources because of the tremendous variation in taste, mixability, cost, and overall acceptance. Many exercising individuals already use protein supplements. There is compelling evidence to indicate that individuals engaged in strenuous exercise should consider protein supplements to maintain or increase muscle mass, especially if there is a desire to lower or prevent an increase of body fat.

Table 10.7 Guidelines for Protein Supplementation

Aerobic Exercise:	Running, cycling, swimming, skiing, rowing, sports events or training lasting longer than 60 minutes
	1. Protein intake (all sources) — maintain 1.8–2.0 g protein/kg/d intake during strenuous training or competition, and 1.0–1.4 g protein/kg/d intake during other periods of training.
	2. Protein supplements — one serving daily (contains 20–60 g of protein, depending upon product serving size and body weight).
Anaerobic Exercise:	Weightlifting, bodybuilding, track and field, maximal intensity events (short-term, repetitive, exhaustive exercise lasting less than 60 minutes, such as football, hockey, wrestling, rowing, cycle sprints, volleyball)
	1. Protein intake (all sources) — 100–200 g per day (2.0–3.0 g protein/kg/d) during strenuous training or competition, and 1.4–1.8 g protein/kg/d during other periods of training.
	2. Protein supplements — one or two servings daily (each serving should contain 20–60 g of protein, depending upon product serving size and body weight).
	3. Weight gain powders — one or two servings daily [should contain protein (25 g per serving), carbohydrate (>25 g per serving), creatine (>3 g per serving), and possibly L-glutamine (2–6 g per serving), taurine (>2 g per serving)]; preferably ingested just after workouts.. May replace or augment protein powder supplements.

ACKNOWLEDGMENTS

The authors wish to thank the following for discussions, reviews, and provision of unpublished information: Vince Andrich, Dan Berg, Chris Busch, Mauro Di Pasquale, Michael Dodson, Dave Ellis, Jeff Feliciano, E.C. Henley, Lee Huffman, Peter Lemon, Drs. Jerzy & George Meduski, Robin Planthaber; Becky O'Reilly, Jeffrey Potteiger, Susan Potter, Michael Rennie, Gale Rudolph, Vince Sciacca, Gunther Schlierkamp, Alan Shugarman, D.G.F. Stoess, Eberbach, Germany; Jim Wright.

REFERENCES

1. Di Pasquale, M., Protein and amino acids in exercise and sports, Ch. 6 in *Macronutrients, Electrolytes, and Macroelements in Sports*, Driskell JA, Wolinsky I, Eds., CRC Press LLC, Boca Raton, FL, 1998, in press.

2. Di Pasquale, M. *Amino Acids and Proteins for the Athlete*, CRC Press LLC, Boca Raton, FL, 1997.

3. Paul, GL, Gautsch, TA, Layman, DK. Amino acid and protein metabolism during exercise and recovery, Ch. 5 in *Nutrition in Exercise and Sport*, 3rd ed., Wolinsky I, Ed., CRC Press LLC, Boca Raton, FL, 1998, 125-158.

4. Bazzarre, TL. Nutrition and strength, Ch. 14 in *Nutrition in Exercise and Sport*, 3rd ed., Wolinsky I, Ed., CRC Press LLC, Boca Raton, FL, 1998, 369-419.

5. Lemon, PWR. Dietary protein requirements in athletes. *J. Nutr. Biochem.* 1997; 8:52-60.

6. Lemon, PWR. Do athletes need more dietary protein and amino acids? *Int. J. Sport Nutr.* 1995; 5:S39-S61.

7. Katch, FI, McArdle, WD, Katch, VL, Freeman, JA. Exercise nutrition: from antiquity to the twentieth century and beyond, Ch. 1 in *Nutrition in Exercise and Sport*, 3rd ed., Wolinsky I, Ed., CRC Press LLC, Boca Raton, FL, 1998, 1-48.

8. Marquart, LF, Cohen, EA, Short, SH. Nutrition knowledge of athletes and their coaches and surveys of dietary intake, Ch. 23 in *Nutrition in Exercise and Sport*, 3rd ed., Wolinsky I, Ed., CRC Press LLC, Boca Raton, FL, 1998, 559-595.

9. *Muscle & Fitness*, 1998; 59(1):1-242.

10. *Flex*, 1998; 15(11):1-254.

11. *Bicycling,* 1998; Dec:1-98. *Runner's World,* 1998; 33(12):1-106. *Running Times,* 1998; Dec(254):1-82. *Triathlete,* 1998; Nov(175):1-82.

12. Bucci, L. Nutritional ergogenic aids — macronutrients, Ch. 2 in *Nutrients as Ergogenic Aids for Sports and Exercise*, CRC Press LLC, Boca Raton, FL, 1993, 16-17.

13. Huffman, LM. Processing whey protein for use as a food ingredient. *Food Technology,* 1996; 50(2):49-52.

14. Forsythe, WA. Soy protein, thyroid regulation and cholesterol metabolism. *J. Nutr.* 1995; 125(3 Suppl):619S-623S.

15. Potter, SM. Soy protein and serum lipids. *Curr. Opin. Lipidol.* 1996; 7(4):260-264.

16. Knight, DC, Eden, JA. A review of the clinical effects of phytoestrogens. *Obstet. Gynecol.* 1996; 87(5 Pt 2):897-904.

17. Tham, DM, Gardner, CD, Haskell, WL. Clinical review 97: Potential health benefits of dietary phytoestrogens: a review of the clinical, epidemiological, and mechanistic evidence. *J. Clin. Endocrinol. Metab.* 1998; 83(7):2223-2235.

18. Young, VR, Wayler, A, Garza, C, Steinke, FH, Murray, E, Rand, WM, Scrimshaw, NS. A long-term metabolic balance study in young men to assess the nutritional quality of an isolated soy protein and beef proteins, *Am. J. Clin. Nutr.,* 1984; 39:8-15.

19. Henley, EC, Kuster, JM. Protein quality evaluation by protein digestibility-corrected amino acid scoring. *Food Technology.* 1994; 48(4):74-77.

20. Dragan, I, Stroescu, V, Stoian, I, Georgescu, E, Baloescu, R. Studies regarding the efficiency of Supro isolated soy protein in Olympic athletes. *Rev. Roum. Physiol.* 1992; 29:63-70.

21. Dragan, I, Georgescu, E, Iosub, I, Baloescu, R. Studies regarding some beneficial effects of Supro® isolated soy protein supply in top swimmers. *Xth FINA World Sport Medicine Congress*, Kyoto, Japan, 1993, 35 [abstract].

22. Stroescu, V, Dragan, I, Georgescu, E. Studies on biological preparation of endurance in top athletes consuming Supro Plus® 675 supplement. *XXVth FIMS World Congress of Sports Medicine*, Athens, Greece, 1994, 81 [abstract #313].

23. Stroescu V, Dragan, I, Simionescu, L, Stroescu, OV. Metabolic and hormonal responses in elite female gymnasts undergoing strenuous training and supplementation with Supro® brand isolated soy protein. *Second International Symposium on the Role of Soy in Preventing and Treating Chronic Disease*, Brussels, Belgium, 1996, 38 [abstract].

24. Husaini, MA. Supplementation of "Supro" beverage powder on body size, iron status and physical performance of growing badminton players. *Scientific Workshop of the 19th SEA Games*, Jakarta, Indonesia, 1997 [abstract].

25. Shilstone, M. Observing the effects of a performance nutrition and conditioning program on professional athletes — a clinical study. *Am. Med. Athletic. Assoc. Quarterly.* 1997; 11(1):6-9.

26. Min, HG. Effects of "Supro" high-energy beverage powder on physiological function of athletes, unpublished data, Protein Technologies International, 1998 [abstract].

27. Wittig de Pena, E, Bunger, A, Sansu, M, Lopez, L, Santana, R. Development of soy-based protein candy bars for athletes. *Arch. Latinoam. Nutr.* 1993; 43(3):241-247.

28. Surawicz, B, Waller, BF. The enigma of sudden cardiac death related to dieting. *Can. J. Cardiol.* 1995; 11(3):228-231.

29. Bucci, L. Dietary substances not required in human metabolism, Ch. 8 in *Nutrients as Ergogenic Aids for Sports and Exercise*, CRC Press LLC, Boca Raton, FL, 1993, 91-92.

30. Reinhold, JG, Clark, JH, Kingsley, GR, Custer, RP, McConnell, JW. Effects of glycine (glycocoll) in muscular dystrophy, with special references to changes in structure and composition of voluntary muscle. *JAMA.* 1934; 102:261-275.

31. Tripoli, CJ and Beard, HH. Muscular dystrophy and atrophy; clinical and biochemical results following oral administration of amino acids. *Arch. Int. Med.* 1934; 53:435-442.

32. Ray, GB, Johnson, JR, Taylor, MM. Effect of gelatine on muscular fatigue. *Proc. Soc. Exp. Biol. Med.* 1939; 40:157-161.

33. Kaczmarek, RM. Effect of gelatin on the work output of male athletes and non-athletes and girl subjects. *Res. Quart.* 1940; 11:4-109.

34. Kaczmarek, RM. Relative influence of exercise, gelatin and sham feeding on work output, heart and pulse rates. *Med. Rec.* 1941; 153:383-391.

35. Maison, GL. Failure of gelatin or aminoacetic acid to increase the work ability. *JAMA.* 1940; 115:1439-1441.

36. Horvath, SM. Knehr, CA, Dill, DB. The influence of glycine on muscular strength, *Am. J. Physiol.*, 1941; 134:469-472.

37. Hellebrandt, FA, Rork, R, Brogdon, E. Effect of gelatin on power of women to perform maximal anaerobic work. *Proc. Soc. Exptl. Biol. Med.* 1940; 43:629-634.

38. Karpovich, PV, Pestrecov, K. Effect of gelatin upon muscular work in man, *Am. J. Physiol.*, 1941; 134:300-309.

39. Pryor, GB and Knapp, ML. Effect of gelatin feeding on strength and weight according to body build. *Lancet.* 1941; 61:484-486.

40. Robinson, S and Harmon, PM. The effects of training and of gelatin upon certain factors which limit muscular work, *Am. J. Physiol.*, 1941; 13:161-169.

41. Gissal, FW and Hall, LK. Analysis of urinary hydroxyproline levels and delayed muscle soreness resulting from high and low intensity step testing under gelatin-free and gelatin-load dietary regimens. *Med. Sci. Sports. Exer.* 1983; 15:165.

42. Prockop, DJ, Sjverdsma, A. Significance of urinary hydroxyproline in man, *J. Clin. Invest.*, 1961; 40:843-849.

43. Grimble, GK. The significance of peptides in clinical nutrition. *Annu. Rev. Nutr.* 1994; 14:419-447.

44. Silk, DBA, Hegarty, JE, Fairclough, PD, Clark, ML. Characterization and nutritional significance of peptide transport in man. *An. Nutr. Metab.* 1982; 26:337-352.

45. Matthews, DM, Payne, JW, Eds. *Peptide Transport in Protein Nutrition.* Elsevier, Amsterdam, 1975.

46. Krug, E. Zur unterstützenden Therapie bei Osteo- und Chondropathien. *Erfahrungsheilkunde Z Arzt Praxis.* 1979; 11:930-938.

47. Goetz, B. Chondropathia patellae. *Arzt Praxis.* 1982; 92:3130-3134.

48. Oberschlep, U. Individuelle Arthrosetherapie ist möglich! *Therapiewoche,* 1985; 44:5094-5097.

49. Seeligmuller, K, Happel, KH. Kann eine Gelatine/L-Cystin-Mischung die Kollagen-und Proteoglykansynthese stimulieren? *Therapiewoche.* 1989; 39:3153-3157.

50. Adam, M. Therapie der Osteoarthrose. Welche Wirkung haben Gelatinepräparate? *Therapiewoche.* 1991; 38:2456-2461.

51. Adam, M. Gelatine. Möglicher medizinischer Einsatz. *Apotheker.* J 1995; 17:18-22.
52. Bucci, LR. Dietary supplements as ergogenic aids, Ch. 13 in *Nutrition in Exercise and Sport*, 3rd ed., Wolinsky I, Ed., CRC Press LLC, Boca Raton, FL, 1998, 315-368.
53. Rowbottom, DG, Keast, D, Morton, AR. The emerging role of glutamine as an indicator of exercise stress and overtraining. *Sports Med.,* 1996; 21(2):80-97.
54. Rennie, MJ, Tadros, L, Khogali, S, Ahmed, A, Taylor, PM. Glutamine transport and its metabolic effects. *J. Nutr.* 1994; 124:1503S-1508S.
55. Kreider, RB, Klesges, R, Harmon, K, Grindstaff, P, Ramsey, L, Bullen, D, Wood, L, Li, Y, Almada, A. Effects of ingesting supplements designed to promote lean tissue accretion on body composition during resistance training. *Int. J. Sport. Nutr.* 1996; 6:234-242.
56. Boirie, Y, Dangin, M, Gachon, P, Vasson, MP, Maubois, JL, Beaufrere, B. Slow and fast dietary proteins differnetially modulate postprandial protein accretion. *Proc. Natl. Acad. Sci.* 1997; 94; 14930-14935.

CHAPTER 11

Creatine Supplementation in Exercise and Sport

Richard B. Kreider

CONTENTS

11.1 INTRODUCTION

During brief explosive exercise lasting several seconds, the energy supplied to rephosphorylate adenosine diphosphate (ADP) to adenosine triphosphate (ATP) depends to a large degree on the amount of phosphocreatine (PCr) stored in the muscle.[1,2] As PCr stores become depleted during explosive exercise, energy availability deteriorates due to the inability to resynthesize ATP at the rate required.[1,2] Consequently, the ability to maintain maximal effort exercise declines. Because the availability of PCr in the muscle may significantly influence the amount of energy generated during brief periods of high-intensity exercise, it has been hypothesized that increasing muscle creatine content via creatine supplements may increase the availability of PCr and allow for an accelerated rate of resynthesis of ATP during and following high-intensity, short duration exercises.[3–6]

Studies investigating this hypothesis have demonstrated that creatine supplementation (15 to 25 g per day for four to seven days) increases total creatine content by 15 to 30% and phosphocreatine stores by 10 to 40%.[4,5,8–22] The increased availability of creatine and phosphocreatine have been reported to maintain ATP levels during high-intensity exercise and facilitate ATP resynthesis following intense exercise.[4,8,15–17,19] Short-term creatine supplementation has been reported to improve maximal power/strength, work performed during sets of maximal effort muscle contractions, single-effort sprint performance, and work performed during repetitive sprint performance. Moreover, long-term supplementation of creatine or creatine containing supplements (15 to 25 g per day for five to seven days and 2 to 25 g per day thereafter for seven to 84 days) have been reported to promote significantly greater gains in strength, sprint performance, and fat-free mass during training compared with matched-paired controls. Although not all studies report ergogenic benefits, most indicate that creatine is an effective and safe nutritional supplement. Consequently, creatine has become one of the most popular nutritional supplements marketed to athletes in recent times. The following chapter overviews the available literature regarding the effects of creatine supplementation on muscle bioenergetics, performance, and body composition. In addition, it discusses the side effects and concerns regarding the safety of creatine supplementation. The chapter concludes with a summary of findings and suggested areas for additional research.

11.2 MUSCLE CREATINE CONTENT AND PHOSPHOCREATINE RESYNTHESIS

The total creatine (TCr) content in the body in free and phosphorylated forms is about 120 g for a 70 kg person.[3] Approximately 95% of creatine is stored in skeletal muscle primarily as PCr (~66%). The remaining amount of creatine is found in the heart, brain, and testes.[1–3] The normal daily requirement for creatine is approximately 1.6% of the TCr pool (about 2 g for a 70 kg individual). Of this, about half of the daily needs of creatine are obtained from the diet primarily from meat, fish, and animal products. For example, there is approximately 1 g of creatine in 250 g of raw red meat. The remaining daily need of creatine is synthesized primarily in the liver, kidney, and pancreas from the amino acids glycine, arginine and methionine (refer to Figure 11.1).

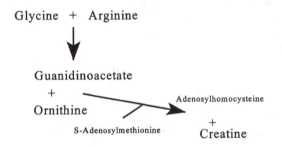

Figure 11.1

Table 11.1 provides a detailed description of studies that have investigated the effects of creatine supplementation on muscle bioenergetics and exercise capacity in humans. The normal muscle TCr concentration ranges between 120 and 125 mmol/kg dry mass muscle.[4,5,8–22] Short-term creatine supplementation (15 to 30 g per day for five to seven days) has been reported to increase TCr by 15 to 30% and PCr stores by 10 to 40%.[4,5,8–22] For example, Harris and co-workers[5] reported that ingesting 20 to 30 g per day of creatine for five, seven, and ten days or on alternate days for 21 days increased TCr by 20% (127 to 149 mmol/kg dry mass) and PCr by 36% (67 to 91 mmol/kg dry mass). Likewise, Balsom and associates[8] reported that creatine supplementation (20 g per day for six days) increased muscle TCr by 18% (129 to 152 mmol/kg dry mass). Studies indicate that the greatest amount of creatine uptake occurs during the first three to five days of supplementation.[5,22] The elevated levels of muscle TCr and PCr can be maintained thereafter by ingesting 2 to 5 g per day thereafter.[13,22] Following cessation of supplementation, TCr and PCr levels return to normal levels in 28 to 35 days.[9,15,22]

Table 11.1 Summary of Studies Investigating the Ergogenic Value of Creatine Supplementation on Muscle Bioenergetics and Exercise Performance

Reference	Subjects/Supplement Dosage	Tests Performed	Results
Greenhaff et al.[4]	Ten male and two female subjects performed pre-testing and then ingested 20 g per day of creatine for five days.	Subjects underwent 20 intense electrically evoked isometric contractions (1.6-s contraction with 1.6-s rest) of the quadriceps or tibialis anterior with limb blood flow occluded. Biopsy samples from the vastus lateralis or ^{31}P MRS were determined prior to and at 40 s and 137 s of recovery.	Creatine supplementation resulted in a 20% increase in recovery muscle PCr determined by biopsy (55 to 67 mmol/kg dry mass) and an 11% higher PCr concentration with MRS (77 to 85 mmol/kg dry mass).
Harris et al.[5]	Twelve male and five female active and inactive subjects ingested between 20 and 30 g per day of creatine for 4.5, 7, 10, or 21 days (taken on alternate days).	Subjects had resting muscle TCr, ATP, and PCr determined prior to and following creatine supplementation. Five subjects performed one-legged cycle ergometry for 60 min so that the effects of exercise following creatine supplementation on TCr, ATP, and PCr could be determined. Blood samples were obtained to determine creatine levels and standard hematological profiles. Urinary creatine excretion was also determined.	Dosages of 5 g of creatine resulted in peak plasma creatine concentrations at 60 min following administration. Repeated doses of 5 g every two hours for eight hours maintained high plasma creatine levels. Creatine supplementation increased TCr by 20% (127 to 149 mmol/kg dry mass), PCr by 36% (67 to 91 mmol/kg dry mass) with no effect on ATP levels. The greatest increases occurred in subjects with lower initial TCr content. Exercise with creatine supplementation resulted in significantly greater muscle TCr (9%). Urinary analysis revealed that creatine uptake was greatest during the first two days. No significant effects were observed in standard clinical blood profiles.
Balsom et al.[8]	Seven male subjects performed pre-supplementation tests and were then administered 20 g per day of creatine for six days.	5 × 6-s cycle ergometer sprints with 30 s rest recovery followed 40 s later with 1 × 10-s maximal effort sprint. Muscle biopsies taken at rest, after the fifth 6-s sprint, and following the 10-s sprint. A series of counter movement squat jumps were performed prior to and following supplementation.	Body mass increased by 1.1 kg. Total muscle creatine content significantly increased (129 to 152 mmol/kg dry wt). Following creatine supplementation, muscle PCr concentration was higher after the fifth sprint (70 vs. 46 mmol/kg dry wt) and muscle lactate was lower (26 vs 44 mmol/kg dry wt) following creatine supplementation. Work output was significantly greater in the 10-s sprint following creatine supplementation. No differences were observed in jump performance.

continued

Table 11.1 (continued) Summary of Studies Investigating the Ergogenic Value of Creatine Supplementation on Muscle Bioenergetics and Exercise Performance

Reference	Subjects/Supplement Dosage	Tests Performed	Results
Febbraio et al.[9]	Six males subjects performed pre-supplementation tests and then ingested 20 g per day of creatine for five days. Subjects then observed a 23-d washout period and began ingesting a placebo for five days.	Subjects performed 4 × 60-s cycle ergometer sprints with 60-s recovery between sprints followed by cycling to exhaustion at a work rate equivalent to 115-120% of $VO_{2\,max}$. Intramuscular TCr, PCr, ATP, ADP, AMP, inosine 5'-monophosphate (IMP), ammonia, lactate and glycogen levels were determined prior to and following exercise.	Creatine supplementation resulted in significant increases in TCr and PCr concentrations with no effect on ATP, ADP, AMP, IMP, NH_3, lactate, or glycogen levels. Creatine supplementation did not affect time to exhaustion during the fifth sprint trial. TCr stores returned to normal within the 28-day washout period.
Green et al.[10]	Twenty-one male subjects ingested 20 g per day of creatine or 20 g per day of creatine with 400 g per day of carbohydrate for five days.	Prior to and following supplementation, TCr and glycogen concentrations were determined.	Creatine supplementation increased TCr by 18% (122 to 143 mmol/kg dry mass) and did not affect glycogen content (365 to 366 mmol/kg dry mass). Ingestion of glucose alone resulted in a 4% decrease in TCr (130 to 124 mmol/kg dry mass) and a 22% increase in glycogen content (338 to 441 mmol/kg dry mass). Ingestion of glucose with creatine resulted in significantly greater increases in TCr (124 to 158 mmol/kg dry mass or 27%). Muscle glycogen content non-significantly increased (331 to 489 mmol/kg dry mass or 48%) but was significantly correlated to changes in TCr.
Green et al.[11]	Twenty-two male subjects were administered (a) a normal diet, no exercise, 20 g per day of creatine with a non-glucose placebo; b) a high-carbohydrate diet, no exercise, 20 g per day of creatine and 93 g per day of carbohydrate; c) a high-carbohydrate, exercise (60 min of cycling at 70% $VO_{2\,max}$), 20 g per day of creatine with 93 g per day of carbohydrate; or d) a normal diet, no exercise, and a placebo.	Plasma creatine, serum insulin, and 24 urinary excretion of creatine were determined on days 1 and 3 of study to evaluate creatine retention.	Results showed that carbohydrate ingestion augmented creatine retention due to a greater increase in insulin levels and that exercise did not provide further benefit.

Reference	Subjects/Supplement Dosage	Tests Performed	Results
Greenhaff et al.[12]	Eight active but not highly trained male subjects ingested 20 g per day of creatine for five days.	Prior to and following supplementation, muscle biopsies were taken at rest and following 0, 20, 60, 120 s recovery from electrically evoked isometric contractions (20 x 1.6-s contractions with 1.6-s rest recovery between contractions).	Subjects had a significant increase in body mass (1.6 kg), resting TCr (15%), and PCr resynthesis was similar at 60-s recovery but 42% greater following 120-s recovery following creatine supplementation. There was some evidence that not all subjects responded to creatine supplementation.
Hultman et al.[13]	Thirty-one male subjects ingested either 20 g per day of creatine for six days followed by ingesting 2 g per day for 22 days or 3 g per day of creatine for 28 days.	Muscle creatine content and urinary excretion of creatine was determined.	Ingesting 20 g per day of creatine for six days resulted in a 20% increase in TCr. Ingesting 2 g per day of creatine thereafter served to maintain muscle TCr levels. However, TCr levels declined within 30 days without ingesting the 2 g per day maintenance dose. Ingesting 3 g per day of creatine resulted in a gradual increase muscle TCr approaching loading levels in 28 days. Urinary excretion paralleled intake.
Kurosawa et al.[14]	Four male and one female subjects consumed 30 g per day of creatine for 14 days.	Subjects performed low- and high-intensity grip exercise in which blood creatine concentration and forearm PCr concentrations were determined using ^{31}P MRS. In addition, muscle biopsies were obtained to measure muscle PCr and ATP concentrations. Subjects then began supplementation and performed grip exercise training with their dominant arm (1 contraction at 30% of maximal voluntary contraction until exhaustion) 6 times per day for 14 days. Pre-tests were then repeated following supplementation.	Creatine supplementation increased blood creatine concentrations (47-fold) and also increased muscle creatine concentration relative to β-ATP levels by 11% in the non-training and 23% in the trained group. Creatine supplementation increased high intensity grip strength performance in non-trained (20%) and trained groups (35%). No significant differences were observed in time to exhaustion during the low intensity muscle contractions although times were increased by 23% and 96% for the untrained and trained arms, respectively.

continued

Table 11.1 (continued Summary of Studies Investigating the Ergogenic Value of Creatine Supplementation on Muscle Bioenergetics and Exercise Performance

Reference	Subjects/Supplement Dosage	Tests Performed	Results
Lemon et al.[15]	Seven active male subjects ingested either 20 g per day of creatine or a placebo for five days. Subjects then observed a 35 day washout period and then repeated the experiment ingesting the alternate supplement.	Subjects performed 20 × 30-s maximal effort isometric muscle contractions (plantar flexion) with 16-s rest recovery following ingesting creatine and the placebo for five days. PCr and ATP concentrations during exercise were determined using ^{31}P MRS. Blood samples were obtained to measure serum creatine.	Creatine supplementation increased body mass by 1.3 kg, PCr/ATP by 8% (p=0.10), total force produced by 11%, and maximal force by 10%. Calculated rates of oxidative phosphorylation and glycolysis were increased with creatine supplementation. In addition, there was some evidence that the 35-day washout was not long enough for TCr levels to return to normal.
Ruden et al.[16]	Five female and four male subjects ingested 20 g per day of creatine and a placebo for four days separated by a 14-day washout period.	Subjects performed a 30-s maximal effort cycle ergometer trial prior to and following supplementation. Muscle TCr and PCr were determined prior to and following exercise.	Muscle TCr was significantly increased following creatine supplementation by 20 to 21 mmol/kg dry mass. No significant differences were observed between groups in gains in PCr (creatine 6.4 vs. placebo 2.5 mmol/kg dry mass). No significant differences were observed between groups in peak power, mean power, or decline in power.
Vandenberghe et al.[17]	Nine male subjects ingested a placebo, 0.5 g/kg/d of creatine, or 0.5 g/kg/d of creatine with 5 mg/kg/d of caffeine for six days.	Prior to and following supplementation, subjects performed three consecutive plantar flexion maximal isometric contractions followed by performing a set of 90, 80 and 50 maximal effort knee extension contractions with a 2-min rest recovery between sets. ^{31}P NMR of the gastrocnemius measured resting and post-isometric contraction ATP and PC concentrations. Dynamic knee extensor torque production was measured using an isokinetic dynamometer.	Creatine supplementation did not significantly affect ATP concentrations. Muscle PCr levels were significantly increased by 4 to 6% in both groups receiving creatine. Muscle torque production was significantly increased by 10-23% in the group ingesting creatine but not in the group ingesting creatine and caffeine.

Reference	Subjects/Supplement Dosage	Tests Performed	Results
Casey et al.[19]	Nine male subjects ingested 20 g per day of creatine for five days.	Prior to and following supplementation, subjects performed two 30-s bouts of cycling. Muscle biopsies were obtained to determine total creatine, ATP, and PCr content.	Creatine supplementation resulted in significant increases in resting PCr in both type I and II fibers. Total creatine content in muscle increased by 23 mmol/kg dry mass. Total work in both exercise bouts increased by 4%. There was 31% less loss in ATP despite producing more work in the creatine group. Changes in resting PCr in type II fibers were positively correlated to changes in PCr during exercise and changes in total work.
Rossiter et al.[20]	In a double-blind manner, 19 competitive rowers ingested either 0.25 g/kg/d of creatine or a placebo for five days.	Total creatine uptake was estimated by monitoring urine creatine output. Subjects performed a 1000-m rowing performance trial to evaluate the ergogenic effects of creatine on rowing performance.	Calculated total creatine uptake over the five day period averaged 35 g with an estimated muscle uptake of 38 mmol/kg dry mass. No change was observed in performance time for the placebo group (214 to 214 s). However, performance time was significantly decreased in the creatine group (211 to 208.7 s). The increase in creatine uptake was non-significantly correlated to performance times ($r=0.43$, $p=0.09$).
Myburgh et al.[21]	In a double-blind and randomized manner, 13 trained cyclists ingested either 20 g per day of creatine or a placebo for seven days and then maintenance doses (2 g per day) of creatine or the placebo during seven days of interval sprint training.	Muscle biopsies and blood samples were obtained prior to and following seven days of supplementation and one day after seven days of sprint training (10 × 10-s sprints with 140-s rest recovery for seven days). In addition, subjects performed a 30-s cycle ergometry Wingate anaerobic power test and a one hour performance time trial.	Muscle creatine content was significantly increased by 21% in the creatine group (121 to 147 mmol/kg dry mass). The increase in total creatine content was significantly correlated to the percentage of type IIb muscle fiber. No significant differences were observed between groups in resting and post-sprint training ATP levels, blood lactate, ammonia, or hypoxanthine levels. In addition, no differences were observed between groups in anaerobic power during the 30-s Wingate test or in one hour time trial performance.

continued

Table 11.1 (continued) Summary of Studies Investigating the Ergogenic Value of Creatine Supplementation on Muscle Bioenergetics and Exercise Performance

Reference	Subjects/Supplement Dosage	Tests Performed	Results
Vanderberghe et al.[22]	In a double-blind and randomized manner, 19 untrained females ingested a placebo or 20 g per day of creatine for four days. Subjects then ingested 5 g per day thereafter for 66 days. A subset of 13 subjects then terminated training while maintaining low dose supplementation. Subjects were then evaluated 28 days following cessation of supplementation.	Prior to and following 4, 35, and 70 days of supplementation, total PCr and the ratio of PCr/ATP were determined using ^{31}P NMR. In addition, strength tests (30 maximal effort arm flexion contractions), training lifting volume, and hydrostatically determined body composition assessments were performed. A subset of 13 subjects were also evaluated at 7, 28, and 70 days of cessation of supplementation and detraining.	NMR determined total PCr and the ratio of PCr/ATP were significantly increased by 6% following four days of supplementation in the creatine group. These values were maintained during the low dose supplementation phase. Urine volume did not differ between groups however creatine supplementation increased creatine. Creatine supplementation resulted in significantly greater increases in maximal strength (20 to 25%), maximal intermittent exercise performance (10 to 25%), and fat free mass (60%) in comparison to the placebo group. After cessation of training, gains in strength and fat free mass were maintained in the creatine group ingesting 5 g per day of creatine. Muscle PCr levels declined after 28 days of cessation of supplementation. However, gains in fat free mass were maintained in the creatine group.
Becque et al.[23]	In a double-blind and randomized manner, 23 male resistance trained athletes ingested either 20 g per day of creatine for seven days and 2 g per day of creatine for 35 days or a sucrose placebo.	Subjects performed 1RM biceps curl strength tests and had body composition determined by hydrostatic weighing prior to and following supplementation.	Subjects ingesting creatine observed a significantly greater gain in 1RM strength (11.9 vs 6.8 kg). Body mass (2 kg), and fat free mass (1.6 kg) were significantly increased in the creatine group while no changes were observed in the placebo group.
Birch et al.[24]	In a double-blind and randomized manner, 14 male subjects ingested either 20 g per day of creatine or an equivalent amount of a placebo for five days.	Subjects performed 3 × 30-s maximal effort isokinetic cycling sprints with 4 min of passive recovery between sprints. Blood samples were obtained prior to and following exercise to determine ammonia and lactate levels.	Peak power output was significantly increased (8%) in the creatine group during sprint 1. Mean power output (~6%) and work performed (~9%) were significantly increased in sprints 1 and 2 following creatine ingestion. No significant differences were observed in sprint 3. Plasma ammonia levels were decreased following creatine supplementation. No differences were observed between groups in lactate levels.

Reference	Subjects/Supplement Dosage	Tests Performed	Results
Earnest et al.[25]	In a double-blind and randomized manner, ten resistance trained male subjects ingested either 20 g per day of creatine or a placebo for 28 days during training.	Prior to and following supplementation, subjects performed 3 × 30-s Wingate cycle ergometer tests with 5-min rest recovery between trials; a 1RM bench press test; a bench press repetition test at 70% 1RM; and had body composition determined by hydrostatic weighing.	Creatine supplementation resulted in significant increases in work performed in the 3 × 30-s Wingate tests (15, 24, & 23%); an 8% increase in 1 RM bench press in the creatine group; a 43% increase in lifting volume; and a 1.7 kg increase in body mass in which FFM accounted for 1.6 kg of the gain (p=0.054).
Greenhaff et al.[26]	In a double-blind and randomized manner, nine male and three female active but not highly trained subjects ingested either 20 g per day of creatine with 4 g per day of glucose or 24 g per day of glucose for five days.	Subjects performed 5 sets of 30 maximal knee extension contractions with 60-s rest between sets on an isokinetic dynamometer. Blood samples were obtained to measure plasma ammonia and blood lactate.	Creatine supplementation resulted in a significant increases in total peak torque during bouts 2 and 3 and approached significance in the 4th set. In addition, total peak torque in the last 10 repetitions of set 1 was significantly greater in the creatine group. Plasma ammonia levels were significantly lower following the 4th and 5th set of exercise in the group receiving creatine. No significant differences were observed between groups in blood lactate levels.
Schnieder et al.[27]	In a single-blind manner, nine untrained males ingested a 30 g per day of a glucose placebo for seven days followed by ingesting 25 g per day of creatine with 5 g per day glucose for seven days.	Prior to and following each supplementation treatment, subjects performed 5 × 15-s cycling sprints with 6-sec rest recovery between sprints. Blood lactate levels were determined 5 min following the 5 × 15-s sprints. A subset of 6 subjects also performed 5 × 60-s sprints with 5-min rest recovery between sprints.	Creatine supplementation significantly increased work performed during each 15-s sprint and total work performed by 7%. No significant differences were observed in post-exercise lactate levels. No significant differences were observed between groups in work performed during the 5 × 60-s sprints.
Stout et al.[28]	In a double-blind and randomized manner, 24 Division II football players ingested either a flavored powder containing 35 g of glucose (G); 5.25 g of creatine with 1 g of glucose in a flavored powder (Cr); or, the G powder containing 5.25 g of creatine (G/Cr). Subjects ingested these supplements four times per day for five days and twice a day for 56 days during off-season resistance training.	Prior to and following supplementation, subjects had body composition determined by dual energy x-ray absorptiometry (DEXA) and performed 1RM bench press, vertical jump, and 100-yd sprints.	Compared with the placebo group, subjects ingesting G/Cr had significantly greater gains in FFM (2.9 kg), bench press 1RM (16 kg), and vertical jump performance (4.3 cm) while decreasing 100 yd dash time by an additional (0.29 s). Subjects ingesting creatine observed greater gains in FFM (2.6 kg), bench press 1RM (4.4 kg), and vertical jump performance (3.8 cm) while decreasing 100 yd dash time by an additional (-0.22 s) in comparison to the placebo group but these differences were not statistically significant due to between-subject variability.

continued

Table 11.1 (continued) Summary of Studies Investigating the Ergogenic Value of Creatine Supplementation on Muscle Bioenergetics and Exercise Performance

Reference	Subjects/Supplement Dosage	Tests Performed	Results
Volek et al.[29]	In a double-blind and randomized manner, 14 resistance-trained male subjects ingested 25 g per day of creatine or a placebo for seven days.	Subjects performed five sets to failure at their 10 RM max for the bench press with 2 min recovery between sets. The next day, subjects performed five sets of ten repetitions of jump squats at 30% of the subjects 1 RM in the squat. Body composition was assessed using skinfolds and blood lactate was determined prior to and following exercise bouts.	Body mass was significantly increased by 1.1 kg with no significant differences observed in sum of skinfold measurements. Creatine supplementation resulted in a significant increase in the number of repetitions performed in all five sets of the bench press and jump squat.
Goldberg et al.[30]	34 Division I-A football and track athletes ingested either 3 g per day of creatine or a placebo for 14 days during training.	Prior to and following supplementation, subjects had body mass, vertical jump, and 40-yd sprint times determined. In addition, subjects performed 1RM bench press, leg sled, and leg extension tests.	Body weight (0.9 kg) and vertical jump performance (2.6%) were significantly increased in the creatine group. No significant differences were observed between groups in 1RM bench press, 40 yd sprint times, leg sled endurance, or leg extension performance.
Bosco et al.[31]	In a double-blind and randomized manner, qualified male sprinters and jumpers ingested either 20 g per day of creatine or a placebo for five days.	Subjects performed a 45-s maximal continuous jumping test and an all-out treadmill run to exhaustion at 20 km/h (lasting about 60 s).	Creatine supplementation promoted a 7% improvement in jumping performance during the first 15 s of the jump test and a 5% improvement in jump performance in the second 15-s segment. Run time to exhaustion was increased by 13% in the creatine group.
Almada et al.[32]	In a double-blind and randomized manner, 41 NCAA Division I-A football players ingested a glucose powder (G), the G with 3 g per day of calcium HMB, or the G/HMB supplement with 15.75 g per day of creatine for 28 days during resistance/agility training.	Subjects performed 12 × 6-s cycle ergometer sprints with 30-s rest recovery, lifting volume in bench press, squat, and power clean.	There was some evidence that subjects administered creatine with the GET/HMB supplement observed greater gains in mean work performed during the repetitive sprint performance (p=0.06) and greater gains in and squat (p=0.08) and power clean (p=0.008) lifting volume.
Hamilton-Ward et al.[33]	In a double-blind and randomized manner, 20 female racquet players ingested either a placebo or 25 g per day of creatine for seven days	Prior to and following supplementation, subjects performed 1RM internal rotation tests and an elbow flexion test to fatigue.	No significant differences were observed between groups in concentric and eccentric 1RM internal rotation force or in elbow flexion to fatigue. There was a non-significant 0.7 kg increase in body mass.
Johnson et al.[34]	In a double-blind and randomized manner, 18 male and female subjects ingested either a placebo or 20 g per day of creatine for six days.	Prior to and following supplementation, subjects performed concentric/eccentric maximal power output knee extension exercises. This was followed by an isotonic muscular fatigue test.	Creatine supplementation resulted in significant increases concentric peak power (6%), eccentric peak power (9%), total concentric work (25%), and total eccentric work (15%).

Reference	Subjects/Supplement Dosage	Tests Performed	Results
Kreider et al.[35]	In a double-blind and randomized manner, 25 Division I-A football players ingested either a glucose, electrolyte, and taurine placebo or this placebo with 15.75 g per day of creatine for 28 days during resistance/agility training.	Prior to and following supplementation, subjects 1) had body weight, total body water, and body composition determined by DEXA; 2) donated fasting blood samples; 3) performed 12 × 6-s maximal effort cycle ergometry sprints with 30-s rest recovery; and 4) performed a maximal repetition test on the isotonic bench press, squat and power clean.	Clinical blood profiles remained within normal for athletes engaged in intense training. However, subjects ingesting creatine observed greater increases in creatinine, CK, LDH, and ALT levels while the ratio of urea nitrogen/creatinine was decreased. In addition, postivie lipid modifying effects were observed. Gains in body mass (2.4 kg) and fat/bone free mass (2.4 kg) in the creatine group were significantly greater than the placebo group. Sprint performance during the first five of 12 × 6-s sprints and overall gains in lifting volume was significantly greater in the creatine group.
Grindstaff et al.[36]	In a double-blind and randomized manner, 11 female and nine male regional and nationally competitive U.S. junior swimmers ingested either 21 g per day of creatine with 4 g per day of maltodextrin or 25 g per day of maltodextrin for nine days during training.	Prior to and following supplementation, subjects had body mass, total body water, and body composition measurements via skinfolds determined. In addition, subjects performed 3 × 100-m competitive freestyle swims with 60-s rest recovery between trials and 3 × 20-s upper extremity isokinetic arm ergometer tests in the prone position with 60-s rest recovery between sprints.	Body mass was non-significantly increased (0.5 kg) in the creatine group. However, there was some evidence that fat mass (p=0.08) and body composition (p=0.09) was decreased in the creatine group. 100-m swim times were significantly faster in the creatine group in heat 1 (1.1-s). In addition, creatine supplementation significantly decreased swim times in the second 100-m heat by 0.93-s. There was some evidence of improved swim times for all three 100-m sprints (p=0.057). Upper extremity work in the creatine group was significantly greater than placebo responses after 20-s sprint trial (7.8%) but was not significantly greater than placebo responses in sprint 2 (5.3%) or sprint 3 (0.5%).
Prevost et al.[37]	Eighteen subjects ingested a calcium chloride placebo for five days days prior to pre-testing. Subjects were then administered in a double-blind and randomized manner either the placebo or 18.75 g per day of creatine for five days prior to post-testing and 2.25 g of creatine each day during post-testing.	Prior to and following supplementation, subjects cycled to exhaustion using a work rate approximating 150% of VO_2 peak under the following conditions: 1) cycle continuously to exhaustion; 2) cycle intermittently for 60 s work/120 s rest recovery; 3) cycle intermittently for 20 s work/40 s rest recovery; or 4) cycle intermittently for 10 s /20 s rest recovery.	Creatine supplementation resulted in significant increases in total work for all exercise bouts with the greatest improvement in work performed on the 10-s work/20-s rest recovery protocol [Protocol 1(23.5%), Protocol 2 (61%), Protocol 3 (62%), Protocol 4 (100%)].

continued

Table 11.1 (continued) Summary of Studies Investigating the Ergogenic Value of Creatine Supplementation on Muscle Bioenergetics and Exercise Performance

Reference	Subjects/Supplement Dosage	Tests Performed	Results
Ziegenfuss et al.[38]	In a double-blind and randomized manner, 33 trained male and female subjects ingested either 0.35 g/kg/d of creatine or a maltodextrin placebo for three days or five days.	Subjects had muscle thigh volume determined by MRI and intra and extracellular water determined by BIA. In addition, subjects performed 6 x 10-s cycle ergometer sprints to determine anaerobic power. Finally, whole body protein turnover ([15N] glycine) was determined in three subjects to evaluate whether creatine affects protein synthesis/catabolism.	Results revealed that total work in the first, and peak power in the last 5 × 10-s sprints were increased in the Cr group. Muscle thigh volume increased by 7% in five of six subjects. Total body and intracellular water increased by 2–3%. Nitrogen status was increased by either increased protein synthesis or a decreased protein breakdown. There were no gender or training mode effects observed.
Balsom et al.[39]	In a double-blind and randomized manner, 18 active to well-trained male subjects ingested either 30 g per day of creatine with 6 g per day glucose or 36 g per day of glucose for six days.	Treadmill time to exhaustion lasting 3–4 min and a 6-km outdoor terrain run. Oxygen uptake was determined during treadmill run. Post-exercise heart rate, lactate, and hypoxanthine levels determined.	Subjects observed a significant increase (0.9 kg) in body mass in the creatine group. No significant differences were observed between groups in time to treadmill exhaustion (placebo +0.21 min, creatine +0.25 min). Significantly greater increases in lactate occurred in the creatine group following treadmill run. There was a significant increase in time to perform the 6-km run presumably due to weight gain.
Dawson et al.[40]	In a double-blind and randomized manner, 18 male subjects (Study I) and 11 male subjects (Study II) performed baseline tests and then ingested either 20 g per day of creatine or glucose for five days.	Study I. Subjects performed one 10-s cycling sprint trial prior to and one and three days following supplementation. Study II. Subjects performed 6 × 6-s cycle ergometer sprints with 30 s rest recovery between sprints.	Study I: No significant differences between pre- and post-supplementation work performed in the 10-s sprint. Study II: Creatine supplementation resulted in significant increases in total work performed during the 6 × 6-s sprints, work completed in sprint 1, and peak power.
Ferreira et al.[41]	In a double-blind and randomized manner, 25 Division I-A football players ingested either a glucose, electrolyte, and taurine placebo or this placebo with 15.75 g per day of creatine for 28 days during resistance/agility training.	Prior to and following supplementation, subjects: 1) performed 12 × 6-s maximal effort cycle ergometry sprints with 30 s rest recovery; and 2) performed a maximal repetition test on the isotonic bench press and squat.	Sprint performance during the first five of 12 × 6-s sprints, bench press lifting volume, and overall gains in lifting volume were significantly greater in the creatine group.
Harris et al.[42]	In a double-blind and randomized manner, 10 trained middle distance male runners ingested either a placebo or 30 g per day of creatine with 5 g per day of glucose for six days.	Prior to and following supplementation, subjects performed 4 × 300-m maximal effort runs with 4 min rest recovery. On the next day, subjects performed 4 × 1000-m runs with 3 min rest recovery.	Creatine supplementation resulted in significant decreases in final 300-m and 1000-m run performance times. In addition, total time to perform the 4 × 1000-m runs was significantly improved in the creatine group. Best 300-m and 1000-m times were significantly reduced by -0.3 s and -2.1 s in the creatine group.

Reference	Subjects/Supplement Dosage	Tests Performed	Results
Kirksey et al.[43]	In a double-blind and randomized manner, 16 male and 20 female track athletes ingested either 0.3 g/kg/d of creatine or a placebo for 42 days during pre-season conditioning.	Prior to and following supplementation, subjects had body composition measured using hydrodensitometry and skinfolds. In addition, subjects performed static and counter movement vertical jumps and 5 × 30-s Wingate cycle ergometer tests.	Creatine supplementation resulted in significantly greater increases in FFM (4.8 vs. 3.5 kg) and average peak power for the Wingate tests (106 vs. 38 W). No group × time × gender effects were observed.
Leenders et al.[44]	In a double-blind and randomized manner, 6 female college swimmers ingested either 20 g per day of creatine or a placebo for 14 days during training.	During training and performance trial sets, subjects performed interval sets of 6 × 50-m swims with 180-s recovery, 10 × 25-m swims with 60-s recovery, and 12 × 100-m swims with 150 s recovery.	No significant differences were observed between groups in 10 × 25-m or 12 × 100-m sprint times. However, swim times to perform the 6 × 50-m set were significantly reduced. In addition, a significant linear trend for increased interval set swim velocity was observed in the creatine group.
Earnest et al.[45]	In a double-blind manner, 8 male and 7 female active subjects ingested either 20 g per day of creatine or a placebo for five days.	Subjects complete familiarization and baseline trials to establish work rates designed to elicit fatigue in 90–600 s. Subjects then performed three experimental trials after five days of supplementation to evaluate the effects of creatine supplementation on time to exhaustion at various work rates.	Subjects ingesting creatine produced significantly greater work due to its effect on extending exercise time primarily at the shorter, higher intensity work rates.
Earnest et al.[46]	In a double-blind and randomized manner, 11 trained male subjects ingested either 20 g per day of creatine with 4 g per day of glucose for four days followed by ingesting 10 g per day of creatine for six days or a placebo.	Prior to and following supplementation, subjects performed two treadmill runs to exhaustion at 214 m/min with a grade determined to elicit fatigue within 90 s. The treadmill runs were separated by an 8 min rest recovery. Blood lactate levels were determined prior to and following exercise.	No significant differences were observed between groups in changes in body mass. Creatine supplementation significantly improved total treadmill time to exhaustion (placebo 166 to 163.8; creatine 176.5 to 182.2-s). The greatest improvement was observed in the second run to exhaustion. Post-exercise blood lactate levels were significantly greater following exercise in the creatine group.
Nelson et al.[47]	Nineteen male and nine female trained runners performed pre-testing and then ingested 20 g per day of creatine for seven to eight days.	Prior to and following supplementation, subjects performed an incremental maximal exercise test to determine maximal VO_2 and ventilatory anaerobic threshold (VANT). In addition, pre- and post-exercise blood lactate and ammonia concentrations were determined.	No significant differences were observed in peak VO_2. However, creatine supplementation resulted in a significant increase in VANT (67% to 74%). In addition, there was a significant decrease in blood lactate and ammonia.

continued

Table 11.1 (continued) Summary of Studies Investigating the Ergogenic Value of Creatine Supplementation on Muscle Bioenergetics and Exercise Performance

Reference	Subjects/Supplement Dosage	Tests Performed	Results
Jacobs et al.[48]	In a double-blind and randomized manner, 26 male and female subjects ingested either 20 g per day of creatine or a placebo for five days.	Subjects exercised to exhaustion at a work rate equivalent to 125% of VO_2 max prior to, following five days of supplementation, and seven days following cessation of supplementation. Time to exhaustion and maximal accumulated oxygen deficit (MAOD) was determined during each trial.	Creatine supplementation significantly increased time to exhaustion at five days following supplementation (130 to 141-s or 8%) and remained increased following seven days of cessation of supplementation (139 s or 7%). In addition, MOAD was significantly increased by 9% after five days and remained elevated by 7% after seven days of cessation of supplementation.
Balsom et al.[49]	In a double-blind and randomized manner, 16 active but not highly trained male subjects ingested either 25 g per day of creatine with 5 g per day of glucose or 30 g per day of glucose for five days.	10 × 6-s cycle ergometer sprints with 30 s rest recovery at 130 and 140 rev/min. Blood samples were taken to determine lactate and hypoxanthine levels. Post-exercise oxygen uptake was also measured.	Subjects ingesting creatine observed a significant increase in body mass (1.1 kg). No differences were observed between groups at the 130 rev/min intensity. Sprint performance during the 4- to 6-s segment in the creatine group was significantly greater in the creatine group in the latter sprints. Blood lactate and hypoxanthine levels were lower in the creatine group despite performing more work. No significant differences in post-exercise oxygen uptake.
Thompson et al.[50]	Ten female swimmers ingested either 2 g per day of creatine or a placebo for 42 days during training.	Resting and exercise (10 to 15 min of submaximal plantar flexion contractions) ATP and PC concentrations were determined using ^{31}P MRS.	No significant differences were observed between groups in resting, exercise, or post-exercise bioenergetics.
Odland et al.[51]	In a double-blind, crossover and randomized manner nine active but untrained male subjects performed a maximal effort sprint test following a three-day control period or ingesting 20 g per day of creatine or a placebo for three days. Treatments were separated by a 14-day washout period.	Prior to and following each treatment period, subjects performed one 30-s maximal effort cycle ergometer anaerobic power test. Muscle biopsies were obtained prior to supplementation as well as prior to each exercise session. Blood lactate was determined 3 min post-exercise.	No significant differences were observed between treatments in resting ATP, PCr, or TCr. The ratio of TCr/ATP was significantly greater in the creatine supplemented group. No significant differences were observed between treatments in peak, mean 10-s, or mean 30-s power, percent fatigue, or post-exercise lactate levels.
Burke et al.[52]	In a double-blind and randomized manner, 18 male and 14 female Australian National Team swimmers ingested 20 g per day of creatine or a sucrose placebo for five days.	Subjects performed single effort swim performance trials at 25-, 50-, and 100-m distances with a 10-min active recovery performed between sprint tests and a 10-s sprint on a cycle ergometer prior to and following supplementation.	No significant differences between groups in swim performance or 10-s cycling sprint performance.

Reference	Subjects/Supplement Dosage	Tests Performed	Results
Cooke et al.[53]	In a double-blind and randomized manner, 12 untrained male subjects ingested either 20 g per day of creatine with 4 g per day of glucose or 24 g per day of glucose for five days.	Subjects performed 2 × 15-s cycle ergometry sprint trials separated by a 20-min rest recovery between sprints.	No significant differences between groups in cycling power or work performed.
Mujika et al.[54]	In a double-blind and randomized manner, nine male and 11 female swimmers ingested either 20 g per day of creatine or a placebo for five days.	Prior to and following supplementation, subjects performed 25-m, 50-m, 100-m sprint trials with 20 to 25 min rest recovery between sprints. Post-exercise blood samples were obtained to determine blood lactate and ammonia concentrations.	Body mass significantly increased by 0.7 kg in the creatine group. No significant differences were observed between groups in performance times or lactate concentrations. Post-exercise ammonia levels were significantly lower at the 50- and 100-m distances in the creatine group.
Redondo et al.[55]	In a double-blind and randomized manner, 14 female college field hockey players and eight male baseball players ingested either 25 g per day of creatine or a placebo for seven days.	Subjects performed three 60-m sprints separated by 5 min resting recovery. Biomechanical analysis of running velocity and stride length were determined at 20 to 30 m, 40 to 50 m, and 50 to 60 m zones.	Body mass non-significantly decreased by -0.8 kg in the creatine group. No significant differences were observed between groups in running velocities or stride length.
Barnett et al.[56]	Seventeen active male subjects were administered 40 g per day of glucose for four days. Subjects were then matched based on sprint performance and were then administered 0.28 g/kg/d of creatine for four days.	Subjects performed 7 × 10-s cycle ergometer sprints with 30 s rest recovery for sprints 1 through 5. Subjects then rested for 5-min and completed sprint 6 and 7 with a 30-s rest recovery between sprints. Blood samples were obtained prior to, after the fifth sprint, before the sixth sprint, and following sprint 7. Post-exercise oxygen uptake was measured for 5 min following sprint 7.	No significant differences were found in multiple sprint performance power output, plasma lactate, blood pH, or post-exercise oxygen uptake.
Terrilion et al.[57]	In a double-blind and randomized manner, 12 trained male runners ingested either 20 g per day of creatine or a placebo for five days.	Prior to and following supplementation, body mass and total body water were determined. In addition, subjects performed two 700-m outdoor runs with 60 min recovery between trials. Blood samples were collected to evaluate changes in blood lactate.	No significant differences were observed between groups in changes in body mass (placebo -0.4; creatine 0.6 kg) or in total body water. No significant differences were observed between groups in changes in performance times for each trial (placebo 0.2, -0.4-s, creatine 0.5, -1.9-s) or in blood lactate concentrations.
Cooke et al.[58]	In a randomized manner, 80 active male subjects were randomly assigned to ingest a placebo or 20 g per day of creatine for five days.	Subjects performed two maximal effort cycle ergometer sprints separated by 30, 60, 90, or 120 s of recovery.	No significant interactions were observed between groups in peak power and absolute time to fatigue in the first or second sprint regardless of rest recovery observed.

continued

Table 11.1 (continued) Summary of Studies Investigating the Ergogenic Value of Creatine Supplementation on Muscle Bioenergetics and Exercise Performance

Reference	Subjects/Supplement Dosage	Tests Performed	Results
Godly et al.[59]	In a double-blind and randomized manner, 13 male and three female well-trained cyclists ingested either 24 g per day of creatine or a placebo for five days.	Prior to and following supplementation, subjects performed a 25-km cycling time trial on their own bike attached to a computerized simulator, interspersed with 15-s all out sprints at 4-km intervals.	No significant differences were observed between groups in changes in total body mass. Performance times in the creatine group decreased from 41.36- to 40.34-min compared to 41.97- to 41.75-min in the placebo group. However, this difference was not statistically significant.
Stroud et al.[60]	Eight males subjects performed pre-testing and then consumed 20 g per day of creatine for five days.	Prior to and following supplementation, subjects performed a continuous incremental exercise test running at 10 km/h at workloads eliciting 50% to 90% of $VO_{2\,max}$ for 6 min each. Respiratory gases and blood lactate were determined at each workload and at 5-min intervals during recovery.	No significant differences were observed in respiratory exchange ratio or blood lactate at each workload.
Kreider et al.[62]	In a double-blind and randomized manner, 41 Division I-A football players ingested either a glucose placebo (G), the G with 3 g per day of calcium HMB (G/HMB), or the G/HMB supplement with 15.75 g per day of creatine (G/HMB/Cr) for 28 days during resistance/agility training.	Prior to and following supplementation, subjects had total body mass, total body water, and body composition determined using DEXA.	Subjects ingesting G/HMB/Cr observed significantly greater increases in body mass (1.2 kg) and FFM (1.3 kg) with no changes in total body water in comparison to subjects ingesting G and the G/HMB supplement.
Kreider et al.[66]	In a double-blind and randomized manner, 52 Division I-A football players ingested near isoenergetic amounts of a maltodextrin placebo, Phosphagain® containing 20 g per day of creatine (P-I), or Phosphagain II® containing 25 g per day of creatine for 35 days during resistance/ agility training.	Prior to and following 35 days of supplementation, subjects had body composition determined using DEXA. In addition, subjects performed 1RM tests at 0.25, 0.99, and 1.54 m/s as well as five sets of 15 maximal effort contractions at 0.25 m/s with 60 s rest recovery between sets on an isokinetic bench press.	Subjects ingesting P-I (2.4 kg) and P-II (3.5 kg) observed significantly greater gains in FFM in comparison to the placebo group (1 kg). In addition, subjects ingesting P-I and P-II observed significantly greater gains in 1RM strength at 0.99 m/s. No significant differences were observed among groups in remaining 1 RM velocities or in gains in mean peak force, average force, or total work performed during the 5 sets of 15 maximal effort contractions at 0.25 m/s.

Reference	Subjects/Supplement Dosage	Tests Performed	Results
Kreider et al.[67]	In a double-blind and randomized manner, 28 resistance-trained male subjects ingested a maltodextrin placebo, a higher calorie carbohydrate/protein weight gain powder (Gainers Fuel 1000®), or Phosphagain® containing 20 g per day of creatine for 28 days during training.	Subjects had total body mass, total body water, and body composition determined using DEXA on days 0, 7, 14, and 28 of supplementation.	Subjects ingesting Phosphagain® observed significantly greater gains in body mass and FFM (1.1 to 1.3 kg) than subjects ingesting the placebo and higher calorie weight gain powder. The greatest gains occurred in the first 14 days of supplementation.
Kreider et al.[68]	In a double-blind and randomized manner, 24 untrained and 26 endurance trained males and females ingested either a glucose placebo (G), 16.5 g per day of creatine, or the G placebo with 15.75 g per day of creatine for 14 days.	Prior to and following supplementation, subjects had total body mass, total body water, and body composition determined via skinfolds.	In both untrained and trained subjects, creatine supplementation resulted in significantly greater increases in body mass and FFM (0.9 kg). No differences were observed between groups ingesting creatine alone or creatine with glucose. There was some evidence that untrained and trained men observed greater gains in FFM in response to creatine supplementation (1.4 kg) than women (0.3 kg).
Sipilä et al.[70]	Two female and five male gyrate atrophy patients performed pre-tests and then were administered 1.5 g per day of creatine for one year.	Prior to and at three-month intervals during the supplementation period, subjects had serum and urinary amino acids, creatine, creatinine, and muscle and liver enzyme levels determined. In addition, muscle biopsies were obtained to determine muscle fiber types and diameter, body mass was measured, and ophthalmologic examinations were performed.	Creatine supplementation resulted in a 10% increase in total body mass. Muscle biopsy analysis revealed that type II fiber diameter increased by 34% with no effect on type I fiber. There were occasional increases in muscle and liver enzyme efflux and serum and urinary creatine and creatinine levels. However, these parameters remained within normal limits. No effects were observed in ophthalmologic exam results. No side effects were reported.
Almada et al.[71]	In a double-blind and randomized manner, 34 untrained men and women (mean of 51 years) subjects ingested either 20 g per day of creatine for five days and 10 g per day of creatine for 51 days or a glucose placebo.	Muscle and liver enzymes changes were measured at zero, four, and eight weeks of supplementation and following four weeks of cessation.	There were no significant differences in AST, ALT, ALP, GGT, LDH, or CK levels between groups. Males ingesting creatine had greater increase in CK levels than females taking creatine (119 to 181 IU)

continued

Table 11.1 (continued) Summary of Studies Investigating the Ergogenic Value of Creatine Supplementation on Muscle Bioenergetics and Exercise Performance

Reference	Subjects/Supplement Dosage	Tests Performed	Results
Earnest et al.[72]	In a double-blind and randomized manner, 18 male and 16 female middle-aged subjects (32-70 yrs) ingested either a placebo or 20 g per day of creatine with 4 g per day of glucose for five days and 10 g per day of creatine with 2 g per day of glucose for 51 days.	Subjects had plasma lipid, lipoprotein, glucose, urea nitrogen, and creatinine profiles determined at 0, 28, and 56 days of supplementation as well as 28 days following cessation of supplementation.	No significant differences were observed between groups in body mass. Creatine supplementation resulted in significant decreases in total cholesterol (-5 and -6% at day 28 and 56 days, respectively), triglycerides (-23 and -22% at 28 and 56 days, respectively). A similar response was observed for VLDL. No significant differences were observed between groups in glucose, creatinine or urea nitrogen. However, women ingesting creatine observed a modest increase in urea nitrogen.
Poortmans et al.[73]	In a double-blind and randomized manner, five subjects ingest either a placebo or 20 g per day of creatine for five days.	Subjects had blood and urine samples determined to creatine, creatinine, total protein, albumin, and urine output.	Creatine supplementation increased arterial (3.7-fold) and urinary excretion of creatine. Blood and urine creatinine levels were not affected by creatine supplementation. The glomular filtration rate (creatinine clearance) and total protein and albumin excretion rates remained within normal limits.
Gordon et al.[79]	In a double-blind and randomized manner, 17 heart failure patients with less than a 40% ejection fraction ingested either 20 g per day of creatine or a placebo for ten days.	Prior to and following supplementation, subjects had ejection fraction determined using radionuclide angiography. In addition, subjects performed symptom-limited one-legged knee extension strength tests and a cycle ergometry performance test. Muscle biopsies were obtained to evaluate TCr and PCr concentrations.	Creatine supplementation significantly increased muscle TCr by 17% and PCr by 12%. Increments were seen only in patients with TCr less than 140 mmol/kg dry mass. Creatine supplementation did not affect resting or post-exercise ejection fraction. Creatine supplementation significantly increased one-legged knee extensor performance (21%), cycle ergometer performance (10%), and peak torque (5%). Gains in peak torque and knee extensor performance were correlated to muscle PCr content.
Tarnapolosky et al.[80]	In a randomized and crossover design, seven mitochondrial cytophatic patients ingested a placebo or 5 g of creatine for 14 days followed by 2 g per day for seven days.	Prior to and following supplementation, subjects were assessed for activities of daily living, ischemic isometric handgrip strength (1 min), lactate, evoked and voluntary contraction strength of the dorsiflexors, ischemic and non-ischemic dorsiflexor torque, and aerobic exercise capacity.	Creatine supplementation increased strength of high-intensity anaerobic and aerobic activities with no effect on submaximal exercise activities.

Some evidence shows that some individuals do not appear to respond as well to creatine supplementation (i.e., observe less than a 20 mmol/kg dry mass change in TCr levels).[5,12] However, more recent studies[10,11] indicate that ingesting creatine (20 g per day) with glucose (380 g per day) for five days increased muscle creatine content by 10% more than when creatine was ingested alone (143 to 158 mmol/kg dry mass). In this case, muscle creatine content increased in all subjects. Moreover, when creatine was ingested with glucose, glycogen content increased by 18% more than when glucose was ingested alone (418 to 489 mmol/kg dry mass). Although this change was not significantly different due to intra-subject variability, gains in glycogen were significantly correlated with gains in TCr, suggesting that the glycogen increases were due in part to creatine. The enhanced creatine uptake was associated with a glucose mediated increase in serum insulin.[11] These data suggest that when creatine was ingested with large amounts of glucose, all subjects may have responded to creatine supplementation. Figure 11.2 presents the average changes in TCr and PCr reported in the literature in response to creatine supplementation with and without glucose.

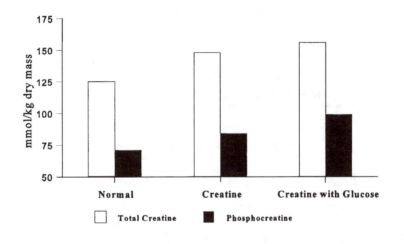

Figure 11.2

Because creatine supplementation may increase intramuscular PCr, several studies have evaluated the effects of creatine supplementation on ATP and PCr resynthesis following high-intensity exercise.[4,8, 9,12,15,17–19] These studies indicate that creatine supplementation does not appear to alter pre-exercise ATP concentrations.[5,9,21] However, the elevated PCr concentrations serve to maintain ATP concentrations to a greater degree during a maximal effort sprint performance.[19] In addition, creatine supplementation has been reported to enhance the rate of ATP and PCr resynthesis following intense exercise.[4,8,15–17,19]

For example, Balsom and colleagues[8] investigated the effects of creatine supplementation (20 g per day for six days) on PCr resynthesis rates following sprint performance (5 × 6-s sprints with 30-s rest recovery between sprints). The results revealed that muscle PCr concentrations were significantly higher after the fifth sprint (70 vs. 46 mmol/kg dry mass) following creatine supplementation. Likewise, Greenhaff and associates[12] reported that creatine supplementation promoted a 42% greater resynthesis rate of PCr following 120 s of recovery from 20 electrically evoked isometric contractions. Collectively, these findings indicate that short-term creatine supplementation may be effective in increasing muscle TCr and PCr concentrations. Further, the increased TCr and PCr serves to help maintain ATP concentrations during high-intensity exercise as well as enhance PCr resynthesis following intense exercise. Theoretically, creatine supplementation may improve performance in single effort and/or repetitive sprints involving the phosphagen energy system (see Figures 11.3 and 11.4).

**Theoretical Effect of Creatine Supplementation on
[ATP] and [PC] During High-Intensity Exercise**

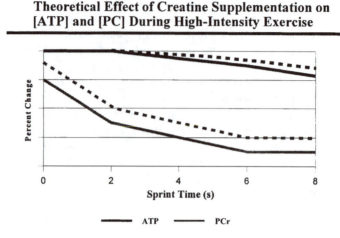

Figure 11.3

**Theoretical Effect of Creatine Supplementation on
Repeated Bouts of High-Intensity Exercise**

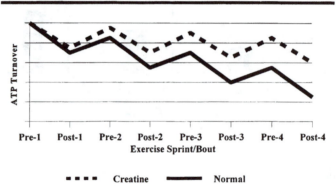

Figure 11.4

11.3 ERGOGENIC EFFECTS OF CREATINE SUPPLEMENTATION

Most studies that have investigated the ergogenic value of short-term (five to seven days) and/or long-term (seven to 140 days) creatine supplementation (20 to 25 g per day for five to seven days and 2 to 25 g per day thereafter) have reported that creatine supplementation significantly increases strength/power, sprint performance, and/or work performed during multiple sets of maximal effort muscle contractions (see Table 11.2). The improvement in exercise capacity has been attributed to increased TCr and PCr content,[4,5,8–22] particularly in type II muscle fiber,[19,21] greater resynthesis of PCr,[4,8,15–17,19] improved metabolic efficiency,[8,19,24,26,47,49] and/or an enhanced quality of training promoting greater training adaptations.[20,24,28,30,32,35,36,41,43,44,62,66] The following analysis evaluates some of the literature supporting the ergogenic benefits of creatine supplementation. Additional information regarding studies investigating the effects of creatine supplementation on exercise performance can be found in Table 11.1.

Table 11.2 Summary of the Types of Exercise and/or Exercise Conditions in Which Creatine Supplementation Has Been Reported to Provide Ergogenic Benefit

Type of Exercise/Performance

One repetition maximum and/or peak power[17,22,23–29,34,38,40,43,66]
Vertical jump[28,30,31]
Multiple sets of maximal effort muscle contractions[14,15,17,22,25,26,29,31–35]
Single sprints lasting 6 to 30 s[8,19,24–28,32,36–38,41]
Repetitive sprints (recovery 0.5 to 5 min)[8,24,25,27,32,35,38,40–44,49]
Exercise lasting 1.5 to 5 min[42,45–47]
Increased ventilatory anaerobic threshold[47]
Increase maximal exercise capacity[48]

11.3.1 Maximum Strength/Power

Several studies have evaluated the effects of short-term and/or long-term creatine supplementation on maximal strength and power.[17,22–31,33,34,38,40,43,66] Creatine supplementation during training has been reported to increase gains in one repetition maximum (1RM) strength performance.[22,23,25,28] For example, Earnest and associates[25] reported that 28 days of creatine supplementation (20 g per day for 28 days) during resistance training promoted a significantly greater gain in 1RM bench press performance (8.2 vs. -2.9 kg). Moreover, Vandenburghe and colleagues[22] reported that creatine supplementation (20 g per day for four days followed by 5 g per day for 66 days) promoted a 20 to 25% greater gain in 1RM strength in untrained women participating in a 70-day resistance-training program. The gains in strength observed were maintained in subjects ingesting creatine during a 70-day detraining period.

Creatine supplementation has also been reported to enhance peak power generated during isokinetic exercise.[24,26,34,38,40,43,79] In this regard, Dawson and co-workers[40] reported that creatine supplementation (20 g per day for five days) significantly increased peak power during the first set of 6 × 6-s sprints. Likewise, Birch and colleagues[24] reported that creatine supplementation (20 g per day for five days) significantly increased peak power output (8%) during three sets of 30 maximal effort cycling sprints. Preliminary reports also suggest that creatine supplementation may increase peak concentric and eccentric power[34] as well as vertical jump performance.[28,30,31] Collectively, these studies suggest that creatine supplementation may improve 1RM strength and power.

11.3.2 Multiple Sets of Maximal Effort Muscle Contractions

Studies have also indicated that creatine supplementation may enhance the amount of work performed during a series of maximal effort contractions.[14,15,17,22,25,26,29,31–35] For example, Bosco et al.[31] found that creatine supplementation (20 g per day for five days) significantly increased jump performance during two 15-s jump tests separated by a 15-s rest recovery. Volek and colleagues[29] reported that creatine supplementation (25 g per day for seven days) resulted in a significant increase in the amount of work performed during five sets of bench press and jump squats compared with a placebo group. Moreover, Earnest and associates[25] found that creatine supplementation (20 g per day for 28 days) significantly increased bench press total lifting volume (43%) when performing a 70% of 1RM bench press repetition test. Finally, Kreider et al.[35] reported creatine supplementation (15.75 g per day for 28 days) promoted a 41% greater gain in combined bench press, squat, and power clean lifting volume. These findings suggest that creatine supplementation may enhance the ability to perform sets of multiple effort muscle contractions.

11.3.3 Sprint Performance

Creatine supplementation has been reported to improve single effort[8,19,24,25,26,28,32,36–38,41] and/or repetitive sprint performance,[8,24,25,32,35-38,40–44,49] particularly in sprints lasting 6 to 30 s with 30 s to 5 min of rest recovery between sprints. For example, Birch et al.[24] reported that creatine supplementation (20 g per day for five days) significantly increased work performed during the first of 3×30-s cycle ergometer sprints with 4 min recovery between sprints. Grindstaff and co-workers[36] reported that creatine supplementation (21 g per day for nine days) significantly improved 3×100-m swim performance with 60-s rest recovery between sprints. Moreover, Kreider and associates[35] reported that 28 days of creatine supplementation (15.75 g per day) during off-season football resistance/agility training resulted in significant improvements in repetitive sprint performance during the first five of 12×6-s sprints with 30-s rest recovery between sprints. Finally, Earnest and colleagues[25] reported that creatine supplementation (20 g per day for 28 days) increased work performed during 3×30-s cycle ergometer sprints with 5-min rest recovery between sprints. Although not all studies indicate that creatine supplementation improves single and/or repetitive sprint performance (see discussion below), these studies suggest that creatine supplementation may improve single and/or repetitive sprint performance.

11.3.4 High-Intensity Exercise

Some investigators have studied the effects of creatine supplementation on high-intensity exercise performance lasting 60 s to 10 minutes.[42,45,46,48] In this regard, Harris and co-workers[42] reported that sprint performance during a series of 300- and 1000-m runs were significantly improved with creatine supplementation (30 g per day for six days). Earnest and colleagues[46] found that creatine supplementation (20 g per day for four days followed by 10 g per day for six days) significantly increased cumulative time to exhaustion when performing two treadmill runs lasting approximately 90 s each separated by an 8-min recovery period (placebo 0.8; creatine 5.7 s). Moreover, Rossiter et al.[20] reported that creatine supplementation (0.25 g/kg/d for five days) significantly decreased time to perform a 1000-m rowing time trial by -2.3 s in an event lasting about 210 s in comparison to a placebo group. Finally, Jacobs and associates[48] reported that creatine supplementation significantly increased time to exhaustion by 8% (130 to 141 s) following five days of creatine supplementation (20 g per day) as well as following seven days cessation of supplementation by 7% (139-s). Although additional research is necessary, these findings suggest that creatine supplementation may provide some ergogenic benefit in events lasting up to 4 to 5 min.

11.4 STUDIES REPORTING NO ERGOGENIC BENEFIT

Although most studies have reported improved exercise performance in response to creatine supplementation, some well-controlled studies have reported no ergogenic benefit from creatine supplementation (see Table 11.3). For example, Odland and co-workers[51] reported that although creatine supplementation (20 g per day for three days) significantly increased the ratio of TCr/ATP, no significant differences were observed in cycling power output during a 30-s sprint compared with control and placebo trials randomly performed, with 14-day washout periods observed between trials. Likewise, Cooke and associates[53] reported that creatine supplementation (20 g per day for five days) did not significantly affect cycling power output or work performed during 2×15-s sprints separated by a 20-min rest recovery. This group also reported[58] that creatine supplementation (20 g per day for five days) did not affect cycling sprint performance when two maximal effort sprints were separated by 30, 60, 90, or 120 s of rest recovery. Similarly, Barnett and colleagues[56] reported that creatine supplementation (0.28 g/kg/d for four days) did not significantly affect repetitive cycling sprint performance (5×10 s with 30 s recovery, 5 min rest, 2×10 s with 30 s recovery).

Table 11.3 Summary of Types of Exercise and/or Exercise Conditions in Which Creatine Supplementation Has Been Reported to Provide No Ergogenic Benefit

Type of Performance

One repetition maximum and/or peak force[33]

Work performed during low-intensity muscle contractions[14,50]

Single sprints lasting 6 to 30 s[16,30,40,51]

Repetitive sprints (recovery 30 to 120 s[51] and 5 to 25 min[27,52-56])

Exercise lasting longer than 60 s[9,21,27,52,57,59]

Several field reports also suggest that creatine supplements may not provide ergogenic benefit. Burke and associates[52] and Mujika et al.[54] reported that creatine supplementation (20 g per day for five days) did not significantly improve 25-, 50-, or 100-m swim performance times with 10 min of active recovery[52] or 20–25 min of passive recovery[54] observed between heats. Moreover, Redondo and co-workers[55] found that creatine supplementation (25 g per day for seven days) did not significantly improve 60-m running velocity or stride length in baseball and field hockey players. Likewise, Terrilion et al.[57] found that creatine supplementation (20 g per day for five days) did not affect repeated 700-m run performance times separated by a 60-min recovery period. Finally, Balsom and colleagues[39] reported that creatine supplementation 30 g per day for six days significantly increased 6-km outdoor run performance apparently due to a 1 kg increase in body mass following creatine supplementation.

It is unclear why creatine supplementation had no ergogenic effect in these studies. It is possible that individual variability in response to creatine supplementation previously discussed may account for the lack of ergogenic benefit reported.[5,12] It is also possible that differences in experimental design may account for some of the differences. In this regard, creatine supplementation appears to be less ergogenic when supplementation regimens are less than 20 g per day for five days[16,51,56] or involve low-dose supplementation regimens (2 to 3 g per day) without an initial higher dose loading period.[26,48] In addition, studies that used relatively small sample sizes (e g., less than six subjects per group) or employed cross-over experimental designs with less than a five-week washout period between trials typically have found no ergogenic benefit.[9,15,16,51] Creatine supplementation may also be less ergogenic, depending on the amount of work performed and rest recovery observed between repetitive exercise trials. Several studies report that creatine supplementation does not effect performance in sprints lasting 6 to 60 s when prolonged recovery periods (5 to 25 min) are observed between sprint trials.[52-55] Creatine supplementation also does not appear to enhance endurance exercise.[21,39,59,60] Consequently, although most studies indicate that creatine supplementation may improve performance, creatine supplementation may not provide ergogenic value for everyone.

11.5 EFFECTS OF CREATINE ON BODY MASS AND COMPOSITION

Table 11.4 lists studies that have evaluated the effects of creatine supplementation on body mass and composition. Most studies indicate that short-term creatine supplementation (20 to 25 g per day for five to seven days) increases total body mass by approximately a 0.7 to 1.6 kg.[12,15,17,35,38,39] In addition, several long-term (7 to 140 days) studies investigating the effects of creatine or creatine containing supplements (20 to 25 g per day for five to seven days and 2 to 25 g per day thereafter) on body composition alterations during training have reported significantly greater gains in total body mass[22,23,25,35,61,66-68] and fat-free mass.[22,23,28,35,43,61,62,66-68] The gains in total body mass and fat-free mass (FFM) observed were typically 0.8 to 3 kg greater than matched-paired controls, depending on the length and amount of supplementation.[22,23,28,35,43,61,62,66-68] For example, Kreider et al.[35] reported that 28 days of creatine supplementation (15.75 g per day) resulted in a 1.1 kg greater gain in FFM in college football players undergoing off-season resistance/agility training. In addition, Vandenburghe and co-workers[22] reported that untrained females ingesting creatine (20 g per day for four days followed by 5 g per day for 66 days) during resistance-training observed significantly greater gains in FFM (1.0 kg) than subjects ingesting a placebo during training. Moreover, the gains in FFM observed were maintained while ingesting creatine (5 g per day) during a 10-week period of detraining as well as following four-weeks cessation of supplementation. Findings like these suggest that creatine supplementation may promote gains in lean body mass during training.

Table 11.4 Effects of Creatine on Body Mass and Composition

Effect
Significant increase in total body mass following short-term supplementation regimens[8,11,12,15,17,29,39,49,54]
No significant effect on total body mass following short-term supplementation regimens[22,33,36,55,57,59,72]
Significant increase in total body mass following long-term supplementation regimens[22,23,25,28,30,43,62,67,68,70]
Significant increase in fat-free mass[22,23,25,28,38,43,62,66-68]

However, the mechanism in which creatine supplementation may affect gains in body mass and/or fat free mass is not currently understood. The two prevailing theories suggest that creatine supplementation may promote water retention and/or enhanced protein synthesis.[3,38,64,65] Although most studies indicate that creatine supplementation does not increase the percentage of total body water,[35,57,62,66,67] there is some preliminary evidence that creatine may affect protein synthesis.[38,63,64] It is also possible that creatine may allow an athlete to maintain a greater training volume, thereby promoting lean tissue accretion during training. However, additional research is necessary to evaluate the effects of creatine supplementation on protein synthesis, fluid retention, training volume, and body composition before definitive conclusions can be drawn.

11.6 EFFECTS OF CREATINE ON MARKERS OF MEDICAL STATUS

Several studies have evaluated the effects of creatine supplementation on markers of clinical status. Serum creatine levels typically increase for several hours following ingestion of a 5 g dose of creatine.[5,15] Creatine uptake into the muscle primarily occurs during the first several days of creatine supplementation.[5,20] Excess creatine ingested thereafter has been reported to be primarily excreted as creatine in the urine with small amounts converted to creatinine and urea.[1,3,5,20] Serum creatinine levels have been reported to be either not affected[71,72] or slightly increased[35,70] following 28,[35] 56,[71,72] and 365 days[70] of creatine supplementation. The increased serum and urinary creatinine have been suggested to reflect an increased release and cycling of intramuscular creatine as a consequence of enhanced myofibrillar protein turnover in response to creatine supplementation and not of pathologic origin.[3,35,72]

Studies investigating the effects of creatine supplementation on muscle and liver enzymes have found either no effect[70,71] or moderate increases in creatine kinase,[35,71] lactate dehydrogenase,[35] and aspartate amino transferase[35] levels following 28 and 56 days of supplementation. The increased CK, LDH, and AST levels reported following creatine supplementation were within normal limits for athletes engaged in heavy training and may reflect a greater concentration/activity of CK and/or ability to maintain greater training volume.[3,35] Interestingly, the athletes ingesting creatine had a lower urea nitrogen/creatinine ratio.[35] Increases in the ratio of urea nitrogen/creatinine are used as a general marker of catabolism. Consequently, these findings suggest that despite modest increases in serum CK, LDH, and AST, subjects ingesting creatine may have experienced less catabolism during training.[35]

Creatine supplementation has also been reported to positively affect lipid profiles in middle-aged male and female hypertriglyceremic patients[72] and trained male athletes.[35] In this regard, Earnest and colleagues[72] reported that 56 days of creatine supplementation resulted in significant decreases in total cholesterol (-5 and -6% at day 28 and 56, respectively) and triglycerides (-23 and -22% at day 28 and 56, respectively) in mildly hypertriglyceremic patients. A similar response was observed with very-low-density lipoproteins (VLDL). In addition, Kreider and co-workers[35] reported that 28 days of creatine supplementation increased high-density lipoproteins (HDL) by 13%, while decreasing VLDL (-13%) and the ratio of total cholesterol to HDL (-7%). Although additional research is necessary, these findings suggest that creatine supplementation may posses health benefits in modifying blood lipids.

Finally, intravenous phosphocreatine administration has been reported to improve myocardial metabolism and reduced the incidence of ventricular fibrillation in ischemic heart patients.[63,74–78] Consequently, there has been interest in determining the effects of oral creatine supplementation on heart function and exercise capacity in patients who have heart disease. Gordon and associates[79] reported that creatine supplementation (20 g per day for ten days) did not improve ejection fraction in heart failure patients with an ejection fraction less than 40%. However, creatine supplementation significantly increased one-legged knee extension exercise performance (21%), peak torque (5%), and cycle ergometry performance (10%). In addition, Tarnapolosky et al.[80] reported that creatine supplementation (5 g per day for 14 days followed by 2 g per day for seven days) significantly increased anaerobic and high-intensity aerobic exercise capacity in patients with mitochondrial cytopathy. Collectively, these findings suggest that phosphocreatine administration and/or oral creatine supplementation may posses some therapeutic value to certain patient populations. Although additional research is necessary to evaluate the long-term effects of creatine supplementation on medical status, available studies suggest that creatine supplementation is medically safe and may provide health benefits when taken at dosages described in the literature.

11.7 SIDE EFFECTS

The only side effect reported from clinical studies investigating dosages of 1.5 to 25 g per day for 3 to 365 days in preoperative and post-operative patients, untrained subjects, and elite athletes has been weight gain.[3] Many concerns about possible side effects of creatine supplementation have been mentioned in lay publications, supplement advertisements, and on Internet mailing lists (see Table 11.5). It should be noted that these concerns emanate from unsubstantiated anecdotal reports

Table 11.5 Unsubstantiated Anecdotal Side Effects/Concerns Reported in the Popular Literature About Creatine Supplementation

A possible suppression of endogenous creatine synthesis.
A possible enhanced renal stress/liver damage.
Anecdotal reports of muscle cramping when exercising in the heat.
Anecdotal reports of muscle strains/pulls.
Unknown long-term effects of creatine supplementation.

and may be unrelated to creatine supplementation. There is no evidence from any well-controlled clinical study that indicates that creatine supplementation causes any of these side effects. However, one must also consider that few studies have directly evaluated the effects of creatine supplementation on side effects. Consequently, discussion about possible side effects is warranted.

Some concern has been raised whether creatine supplementation may suppress endogenous creatine synthesis. Studies have reported that it takes about four weeks after cessation of creatine supplementation for muscle creatine[9] and phosphocreatine[22] levels to return to normal. Although it is unclear whether muscle creatine or phosphocreatine content falls below normal thereafter, there is no evidence that creatine supplementation causes a long-term suppression of creatine synthesis.[3,13]

Because creatine is an amino acid, it has been suggested that creatine supplementation may increase renal stress or cause liver damage. However, no studies have reported clinically significant elevations in liver enzymes in response to creatine supplementation.[35,71] Further, Poortmans and colleagues[73] reported that short-term creatine supplementation (20 g per day for five days) does not affect markers of renal stress. Consequently, there is no evidence that creatine supplementation increases renal stress when taken at recommended dosages.

There have also been some anecdotal claims that athletes training hard in hot or humid conditions may experience a greater incidence of severe muscle cramps and/or muscle injury when taking creatine. However, no study has reported that creatine supplementation causes cramping, dehydration, changes in electrolyte concentrations, or increased susceptibility to muscle strains/pulls even though some of these studies have evaluated highly trained athletes undergoing intense training[20,28,29,35,36,42-45,50,52,54,59,62,66-68] in hot/humid environments.[28,35,59,62,66,68]

Concern has also been expressed regarding unknown long-term side effects. Although long-term (greater than one year) well-controlled clinical trials have yet to be performed, it should be noted that athletes have been using creatine as a nutritional supplement for more than ten years. Yet, this author is not aware of any significant medical complications that have been directly linked to creatine supplementation. Consequently, from the literature available, creatine supplementation appears to be a medically safe practice when taken at dosages described in the literature.

11.8 SUMMARY AND CONCLUSIONS

Based on available research, short-term creatine supplementation may improve maximal strength/power by 5 to 15%, work performed during sets of maximal effort muscle contractions by 5 to 15%, single-effort sprint performance by 1 to 5%, and work performed during repetitive sprint performance by 5 to 15%. Moreover, long-term supplementation of creatine or creatine containing supplements (15 to 25 g per day for five to seven days and 2 to 25 g per day thereafter for 7 to 140 days) may promote significantly greater gains in strength, sprint performance, and fat-free mass during training compared with matched-paired controls. However, not all studies have reported ergogenic benefit possibly due to differences in subject response to creatine supplementation, length of supplementation, exercise criterion evaluated, and/or the amount of recovery observed during repeated bouts of exercise. The only side effect reported in the scientific literature from creatine supplementation has been weight gain. Consequently, creatine supplementation appears to be a safe and effective nutritional strategy to enhance exercise performance.

Additional research involving creatine supplementation should 1) include protein turnover, creatinine kinetics, muscle and liver enzyme efflux, lipid and cholesterol metabolism, fluid retention, and lean tissue accretion, 2) determine the therapeutic value and medical safety of creatine supplementation, 3) measure the effects of creatine supplementation on training volume/intensity and performance in a variety of sports events, and 4) determine whether there is any validity to anecdotal reports of increased incidence of muscular cramping and/or musculoskeletal injuries in athletes taking creatine during training.

ACKNOWLEDGMENTS

The author would like to thank the many subjects, students, research assistants, and colleagues at The University of Memphis who have contributed to studies investigating the ergogenic value and medical safety of creatine supplementation.

REFERENCES

1. Chanutin, A. The fate of creatine when administered to man. *J. Biol. Chem.* 1926;67:29-41.
2. Hultman, E, Bergstrom, J, Spriet, L, Söderlund, K. Energy metabolism and fatigue. In: Taylor, A, Gollnick, P, Green, H, editors. *Biochemistry of Exercise VII*. Champaign, IL: Human Kinetics, 1990:73-92.
3. Balsom, P, Söderlund, K, Ekblom, B. Creatine in humans with special references to creatine supplementation. *Sports Med.,* 1994;18:268-80.
4. Greenhaff, P, Bodin, K, Harris, R, Hultman, E, Jones, D, McIntyre, D, Soderlund, K, Turner, DL. The influence of oral creatine supplementation on muscle phosphocreatine resynthesis following intense contraction in man. *J. Physiol.* 1993;467:75P.
5. Harris, R, Söderlund, K, Hultman, E. Elevation of creatine in resting and exercised muscle of normal subjects by creatine supplementation. *Clin. Sci.* 1992;83:367-74.
6. Tullson, P, Rundell, K, Sabina, R, Terjung, R. Creatine analogue beta-guanidinopropionic acid alters skeletal muscle AMP deaminase activity. *Am. J. Physiol.* 1996;270:C76-85.
7. Kreider, R. Effects of creatine loading on muscular strength and body composition. *Str. Cond.* 1995;Oct:72-3.
8. Balsom, P, Söderlund, K, Sjödin, B, Ekblom, B. Skeletal muscle metabolism during short duration high-intensity exercise: influence of creatine supplementation. *Acta. Physiol. Scand.* 1995;1154:303-10.
9. Febbraio, M, Flanagan, T, Snow, R, Zhao, S, Carey, M. Effect of creatine supplementation on intramuscular TCr, metabolism and performance during intermittent, supramaximal exercise in humans. *Acta. Physiol. Scand.* 1995;155:387-95.
10. Green, A, Sewell, D, Simpson, L, Hulman, E, Macdonald, I, Greenhaff, P. Creatine ingestion augments muscle creatine uptake and glycogen synthesis during carbohydrate feeding in man. *J. Physiol.* 1996;491:63.
11. Green, A, Simpson, E, Littlewood, J, Macdonald, I, Greenhaff, P. Carbohydrate ingestion augments creatine retention during creatine feedings in humans. *Acta. Physiol. Scand.* 1996;158:195-202.
12. Greenhaff, P, Bodin, K, Söderlund, K, Hultman, E. Effect of oral creatine supplementation on skeletal muscle phosphocreatine resynthesis. *Am. J. Physiol.* 1994;266:E725-30.
13. Hultman, E, Söderlund, K, Timmons, J, Cederblad, G, Greenhaff, P. Muscle creatine loading in man, *J. Appl. Physiol.,* 1996;81:232-7.
14. Kurosawa, Y, Iwane, H, Hamaoka, T, Shimomitsu, T, Katsumura, T, Sako, T, Kuwamon, M, Kimura, N. Effects of oral creatine supplementation on high-and low-intensity grip exercise performance. *Med. Sci. Sport Exerc.* 1997;29:S251.
15. Lemon, P, Boska, M, Bredle, D, Rogers, M, Ziegenfuss, T, Newcomer, B. Effect of oral creatine supplementation on energetic during repeated maximal muscle contraction. *Med. Sci. Sport Exerc.* 1995;27:S204.
16. Ruden, T, Parcell, A, Ray, M, Moss, K, Semler, J, Sharp, R, Rolfs, G, King, D. Effects of oral creatine supplementation on performance and muscle metabolism during maximal exercise. *Med. Sci. Sport Exerc.* 1996;28:S81.
17. Vandenberghe, K, Gillis, N, Van Leemputte, M, Van Hecke, P, Vanstapel, F, Hespel, P. Caffeine counteracts the ergogenic action of muscle creatine loading. *J. Appl. Physiol.* 1996;80:452-7.
18. Brannon, T. Effects of creatine loading and training on running performance and biochemical properties of rat muscle. *Med. Sci. Sport Exerc.* 1997;29:489-95.
19. Casey, A, Constantin-Teodosiu, D, Howell, D, Hultman, E, Greenhaff, P. Creatine ingestion favorably affects performance and muscle metabolism during maximal exercise in humans, *Am. J. Physiol.,* 1996;271:E31-7.
20. Rossiter, H, Cannell, E, Jakeman, P. The effect of oral creatine supplementation on the 1000-m performance of competitive rowers. *J. Sports Sci.* 1996;14:175-9.
21. Myburgh, K, Bold, A, Bellinger, B, Wilson, G, Noakes, T. Creatine supplementation and sprint training in cyclists: metabolic and performance effects. *Med. Sci. Sport Exerc.* 1996;28:S81.
22. Vanderberghe, K, Goris, M, Van Hecke, P, Van Leeputte, M, Vangerven, L, Hespel, P. Long-term creatine intake is beneficial to muscle performance during resistance-training. *J. Appl. Physiol.* 1997;83:2055-63.

23. Becque, B, Lochmann, J, Melrose, D. Effect of creatine supplementation during strength training on 1RM and body composition. *Med. Sci. Sport Exerc.* 1997;29:S146.

24. Birch, R, Noble, D, Greenhaff, P. The influence of dietary creatine supplementation on performance during repeated bouts of maximal isokinetic cycling in man. *Eur. J. Appl. Physiol.* 1994;69:268-70.

25. Earnest, C, Snell, P, Rodriguez, R, Almada, A, Mitchell, T. The effect of creatine monohydrate ingestion on anaerobic power indices, muscular strength and body composition. *Acta. Physiol. Scand.* 1995;153:207-9.

26. Greenhaff, P, Casey, A, Short, A, Harris, R, Söderlund, K, Hultman, E. Influence of oral creatine supplementation of muscle torque during repeated bouts of maximal voluntary exercise in man. *Clin. Sci.* 1993;84:565-71.

27. Schneider, D, McDonough, P, Fadel, P, Berwick, J. Creatine supplementation and the total work performed during 15-s and 1-min bouts of maximal cycling. *Aust. J. Sci. Med. Sport.* 1997;29(3):65-8.

28. Stout, J, Eckerson, J, Noonan, D, Moore, G, Cullen, D. The effects of a supplement designed to augment creatine uptake on exercise performance and fat-free mass in football players. *Med. Sci. Sport Exerc.* 1997;29:S251.

29. Volek, J, Kraemer, W, Bush, J, Boetes, M, Incledon, T, Clark, K, Lynch, J. Creatine supplementation enhances muscular performance during high-intensity resistance exercise. *J. Am. Diet. Assoc.* 1997;97:765-70.

30. Goldberg, P, Bechtel, P. Effects of low dose creatine supplementation on strength, speed and power by male athletes. *Med. Sci. Sport Exerc.* 1997;29:S251.

31. Bosco, C. Tihanyi, J, Pucspk, J, Kovacs, I, Gobossy, A, Colli, R, Pulvirenti, G, Tranquilli, C, Foti, C, Viru, M, Viru, A. Effect of oral creatine supplementation on jumping and running performance. *Int. J. Sports Med.,* 1997;18:369-72.

32. Almada, A, Kreider, R, Ferreira, M, Wilson, M, Grindstaff, P, Plisk, S, Reinhardy, J, Cantler, E. Effects of calcium β-HMB supplementation with or without creatine during training on strength and sprint capacity. *FASEB J.* 1997;11:A374.

33. Hamilton-Ward, K, Meyers, M, Skelly, W, Marley, R, Saunders, J. Effect of creatine supplementation on upper extremity anaerobic response in females. *Med. Sci. Sport Exerc.* 1997;29:S146.

34. Johnson, K, Smodic, B, Hill, R. The effects of creatine monohydrate supplementation on muscular power and work. *Med. Sci. Sport Exerc.* 1997;29:S251.

35. Kreider, R, Ferreira, M, Wilson, M, Grindstaff, P, Plisk, S, Reinhardy, J, Cantler, E, Almada, A. Effects of creatine supplementation on body composition, strength and sprint performance. *Med. Sci. Sport Exerc.* 1998;30:73-82.

36. Grindstaff, P, Kreider, R, Bishop, R, Wilson, M, Wood, L, Alexander, C, Almada, A. Effects of creatine supplementation on repetitive sprint performance and body composition in competitive swimmers. *Int. J. Sport Nutr.* 1997;7:330-46.

37. Prevost, M, Nelson, A, Morris, G. The effects of creatine supplementation on total work output and metabolism during high-intensity intermittent exercise. *Res. Q. Exerc. Sport.* 1997;68:233-40.

38. Ziegenfuss, T, Lemon, P, Rogers, M, Ross, R, Yarasheski, K. Acute creatine ingestion: effects on muscle volume, anaerobic power, fluid volumes, and protein turnover. *Med. Sci. Sport Exerc.* 1997;29:S127.

39. Balsom, P, Harridge, S, Söderlund, K, Sjodin, B, Ekblom, B. Creatine supplementation per se does not enhance endurance exercise performance. *Acta. Physiol. Scand.* 1993;149:521-3.

40. Dawson, B, Cutler, M, Moody, A, Lawrence, S, Goodman, C, Randall, N. Effects of oral creatine loading on single and repeated maximal short sprints. *Aust. J. Sci. Med. Sport.* 1995;27:56-61.

41. Ferreira, M, Kreider, R, Wilson, M, Grindstaff, P, Plisk, S, Reinhardy, J, Cantler, E, Almada, A. Effects of ingesting a supplement designed to enhance creatine uptake on strength and sprint capacity. *Med. Sci. Sport Exerc.* 1997;29:S146.

42. Harris, R, Viru, M, Greenhaff, P, Hultman, E. The effect of oral creatine supplementation on running performance during maximal short term exercise in man. *J. Physiol.* 1993;467:74P.

43. Kirksey, K, Warren, B, Stone, M, Stone, M, Johnson, R. The effects of six weeks of creatine monohydrate supplementation in male and female track athletes. *Med. Sci. Sport Exerc.* 1997;29:S145.

44. Leenders, N, Lesniewski, L, Sherman, W, Sand, G, Sand, S, Mulroy, M, Lamb, D. Dietary creatine supplementation and swimming performance. Overtraining and Overreaching in Sport Conference Abstracts. 1996;1:80.

45. Earnest, C, Stephens, D, Smith, J. Creatine ingestion affects time to exhaustion during estimation of the work rate-time relationship. *Med. Sci. Sport Exerc.* 1997;29:S285.

46. Earnest, C, Almada, A, Mitchell, T. Effects of creatine monohydrate ingestion on intermediate duration anaerobic treadmill running to exhaustion. *J. Str. Cond. Res.* 1997;11:234-8.

47. Nelson, A, Day, R, Glickman-Weiss, E, Hegstad, M, Sampson, B. Creatine supplementation raises anaerobic threshold. *FASEB J.* 1997;11:A589.

48. Jacobs, I, Bleue, S, Goodman, J. Creatine ingestion increases anaerobic capacity and maximum accumulated oxygen deficit. *Can. J. Appl. Physiol.* 1997;22:231-43.

49. Balsom, P, Ekblom, B, Sjodin, B, Hultman, E. Creatine supplementation and dynamic high-intensity intermittent exercise. *Scand. J. Med. Sci. Sport.* 1993;3:143-9.

50. Thompson, C, Kemp, G, Sanderson, A, Dixon, R, Styles, P, Taylor, D, Radda, G. Effect of creatine on aerobic and anaerobic metabolism in skeletal muscle in swimmers. *Br. J. Sports Med.,* 1996;30:222-5.

51. Odland, L, MacDougall, J, Tarnopolsky, M, Elorriage, A, Borgmann, A. Effect of oral creatine supplementation on muscle [PCr] and short-term maximum power output. *Med. Sci. Sport Exerc.* 1997;29:216-219.

52. Burke, L, Pyne, D, Telford, R. Effect of oral creatine supplementation on single-effort sprint performance in elite swimmers. *Int. J. Sport Nutr.* 1996;6:222-33.

53. Cooke, W, Grandjean, P, Barnes, W. Effect of oral creatine supplementation on power output and fatigue during bicycle ergometry. *J. Appl. Physiol.* 1995;78:670-3.

54. Mujika, I, Chatard, J, Lacoste, L, Barale, F, Geyssant, A. Creatine supplementation does not improve sprint performance in competitive swimmers. *Med. Sci. Sport Exerc.* 1996;28:1435-41.

55. Redondo, D, Dowling, E, Graham, B, Almada, A, Williams, M. The effect of oral creatine monohydrate supplementation on running velocity. *Int. J. Sport Nutr.* 1996;6:213-21.

56. Barnett, C, Hinds, M, Jenkins, D. Effects of oral creatine supplementation on multiple sprint cycle performance. *Aust. J. Sci. Med. Sport.* 1996;28:35-9.

57. Terrilion, K, Kolkhorst, F, Dolgener, F, Joslyn, S. The effect of creatine supplementation on two 700-m maximal running bouts. *Int. J. Sport Nutr.* 1997;7:138-43.

58. Cooke, W, Barnes, W. The influence of recovery duration on high-intensity exercise performance after oral creatine supplementation. *Can. J. Appl. Physiol.* 1997;22:454-67.

59. Godly, A, Yates, J. Effects of creatine supplementation on endurance cycling combined with short, high-intensity bouts. *Med. Sci. Sport Exerc.* 1997;29:S251.

60. Stroud, M, Holliman, D, Bell, D, Green, A, MacDonald, I, Greenhaff, P. Effect of oral creatine supplementation on respiratory gas exchange and blood lactate accumulation during steady-state incremental treadmill exercise and recovery in man. *Clin. Sci.* 1994;87:707-10.

61. Kreider, R, Ferreira, M, Wilson, M, Grindstaff, P, Plisk, S, Reinhardy, J, Cantler, E, Almada, A. Effects of ingesting a supplement designed to enhance creatine uptake on body composition during training. *Med. Sci. Sport Exerc.* 1997;29:S145.

62. Kreider, R, Ferreira, M, Wilson, M, Grindstaff, P, Plisk, S, Reinhardy, J, Cantler, E, Almada, A. Effects of calcium β-HMB supplementation with or without creatine during training on strength and sprint capacity. *FASEB J.* 1997;11:A374.

63. Pauletto, P, Stumia, E. Clinical experience with creatine phosphate therapy. In Conway, M and Clark J., editors. *Clinicial and Creatine Phosphate: Scientific and Clinical Perspectives.* San Diego, CA: Academic Press, 1996:185-98.

64. Bessman, S, Savabi, F. The role of the phosphocreatine energy shuttle in exercise and muscle hypertrophy. In: Taylor A, Gollnick P, Green H, editors. *International Series on Sport Sciences: Biochemistry of Exercise VII*: Champaign, IL: Human Kinetics, 1988:167-78.

65. Ingwall, J. Creatine and the control of muscle-specific protein synthesis in cardiac and skeletal muscle. *Circ. Res.* 1976;38:I115-23.

66. Kreider, R, Grindstaff, P, Wood, L, Bullen, D, Klesges, R, Lotz, D, Davis, M, Cantler, E, Almada, A. Effects of ingesting a lean mass promoting supplement during resistance training on isokinetic performance. *Med. Sci. Sport Exerc.* 1996;28:S36.

67. Kreider, R, Klesges, R, Harmon, K, Grindstaff, P, Ramsey, L, Bullen, D, Wood, L, Li, Y, Almada, A. Effects of ingesting supplements designed to promote lean tissue accretion on body composition during resistance exercise. *Int. J. Sport Nutr.* 1996;6:234-46.

68. Kreider, R, Ferreira, M, Wilson, M, Almada, A. Effects of creatine supplementation with and without glucose on body composition in trained and untrained men and women. *J. Str. Cond. Res.* 1997;11:283.

69. Clark, J, Odoom, J, Tracey, I, Dunn, J, Boehm, E, Paternostro, G, Radda, G. Experimental observations of creatine and creatine phosphate metabolism. In Conway, M, Clark, J, editors. *Creatine and Creatine Phosphate: Scientific and Clinical Perspectives.* San Diego, CA: Academic Press, 1996:33-50.

70. Sipila, I, Rapola, J, Simell, O, Vannas, A. Supplementary creatine as a treatment for gyrate atrophy of the choroid and retina. *New. Eng. J. Med.* 1981;304:867-70.

71. Almada, A, Mitchell, T, Earnest, C. Impact of chronic creatine supplementation on serum enzyme concentrations. *FASEB J.* 1996;10:A4567.

72. Earnest, C, Almada, A, Mitchell, T. High-performance capillary electrophoresis-pure creatine monohydrate reduces blood lipids in men and women. *Clin. Sci.* 1996;91:113-18.

73. Poortmans, J, Auquier, H, Renaut, V, Durassel, A, Saugy, M, Brisson, G. Effect of short-term creatine supplementation on renal responses in men, *Eur. J. Appl. Physiol.*, 1997;76:566-7.

74. Constantin-Teodosiu, D, Greenhaff, P, Gardiner, S, Randall, M, March, J, Bennett, T. Attenuation by creatine of myocardial metabolic stress in Brattleboro rats caused by chronic inhibition of nitric oxide synthase. *Br. J. Pharmacol.* 1995;116:3288-92.

75. Conway, M, Clark, J, editors. *Creatine and Creatine Phosphate: Scientific and Clinical Perspectives.* San Diego, CA: Academic Press, 1996.

76. Saks, V, Stepanov, V, Jaliashvili, I, Konerev, E, Kryzkanovsky, S, Strumia, E. Molecular and cellular mechanisms of action for cardioprotective and therapeutic role of creatine phosphate. In Conway, M, Clark, J, editors. *Creatine and Creatine Phosphate: Scientific and Clinical Perspectives.* San Diego, CA: Academic Press, 1996:91-114.

77. Wakatsuki, T, Ohira, Y, Nakamura, K, Asakura, T, Ohno, H, Yamamoto, M. Changes of contractile properties of extensor digitorum longus in response to creatine-analogue administration and/or hind-limb suspension in rats. *Jpn. J. Physiol.* 1995;45:979-89.

78. Wakatsuki, T, Ohira, Y, Yasui, W, Nakamura, K, Asakura, T, Ohno, H, Yamamoto, M. Responses of contractile properties in rat soleus to high-energy phosphates and/or unloading. *Jpn. J. Physiol.* 1994;44:193-204.

79. Gordon, A, Hultman, E, Kaijser, L, Kristgansson, S, Rolf, C, Nyquist, O, Sylven, C. Creatine supplementation in chronic heart failure increases skeletal muscle creatine phosphate and muscle performance. *Cardiovasc. Res.* 1995;30:413-18.

80. Tarnapolosky, M, Roy, B, MacDonald, J. A randomized controlled trial of creatine monohydrate in patients with mitochondrial cytopathies. *Muscle Nerve* 1997;20:1502-9.

Physiological Aspects
of Energy Management

CHAPTER 12

Nutritional Implications of Gender Differences in Energy Metabolism

Mark Tarnopolsky

CONTENTS

12.1 GENERAL INTRODUCTION

Much of the research in the area of muscle metabolism, nutrition and exercise physiology has been conducted using, primarily or exclusively, male participants. As a result, the conclusions and recommendations may have an inherent gender bias. In addition to the inequality of such an approach, the applicability of some the conclusions to females lacks scientific validation. For example, most of the studies that have examined the practice of carbohydrate loading have been conducted using participants who were predominantly or exclusively male.[1-4] Research from my laboratory[5] showed that males increased muscle glycogen by about 45%, which corresponded to an increase in endurance performance. On the other hand, females did not increase muscle glycogen nor time to exhaustion in response to the same carbohydrate loading protocol (four-day increase in carbohydrate to 75% of energy intake).[5]

Clearly the question of gender differences in energy metabolism is controversial, and some studies have concluded that there are no gender differences, whereas others have found significant differences. Only in recent exercise physiology textbooks has there even been a comment about the potential for gender differences in the metabolic response to exercise.[6] With careful gender matching, several studies have found that females oxidize more lipid and less protein and carbohydrate during endurance exercise as compared to equally trained males (Table 12.1).

Table 12.1 Energy and Substrate Utilization During Exercise in Males and Females

		kcal/h	kcal/kg/h	kcal/kg LBM/h	CHO(%)	FAT(%)	PRO(%)
Tarnopolsky, L.	6 ♂	797	11.9	14	81	10	9
et al., 1991	6 ♀	620	10.1	13.5	61	41	0
Phillips, S. M.	6 ♂	729	11.4	12.7	47	49	3
et al., 1993	6 ♀	590	10.2	12.5	35	61	2
Tarnopolsky,	7 ♂	1019	13.6	15.9	83	8	6
M. A. et al.,	8 ♀	666	11.6	14.2	72	24	1
1995							
Tarnopolsky,	8 ♂	806	11.1	12.5	75	23	2
M. A. et al.,	8 ♀	616	10.1	13.0	68	29	3
1997							
Total Mean	28 ♂	838(126)**	12(1)*	13.7(1.6)+	72(17)**	22(19)**	5(3)**
(±SD)	27 ♀	623(32)	10.5(0.7)	13.3(0.7)	59(17)	39(16)	2(1)

**p≤0.001; *p≤0.05; values are mean (SD); +=NS

The potential mechanism(s) behind a gender difference in metabolism is not clear, but they may relate to the presence of the female hormone, 17-β-estradiol (E_2). For example, provision of E_2 to rats resulted in an increase in lipid oxidation and a decrease in carbohydrate oxidation in both males and ovariectomized (OVX) females.[7-9] Alternatively, or perhaps in combination with E_2, a restricted energy intake in females may be a contributing factor. The latter point is somewhat controversial, and the question of energy conservation in females is still being debated.[10,11] From an anthropological point of view, the propensity for females to have a higher body fat may be linked to a sexual dimorphism arising out of evolutionary pressures for energy conservation in times of starvation.[12] Although energy conservation may be of phylogenetic advantage during starvation, during times of food abundance, it may lead to a propensity towards obesity. An enhanced energy conservation in females may, in part, explain the observation of reduced energy intake in female athletes that we (Table 12.2), and others[11,13] have demonstrated. Enhanced energy conservation may also explain the greater percent body fat in equally trained female as compared to male runners (Table 12.3).

This chapter explores the potential for a gender difference in the metabolic response to endurance exercise. It also includes some practical examples of study design issues and some ideas for future research studies.

Table 12.2 Habitual Energy and Macronutrient Intake in Male and Female Athletes

		Energy (kcal/d)	Energy (kcal/kg LBM)	%FAT	%PRO	%CHO
Tarnopolsky, L.	6 ♂	3475(214)	61	30	15	55
et al., 1991	6 ♀	2308(178)	50	30	15	55
Phillips, S. M.	6 ♂	3233(216)	57	31	15	53
et al., 1993	6 ♀	1809(133)	38	32	13	56
Tarnopolsky, M. A.	7 ♂	3372(323)	53	24	15	59
et al., 1995	8 ♀	1866(318)	40	27	12	59
Tarnopolsky, M. A.	8 ♂	3218(1328)	50	31	17	52
et al., 1997	8 ♀	2059(363)	44	26	14	60
Total Mean (±SD)	28 ♂	3325(106)	55(4)	29(3)	16(1)	55(3)
	27 ♀	2010(195)	43(5)	29(2)	14(1)	58(2)

Values are mean (SD). *p < 0.01 between groups.

Table 12.3 Body Composition in Male and Female Athletes

		Weight (kg)	Height (cm)	Lean Mass (kg)	Body Fat %
Tarnopolsky, L.	6 ♂	70(2)	175(2)	57(2)	15(1)
et al., 1991	6 ♀	58(2)	168(2)	46(2)	22(1)
Phillips, S. M.	6 ♂	64(5)	173(5)	57(5)	11(2)
et al., 1993	6 ♀	58(5)	168(5)	47(2)	19(1)
Tarnopolsky, M. A.	7 ♂	75(3)	179(4)	64(4)	14(2)
et al., 1995	8 ♀	58(8)	166(5)	47(5)	18(4)
Tarnopolsky, M. A.	8 ♂	73(5)	NA	65(5)	11(3)
et al., 1997	8 ♀	61(9)		47(4)	22(6)
Total Mean (±SD)	28 ♂	71(4)*	176(3)*	61(4)*	13(1)*
	27 ♀	59(1)	167(1)	47(0)	20(2)

Values are mean (SD); *All between group comparisons were significantly different (p≥0.05).

12.2 STUDY DESIGN ISSUES

12.2.1 Matching the Genders in Comparative Studies

One of the most important (and difficult) issues in comparing the metabolic response of males and females is that of equality of comparison between the groups. It is obvious why most researchers try to control for age, weight, height, and exercise training status in between-group comparative research studies. Thus, it is surprising that few studies have controlled for gender. This may have arisen from a lack of consensus as to the optimal criteria for such comparisons and/or the time required for matching.

Habitual endurance exercise training results in significant physiological adaptations (see below). Inequality between groups in training status would lead to erroneous conclusions, for some of the potential gender differences (i.e., increased intramuscular triglycerides) are directionally similar to the effects of training. Therefore, gender-based metabolic studies need to address the issue of between-group comparisons in training status. A commonly accepted indicator of aerobic power is the maximal oxygen uptake ($\dot{V}O_{2\,max}$), and this is a critical variable to measure in between-group designs.

As seen in Table 12.3, a summary of four gender difference studies conducted in our laboratory, showed that comparably trained females have a lower body and lean mass weight and a higher percentage of body fat (% BF) compared with males. Thus, comparison between genders based upon absolute $\dot{V}O_{2\,max}$ would lead to the selection of females who were heavier than the males. Even when expressed relative to body weight (mL/kg/min), comparably trained females will have a lower $\dot{V}O_{2\,max}$ than males, or the females may be excessively lean and may have menstrual abnormalities.

Because of the aforementioned concerns, it has been suggested that both training status and $\dot{V}O_{2\,max}$/kg lean body mass (LBM) be used in comparative studies. Sparling[14] suggested a gender matching scheme based upon careful assessment of habitual activity in the year before the testing. Cureton[15] presented convincing arguments for comparing the genders based upon training history for trained individuals and as $\dot{V}O_{2\,max}$ expressed relative to lean mass in untrained individuals. The only way to compare between genders in human studies is to match the groups based upon assessment of both training history and aerobic capacity expressed relative to lean body mass (mL/O_2/kg LBM). Furthermore, in studies using well-trained athletes, it is important to test at intensities at/or below 75% of $\dot{V}O_{2\,max}$ such that potential differences in lactate threshold (LT) do not alter the results. Using a selection criteria, the LT is about 80% for well-trained males and females (males = $79.4 \pm 1.4\%$; females $80.1 \pm 2.7\%$).[15] This combined matching approach takes into account both the genetic ($\dot{V}O_{2\,max}$ potential) and environmental (training status) factors contributing to $\dot{V}O_{2\,max}$ and expresses them relative to the mass of metabolically active tissues. This matching process takes a lot of time, yet it is critical in between-group studies (Table 12.4).

Table 12.4 Factors to Control in Between-Gender Comparative Studies for Endurance Exercise

1. Age
2. $\dot{V}O_{2\,max}$ (mL/kg LBM/min)
3. Timing of:
    a) Menstrual cycle
    b) Testing (am or pm)
    c) Diet (fed vs. fasted)
    d) Exercise status (? Rest day prior to testing)
4. Training status:
    a) Years of training
    b) Frequency (times/week)
    c) Duration (hours/week)
5. Testing intensity:
    a) Well trained $\Rightarrow \leq 75\%$ $\dot{V}O_{2\,max}$.
    b) Untrained $\Rightarrow$ determine LT $\Rightarrow$ exercise $\leq 70\%$ $VO_{2\,max}$.
6. Diet:
    a) Measure habitual intake
        i)   Checklist diet
        ii)   Pre-packaged diet
        iii) Metabolic ward(Gold Standard)
7. Menstrual status:
    a) Follicular vs. luteal
    b) Eumenorrhea, oligoamenorrhea vs. amenorrhea

It is also important to consider the phase of the menstrual cycle in gender comparative studies. In eumenorrheic females, E_2 and progesterone start at low concentrations at the beginning of the cycle, and E_2 progressively increases until about day 14 (ovulation). This initial phase is called the follicular phase and the phase after ovulation until the onset of menses (day 14–28) is termed the luteal phase. During the luteal phase both E_2 and progesterone are at high concentration. It is important to control for the phase of the menstrual cycle for substrate metabolism differs. For example, muscle glycogen concentration is higher,[16] and protein oxidation is greater,[17] during the luteal compared with the follicular phase.

12.2.2 Models to Study Gender Differences in Metabolism

12.2.2.1 Human Models

The most frequently used model to examine for gender differences in metabolism is the cross-sectional, between-group, comparative design in which males and females are matched according to the above-mentioned criteria. Subjects are then exposed to an intervention (i.e., running on a treadmill, cycling, etc.), with certain variables measured (i.e., muscle glycogen, $\dot{V}O_{2\,max}$, etc.). This approach also requires that many other factors be strictly controlled (Table 12.4).

This design is probably the only way to truly compare between males and females because it takes into account both the genetic and developmental aspects of being male or female.

It is likely that many of the differences in metabolism and physical characteristics between males and females are due to the influence of the sex hormones. For this reason, another model may be used for "gender comparison" studies involving either the withdrawal or provision of sex hormones. These approaches are not truly gender comparative, instead they examine the effect of adding or removing sex hormones. An approach would be to study males and females before sexual maturity (pre-pubertal); however, this is limited in terms of the invasiveness of the testing for metabolic studies in this age group. A similar model would be the study of pre- and post-menopausal females; however, age would be a confounding variable. Another possibility would be to compare amenorrheic to eumenorrheic females.[18] A problem with this latter approach is that there are probably several other confounding variables that could account for the amenorrhea (i.e., dietary intake, amount and/or intensity of exercise, other psychological stressors, endogenous hypothalamic set-point, etc.).

The provision of exogenous hormones provides an opportunity for longitudinal studies within a given subject group. The advantage of this approach is that the randomized, cross-over study design controls for many intrinsic and extrinsic variables inherently improve statistical power. One example is to provide hormone replacement to post-menopausal[19] or amenorrheic females.[20] Researchers have been interested in the metabolic effects of E_2 and have been exploring the potential for a model of E_2 administration to males. The first few attempts consisted of the provision of E_2 by a transdermal patch (Estraderm, Ciba-Geigy, Summit, NJ). We used several doses and administration durations but did not attain testosterone concentrations that were in the female range and got the E_2 mutations only into the early-follicular range. The only side effects were skin irritation from the patch (40%) and a slight propensity for headaches. More recently, we have tried an oral preparation (Estrace, Roberts Pharmaceutical, Mississauga, Ontario) for a longer duration and found few side effects (one person had a slight headache) and were able to get E_2 concentrations that were equivalent to those in the luteal phase of the menstrual cycle. We are currently studying the metabolic effects of this E_2 delivery method in males using stable isotopes of glucose and glycerol.

One problem with the provision of an exogenous hormone is that it does not mimic all of the factors that distinguish being male from female. For example, the pulsatility of hormone release and interactions with progesterone may be important to metabolism. Additionally, it is possible that long hormonal exposure duration may be required to observe the phenotypic expression(s) relevant to metabolism. There are obvious ethical constraints to such an approach in males.

Another powerful design would be to start with untrained males and females and study the acute and chronic metabolic adaptations during a long-term, longitudinal training study. The advantage is that training equivalence could be ensured and the repeated measures design would increase statistical power.

To date, there has been only one gender comparative study that has taken this approach.[21] This group started with untrained males (N = 60) and females (N = 18) and trained them such that they could complete a marathon after 20 months.[21] They found that 1) Females had a greater percentage of body fat before and after training; 2) Post-exercise plasma urea was greater for males; 3) Females preserved LBM loss due to training better than males; 4) Plasma creatine kinase (CK) activity rise was lower for females following the marathon; and 5) Hemoglobin, hematocrit, and ferritin were higher in males. In spite of the rigorous design, it was unfortunate that for many of the muscle metabolite and substrate measurements there was a variable period between the completion of exercise and obtaining the tissue (range = 30 min. $\Rightarrow$ 7 h). Further studies need to use this rigorous design in trying to answer the question of gender differences in metabolism.

12.2.2.2 Animal Models

As with humans, between gender comparisons can be made in animal studies. With animals, it is much easier to rigorously control for environmental and dietary parameters. Most studies in the area of gender differences in metabolism have been performed using rats. With most animals, matching issues do arise because the female is lighter than the male rat throughout the life cycle. This, however, could be considered a gender difference per se, which may be related to gender differences in metabolism.

As mentioned above in human studies, several studies have provided exogenous hormones to male and OVX female rats.[7-9] These models look at the hormonal contribution to potential metabolic differences during exercise and, at least in the short term (less than seven days), there are no effects on body weight.[7,8] A major advantage of the animal model is that many tissues are potentially available for study (i.e., heart, brain, gut, etc.), as opposed to the human where muscle and blood are the main sources of sampling.

In the future, researchers will use transgenic (i.e., over-expression of estrogen receptor gene in a male rat), knockout (i.e., removal of estrogen receptor in female rat), and clonal (i.e., genetically identical animals exposed to differing hormonal stimuli during development) animal models to study gender relevant questions.

12.3 OVERVIEW OF SUBSTRATE METABOLISM DURING ENDURANCE EXERCISE

12.3.1   Acute Effects of Endurance Exercise

During endurance exercise at between 60–75% of $\dot{V}O_{2\,max}$ most of the energy is derived from the oxidation of carbohydrate (see Table 12.1). About 2–5% of the energy may be derived from amino acid oxidation. The proportion of fat, carbohydrate, and protein that is oxidized during endurance exercise depends upon the intensity and duration of exercise. As the intensity of exercise increases, there is a progressive decrease in the proportion of energy derived from fat and an increase in the contribution from carbohydrate. As exercise intensity approaches $\dot{V}O_{2\,max}$, free fatty acid (FFA) cannot supply energy fast enough to keep up with energy demand, and muscle glycogen and blood glucose provide a proportionately greater amount of energy.[22-24] This well-known phenomenon has been referred to as the "cross-over concept" by George Brooks[6] (Figure 12.1). As the exercise continues, muscle glycogen progressively declines and energy derived from fat[23,25] and protein increases proportionately.[26]

In addition to intensity-dependent alterations in the ratio of fat:carbohydrate, there are intensity-dependent differences in the proportional ratios of the substrate source. For example, at an exercise intensity of about 25% $\dot{V}O_{2\,max}$, peripheral lipolysis of triglyceride (TG) more than free fatty acid (FFA) provides the largest proportion of energy, and at 60–65% $\dot{V}O_{2\,max}$, intra-muscular triglyceride (IMTG) lipolysis is more predominant.[27] With respect to carbohydrate metabolism, there is a progressively greater proportion of energy derived from intra-muscular glycogenolysis as exercise intensity increases.[28] Protein catabolism increases with higher exercise intensities; however, the proportional contribution from the different amino acid sources is unknown.

The increase in amino acid oxidation during exercise relates to an increase in the active form of the rate-limiting enzyme in branched-chain amino acid oxidation (namely, branched-chain keto

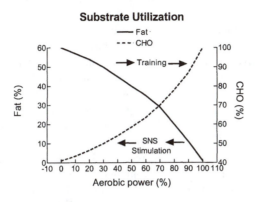

Figure 12.1 Cross-over concept as redrawn from Dr. G. Brooks.[6] This graph shows the interaction of fat:carbohydrate contributions during endurance exercise.

acid dehydrogenase (BCKAD)). BCKAD is activated by glycogen depletion, and thus amino acid and glycogen catabolism are inversely proportional. An increase in amino acid oxidation is probably important as carbohydrate stores are depleted in order to supply carbon skeletons for anapleurosis of the TCA cycle.[29]

12.3.2 Chronic Effects of Exercise Training

In response to endurance exercise training, there is a sparing of glycogen utilization and a proportionate increase in FFA oxidation.[24,30–32] The increased FFA oxidation is primarily derived from the IMTG pool.[23,30,31] As expected, there is an increase in IMTGs to support this increased utilization (IMTG).[31] [The enzymatic capacity for intra-muscular β-oxidation (β-OH-acyl-CoA-dehydrogenase (HAD))[30,33] and FFA transport (fatty acid binding protein (FABP), carnitine palmitoyl transferase (CPT)[34,35]) are increased in response to endurance training (Table 12.5).]

In addition to training-induced increases in enzymatic and substrate capacity, the lipolytic sensitivity to catecholamines also increases.[23,36] However, peripheral lipolysis and catecholamine concentrations are significantly lower at the same absolute exercise intensity following endurance training.[23] At the same time, the contribution from IMTG to total energy expenditure is increased two- to three-fold.[23,30] Thus, following endurance training, the capacity for adipocyte lipolysis increases; however, its relative contribution to energy delivery is reduced relative to IMTG oxidation (see below). Interestingly, LPL gene expression is increased in skeletal muscle and not adipocytes following endurance exercise training, suggesting an enhancement of FFA delivery to skeletal

Table 12.5 Adaptations in Fat Oxidation Consequent to Endurance Training

Variable	Adaptation
1. Muscle transport/storage:	↑ FABP, ↑ IMTG, ↑ mitochondria.
2. Muslce enzyme capacity:	↑ HAD and CPT activity.
3. Whole body oxidation:	↓ peripheral lipolysis.
	↑ lipolytic sensitivity to catecholamines.

FABP	fatty acid binding protein
IMTG	intra-muscular triglycerides
HAD	β-OH-acyl-CoA-dehydrogenase
CPT	carnitine palmitoyl transferase
TG	triglyceride

muscle.[37] This observation is consistent with the observation that IMTG concentration increases following endurance training.[31]

With respect to carbohydrate metabolism, the muscle glucose transporters (GLUT 4)[38] and total glycogen concentration increase. Corresponding to the increase in GLUT 4 is a greater capacity for trained individuals to glycogen load and for a persistence of the elevated glycogen concentrations after such a load.[39] The link between an enhanced FFA oxidation and an attenuation of carbohydrate oxidation is controversial and the locus of control is hotly debated.[40–43]

For protein catabolism, the story is more controversial. Three studies, using the rodent model, yielded conflicting results.[44–46] Two found that the muscle from trained rats oxidized more leucine as compared to untrained animals.[44,45] In another study, using a perfused rat hind-limb model, Hood and Terjung[46] found that endurance training reduced the proportional contribution of leucine to total energy consumption. We have recently completed a study to examine the effects of chronic endurance training on the activation of BCKAD in six males and six females.[46a] We measured the percent of BCKAD in the active form (de-phosphorylated) before and after endurance exercise at 65% $\dot{V}O_{2\,max}$ prior to and following (tested at both the absolute and relative intensity) a 30-day endurance training program. Acute exercise increased the fraction of BCKAD in the active form in the untrained state from 7.6 to 25%. There was also a significant attenuation of the post-exercise activation following training for both males and females at both the absolute (10.5%) and relative (12.7%) intensities.[46a] These findings suggest a "metabolic logic" by the body in that it is not of phylogenetic advantage to continue to oxidize structural and regulatory proteins for energy under periods of metabolic stress (i.e., exercise).

In addition to the changes induced by exercise training per se, the habitual diet is important in determining the adaptation in intra-muscular substrate.[47] A high-carbohydrate diet consumed during endurance exercise training results in an increase in intra-muscular glycogen concentration, whereas consumption of a high-fat diet results in no changes in glycogen and large increases in IMTG.[47] The body adapts to whatever fuel is predominant during the period of exercise training.

In summary, most of the energy for endurance exercise at 60–75% $\dot{V}O_{2\,max}$ comes from carbohydrate, followed by fat, with only small contributions coming from protein oxidation. With higher intensities of exercise, the proportion of carbohydrate and protein increases, while fat contribution decreases. With chronic endurance training, there is a sparing of glycogen utilization and an enhancement of its re-synthesis. Furthermore, there is an up-regulation of the metabolic pathways involved in fat oxidation and a proportional increase in its contribution to energy supply. Less is known about the effects of endurance exercise training upon protein metabolism. However, preliminary evidence suggests an attenuation of BCKAD activation, which should lead to attenuated amino acid oxidation. As stated earlier, most of this work has been conducted using primarily or exclusively male participants. The remainder of the chapter discusses the potential for a gender-specific difference in these substrate metabolic pathways.

12.4 GENDER DIFFERENCES IN FAT METABOLISM

12.4.1 Capacity for Fatty Acid Oxidation

One of the most consistent findings relevant to the potential capacity for FFA oxidation is that the percentage body fat is greater for females than for males. During exercise, however, body fat content is not rate limiting to performance, for even the leanest of male athletes (4% body fat) would still have enough lipid reserve to last for over 30 hours of continuous exercise at 75% $\dot{V}O_{2\,max}$ even with no exogenous food intake (clearly an impossible feat). Aside from providing for a metabolic reserve during starvation, a higher percentage of body fat does not provide female endurance athletes with many advantages, except perhaps added buoyancy in an ultra-swimmer.

More relevant to an endurance athlete is the observation that females have higher IMTG than males. One study of males and females aged 19–85 found that the total fat content of female muscle was 58g/kg and 23g/kg for males.[48] In untrained females, there appears to be an increase in interfascicular fat that was not seen in trained females nor in males (no IMTG measurements were made).[49] We measured the IMTG content of skeletal muscle in six male and six female well-trained endurance athletes from a previous study[5] and found that females had a higher IMTG content (female = 38 mmol/kgdm; male = 32 mmol/kgdm; $P < 0.05$).[50] It remains to be seen whether this gender difference is true IMTG or whether it is from adipocytes in the endo- and peri-mysial space around fibers and fascicles.

The IMTG content per se could enhance FFA oxidation directly for its hydrolysis bypasses peripheral lipolysis, plasma transport, and sarcolemmal uptake that are required for peripheral FFA utilization. Furthermore, endurance training increases IMTG content[31] and proportional oxidation,[23] which indirectly implies that IMTG oxidation is a preferred fuel source during exercise. If females do have an increased IMTG concentration, the potential mechanism for this is unclear. It is possible that E_2 may increase IMTG deposition directly. In rat liver, the administration of E_2 increased FFA synthase and acyl CoA carboxylase (ACC) activity.[51]

In addition to IMTG storage, there is evidence that the enzymatic capacity for fat oxidation is different between the genders. Several studies in rats have found that E_2 treatment decreased adipocyte lipoprotein lipase (LPL) activity.[52–56] In contrast, progesterone has little,[54,57] or modest stimulatory[58,59] effects upon adipocyte LPL activity. Skeletal muscle LPL activity either decreases after a more prolonged period of E_2 exposure as compared to adipocyte LPL activity[52] or it significantly increases.[55,56] Ellis and colleagues[56] showed that five days of E_2 administration to male rats increased both basal and post-exercise LPL activity in red and white vastus and heart.[56] Together, these data suggest that E_2 treatment in rodent models induces a greater propensity for the flux of plasma borne TG-derived FFA toward muscle. Whether the available FFA is shunted into oxidative or synthetic pathways likely depends on the prevailing hormonal milieu and acute and chronic exercise status. It may be that estrogen induces much greater oscillations in the balance between synthesis and oxidation.[60] Female rat adipocytes have greater insulin binding than male adipocytes and fatty acid synthase is four times greater.[61] This enhanced insulin sensitivity for females has also been demonstrated in human skeletal muscle.[62]

It may be that in the post-prandial phase (high insulin), females shunt more FFA into storage due to an increased insulin sensitivity, whereas during exercise fat oxidation is enhanced (see below). In studying the lipolysis of human adipocytes, it is important to note that the fat deposit location influences both LPL activity and lipolysis.[57,63] For example, females have more α_2 receptors (decreased lipolysis) in the gluteal region as compared to males and as compared with their abdominal region.[63] Furthermore, adipocyte LPL activity is greater in the femoral/gluteal region than in the abdominal region.[64] This likely explains the propensity for females to accumulate adipose tissue in the femoral-gluteal region. It is also an important factor to consider in gender comparative work, for the fat biopsy location could alter the results of a study examining LPL activity or lipolysis.

In humans there is some discrepancy in results of lipolytic rates obtained from biopsied adipocytes.[64,65] Despres and colleagues[65] found that males had a higher basal and epinephrine-stimulated lipolytic rate than females. On the other hand, Crampes et al.[64] found that females had a greater lipolytic response to elevated concentrations of both epinephrine and isoproterenol as compared to males, and this was accentuated in the trained vs. untrained state. The differences may relate to the sampling site, as the former study (males greater than females) sampled from the supra-iliac region (perhaps more α_2 receptors) and the latter from the peri-umbilical region (where female and male β-receptor numbers are similar). Furthermore, the gender difference seen by Crampes et al.[64] was predominantly seen in the endurance-trained subjects, which may indicate that female adipocyte lipolysis is more inducible in response to exercise training. It should be noted that for adipocytes, LPL activity and lipolytic rates trend in opposite directions.[57] To date, I am not aware of any studies that have reported gender differences in hormone-sensitive lipase activity.

With respect to FFA transport, there have been two reports demonstrating that females have a higher hepatic FABP concentration in liver than males.[66,67] In rat skeletal muscle, there is indirect evidence that E_2 increased FABP content.[68] Whether this gender difference is present in human skeletal muscle remains to be seen. But if it does exist, then the diffusive flux for FFA may be enhanced in females.

Long-chain FFA transport into the mitochondria is mediated by the carnitine carrier system. The first step is the malonyl-CoA regulated step catalysed by CPT I. An earlier study by Costill and colleagues[34] found no significant gender difference in CPT activity in whole muscle homogenates from male and female athletes.[34] Furthermore, a recent study by Spriet and colleagues isolated mitochondria from male and female athletes, used malonyl-CoA inhibition to confirm the CPT I specific fraction, and found no gender difference in CPT I activity (L. Spriet, personal communication, 1998). Furthermore, there does not appear to be a gender difference in muscle total carnitine content.[69] In summary, there does not appear to be a gender difference in muscle CPT I activity nor total carnitine.

Once within the mitochondrial matrix, the FFA-CoA enters the β-oxidation pathway. None of the following enzymes have been measured in gender-comparative studies: acyl-CoA dehydrogenase, crotonase, or thiolase. Several studies have examined HAD activity between the genders.[70–72] Green and colleagues[71] found that the ratio of HAD/SDH was higher for active females (N = 17) than males (N = 16).[71] They also showed that the PFK/HAD ratio was higher in males as compared to females (indicating a higher glycolytic/fat oxidation potential).[71] There has been only one longitudinal study that examined potential gender differences in HAD activity with altered contractile function (electrical stimulation).[70] Although they did not find a gender difference in HAD activity, the activity increased to a greater extent for the females (+ 30%; P < 0.01) as compared to the males (+ 12%; P < 0.05).[70] Taken together, these data indicate that females may have a greater induction of HAD than males and that the activity of HAD relative to the TCA cycle capacity may be slightly greater. Future studies should examine the activity of the thiolysis step, as it is a non-equilibrium step that is thought to be rate limiting.

In summary, there are greater subcutaneous adipose stores and probably IMTG stores for females as compared to males. This may be related to greater insulin sensitivity in females. LPL activity in adipocytes appears to be higher in males than in females, and this is correlated with E_2 concentration. Epinephrine- and isoproterenol-stimulated lipolysis seems to be higher in trained females than in males. Data exist to suggest that FABP is greater in female muscle; however, no direct studies have been conducted in humans. There are no gender differences in CPT I or in total muscle carnitine. Finally, the HAD/TCA potential may be slightly greater in females and more responsive to exercise induced induction.

12.4.2 Studies of Fat Metabolism During Exercise

As above, there is a lower RER during endurance exercise in females than in males. These results indicate a greater reliance on fat for energy under these circumstances for females than for males. By combining the results from the studies listed in Table 12.1 (N = 52 males; N = 52 females), there is a lower RER for females by about 5% (males = 0.91 (0.06); females = 0.87 (0.05)). This amounts to a 70% higher fat oxidation for females (~39% of total energy for females vs. ~22% of total energy expenditure for males) during endurance exercise at about 65% $\dot{V}O_{2\,max}$. Others have not found a gender difference in fat oxidation during endurance exercise.[34,73] In one of these studies, the RER values were not reported and the untrained subjects were exercised at 75% $\dot{V}O_{2\,PEAK}$, while the trained subjects were exercised at 80% $\dot{V}O_{2\,PEAK}$.[73] Clearly, some of the subjects would have been close to, or over, their anaerobic threshold. Furthermore, it is likely that females will show only enhanced fat oxidation at intensities around 65% $\dot{V}O_{2\,PEAK}$, as this is the intensity where IMTG oxidation contribution is maximal. In the other study that reported no gender differences in fat oxidation during endurance exercise, there were matching issues that may have confounded the interpretation.[34] First, the female athletes were much younger than the males (23 vs. 35, respectively), and more importantly, there is no mention of menstrual status or the phase of the menstrual cycle during which testing took place.[34] It was unlikely that many of the females were eumenorrheic while running 80–115 km per week. Overall, the bulk of the data in humans shows that the RER is lower for females as compared to males during sub-maximal endurance exercise. There have only been two studies using metabolic tracers to examine the question of potential gender differences in the metabolic response to exercise.[74] One reported no differences in palmitate rate of appearance (Ra) between the genders in response to endurance exercise. Unfortunately, there were only four subjects per group and glycerol Ra was not determined.[74]

A recent study has examined the effect of E_2 upon glucose and glycerol turnover during exercise.[75] This group studied six amenorrheic females following each of three treatments (C72 = 72 h placebo patch; E_2 72 = 72 h of 17-β-estradiol patch; and E_2 144 = 144 h of E_2 patch).[75] Plasma [FFA] was greater for both E_2 trials vs. placebo and reported a trend toward slightly lower RER values later in exercise (data not shown).[75] There was no effect of treatment upon glycerol Ra, and glucose Ra was attenuated during both E_2 treatments.[75] Furthermore, there was a significant attenuation in the post-exercise catecholamine concentration for the E_2 treatment trials.[75] Our group has also used an E_2 patch protocol in males and also found no effect on the RER during endurance exercise and no attenuation of muscle glycogen utilization.[76] Unfortunately, although the E_2 patch allowed for a within-group design, it does not mimic all of the differences between males and females but, rather, changes only one parameter (i.e., estradiol). For example, in both of these studies the plasma E_2 concentration was increased by only approximately 100%, whereas a eumenorrheic female has peak E_2 concentrations (luteal phase) that are about 700% greater than basal levels. The model also does not consider the other female sex hormone, progesterone, that may also be an important factor in determining "male" from "female" metabolic responses to endurance exercise.

In the rat model, there is convincing evidence for an effect of 17-β-estradiol to influence metabolism during endurance exercise.[7,9,56] An early study found that eight days of E_2 administration to OVX rats resulted in a significantly lower $^{14}CO_2$ evolution from labeled glucose and a significantly greater $^{14}CO_2$ evolution from labeled palmitate.[9] This suggests that fat oxidation was enhanced and glucose oxidation inhibited by E_2. Similar results were also found with a five-day E_2 treatment protocol in male rats, where both pre- and post-exercise FFA concentrations were elevated as compared to placebo oil injected rats.[7] In this latter study, there was a significant attenuation of muscle and liver glycogen utilizutilizationation, and it was suggested that this was secondary to the increase in fat availability.[7] This same group went on to explore the effect of E_2 on fat oxidation by administering E_2 to male rats for five days and measuring plasma FFA, glycerol and TG as well as muscle, heart, and adipose LPL activity.[7] They found that E_2 treatment resulted in an increased resting glycerol and FFA and a lower TG, which corresponded to a decrease in adipocyte-LPL activity and an increase in muscle- and heart-LPL activity.[56] The ratio of muscle/adipocyte LPL activity was 4.65 for the E_2 group and 1.15 for the placebo group. They suggested that this indicated an E_2 mediated distribution of plasma TG-FFA towards heart and skeletal muscle.[56]

There appears to be significant gender differences in both the storage and utilization of fats. Females have more sub-cutaneous adipose tissue and probably IMTG than males. During sub-maximal endurance exercise there is a greater fat oxidation for females as compared to males, and this may lead to glycogen and protein "sparing" (see below). E_2 appears to be a major mediator of the aforementioned metabolic effects, particularly when one considers work from the rat model.

12.5 GENDER DIFFERENCES IN CARBOHYDRATE METABOLISM

12.5.1 Capacity for Oxidation

There is no evidence that there are any gender differences in basal glycogen concentrations that could account for a greater carbohydrate use by males. Muscle glycogen concentration does not appear to change across the menstrual cycle.[16] From an enzymatic standpoint, Green and colleagues[71] have shown that phosphorylase activity is greater in males than in females. This may partially explain a greater glycogen utilization by males.

It also appears that there may be a gender difference in the ability to carbohydrate load, with males showing an enhanced ability. In one study, Tarnopolsky and colleagues[5] studied the ability of male and female athletes to increase muscle glycogen in response to a four-day period of elevated dietary carbohydrate (55–60% → 75% of energy intake). It was found that males increased muscle glycogen by 41% and performance time increased by 45%, whereas females showed no increase in glycogen (0%) and no increase in performance time (5%).[5] It was possible that these findings were due to the fact that the females were tested in the follicular phase of the menstrual cycle (where glycogen re-synthesis is relatively attenuated), or that the low energy intake by the females resulted in a sub-optimal carbohydrate intake when expressed as a relative percent. However, in a subsequent study by Walker and colleagues,[77] the ability of females to carbohydrate load was tested during the luteal phase and dietary carbohydrate was given in equivalent dose to those in studies conducted in males (~8g/kg). They found a very modest increase in muscle glycogen under these conditions and concluded that the increase was "smaller than that reported for men."[77] Even this modest increase was likely exaggerated compared with that normally seen for the "medium-carbohydrate" diet supplied only 48% carbohydrate, which is lower than the habitual intake for most female runners. A recent study found that during the first four hours after endurance exercise, glycogen repletion is the same for males and females if the carbohydrate source is provided immediately after exercise.[78] This may be a practical nutritional strategy for females trying to carbohydrate load.

The mechanism behind a lesser ability for females to carbohydrate load is not clear, and it appears paradoxical when one considers the enhanced insulin sensitivity mentioned previously. It is clear that although insulin sensitivity is greater in females, much of the insulin-stimulated glucose uptake in adipose tissue is diverted into FFA synthetic pathways.[61] If this holds true in skeletal muscle, it may explain the higher IMTG seen in females. To date, no human studies have looked at potential differences in muscle GLUT 4 concentration (insulin and contraction stimulated glucose transport). After GLUT 4 mediated transport, the next step in glycogenosis is phosphorylation by hexokinase (HK), and it appears that HK activity is lower in females.[71,72] Clearly, more work is needed to explain an attenuated ability for females to carbohydrate load, including an examination of glycogen synthase activity.

12.5.2 Studies During Exercise

As demonstrated in Table 12.1, males use more carbohydrate during endurance exercise than females. At 65% $\dot{V}O_{2\,max}$, there appears to be a sparing of muscle glycogen use for female as compared to male runners.[79] At higher intensities of cycling (75% $\dot{V}O_{2\,max}$), there does not appear to be a gender difference in glycogen utilization, yet RER was still lower for the females.[5] This suggests that, at least at higher intensities of endurance exercise, the lower overall carbohydrate oxidation is not necessarily from muscle glycogen. Ruby and co-workers[75] used a [6,6 ^{2}H]-glucose tracer to study plasma glucose kinetics during exercise in response to E_2 administration in amenorrheic female athletes. They found that E_2 administration resulted in a reduction in glucose Ra and Rd and interpreted this to indicate that gluconeogenesis and glucose uptake were attenuated.[75]

Clearly, further studies combining both tracer methodology and direct muscle measurements are required to more clearly answer this question.

The results with rat studies are consistent with the hypothesis that females oxidise less carbohydrate during endurance exercise. One study gave rats either placebo oil or E_2 injections and measured heart and muscle glycogen before and after strenuous exercise.[7] The rats treated with E_2 ran farther and exhibited a sparing of heart and skeletal muscle glycogen utilization. Further research by this same group essentially replicated these findings and also linked the glycogen sparing to an enhanced lipid oxidation consequent to E_2 administration.[8] Another study found that ^{14}C-glucose oxidation during exercise was lower for E_2 as compared with placebo treated rats.[9] This was inversely correlated to an increase in ^{14}C-palmitate oxidation, again demonstrating a link between an enhanced lipid oxidation and attenuated carbohydrate oxidation. As will be seen below, the sparing of carbohydrate oxidation is likely important in a "sparing" of protein oxidation.

12.6 GENDER DIFFERENCES IN PROTEIN METABOLISM

12.6.1 Capacity for Oxidation

There have been no reported gender differences in the "capacity" for amino acid oxidation in humans. Certainly, the LBM is greater for males than for females (as mentioned previously). However, it is difficult to envision how this fact per se could account for the greater protein oxidation in males (see below). For this reason, we have measured muscle branched chamketo acid dehydrogenase (BCKAD) activity in both males and females before and after endurance exercise training.[46a] There was a significantly lower BCKAD in the active resting and exercise (90 min at 60% $\dot{V}O_2$ peak) leucine oxidation was lower before and after exercise for females than for males at all time points ($P < 0.05$).[46a] These results were similar to our earlier observations of a lesser leucine oxidation for females than for males.[80] Because the percent of BCKAD in the active form was similar for both males and females, the difference in leucine oxidation might have been due to hepatic BCKAD differences. Therefore, females should have lower protein requirements than males (see below).

12.6.2 Studies During Exercise

There have been only a few direct gender comparative studies examining protein metabolism during exercise.[79–81] One study found that plasma urea concentrations increased in male runners after 10-, 25-, and 42-km runs, yet there were no changes for the females.[81] Our group measured urinary urea excretion in six male and six female runners over a 24-hour rest and 24-hour exercise day (run 15.5 km).[79] There were no exercise-induced increases in urea excretion for the females, whereas the males increased urea excretion by 30%. Using the urinary urea excretion measurements and RER from four studies, I have calculated that protein contributed 5% and 1.5% to the total energy requirements in males and females, respectively, during endurance exercise at between 65 and 75% $\dot{V}O_{2\,max}$ for 60–90 minutes.[5,78–80]

Using stable isotope methodology, a subsequent study measured leucine oxidation in males and females cycling for 90 minutes at 65% $\dot{V}O_{2\,max}$.[80] In addition, nitrogen balance studies were completed to determine the adequacy of the Canadian Nutrient Intake for protein (0.86 g/kg/d). We found that leucine oxidation was lower for females than for males, which corresponded to a lower calculated protein contribution (based upon urine urea measurements). Nitrogen balance was negative for both groups, and in spite of the nitrogen intake being lower for the females, the magnitude of the negative nitrogen balance was less.[80]

The influence of the menstrual cycle must also be considered in gender-comparative protein oxidation studies. A study by Lamont and colleagues[17] found that urea excretion was higher during the luteal phase as compared to the follicular phase. Another study found that whole body proteolysis was higher during the mid-luteal phase as compared to the mid-follicular phase.[82] Together, these findings suggest that an elevated progesterone/E_2 ratio may enhance proteolysis and amino acid oxidation. The potential link between the sex hormones and BCKAD activation needs to be explored.

In summary, females appear to oxidize less protein than males during sub-maximal endurance exercise. Although strenuous endurance exercise may slightly elevate dietary protein requirements, the magnitude of that increase would be expected to be less for females from the available data. Future studies need to examine the effects of the sex hormones upon leucine oxidation and dietary protein requirements.

12.7 RECOMMENDATIONS

Perhaps the most prudent recommendation is that there is a great need for further research into potential gender differences in metabolism. Based upon the paucity or current findings, it appears that a few gender-specific nutritional recommendations can be made. First, protein requirements for very well-trained endurance athletes are greater than Canadian and U.S. recommendations for the general population. However, these modest increases are not as significant for females as compared to males. Second, females appear to have a lesser capacity to glycogen load as compared to males. It remains to be seen if this impairment can be overcome by early post-exercise supplementation and/or increase in total energy.

From a metabolic perspective, females may be even better suited to ultra-endurance sports and should not be excluded from such events.

12.8 CONCLUSIONS

There appears to be significant gender differences in endurance exercise metabolism characterized by higher fat oxidation and lower protein and carbohydrate oxidation for females as compared to males. Animal studies have replicated these findings through the provision of exogenous E_2, suggesting that it is the main determinant of gender differences in metabolism. It appears that fat oxidation is the primary process being regulated and that the other metabolic substrates follow. For example, E_2 increases IMTG (storage), FABP (transport), and HAD (oxidation capacity). Thus, carbohydrate oxidation would be lower due to the increased fat utilization, and the "sparing" of muscle glycogen should result in a lower BCKAD activation (lower protein oxidation).

The potential implications of some of the aforementioned observations are unclear and await further direct testing. With respect to carbohydrate loading, it may be that females have a reduced capacity to load. However, by increasing total carbohydrate and energy intake and by consuming carbohydrates immediately after exercise, females are likely to be able to increase muscle glycogen. Whether this is enough to improve performance remains to be answered. With respect to dietary protein requirements, it appears that any increase in requirement induced by rigorous training will be about 20–25% less for females. It is hoped that this chapter provides at least the groundwork for future researchers to consider the potential for gender differences in metabolism and to include equal numbers of both male and female participants.

From a performance aspect, it is unlikely that females will outperform males in strength and/or power events due to their smaller body mass. However, in the ultra-endurance sports, an enhanced lipid oxidation and glycogen sparing[5,12–14] may favor the female athlete. Because most of the metabolic fuel for the completion of a marathon (42 km) comes from carbohydrate oxidation, it is likely that males will have a slight metabolic advantage up to this distance. But as the distance exceeds 42 km, females should have an increasing advantage over males.

These concepts have been examined by Speechley and colleagues[83] in 1996. They found that equally trained males and females performed identically over a distance of 42 km, yet the females outperformed the males over 90 km. They claimed (accurately) that this was not due to a greater maximal aerobic capacity, training history, or running economy. However, they erroneously claimed that it was not due to differences in lipid oxidation (based upon plasma free fatty acid concentration measurements only). Another study from South Africa[84] matched males and females for performance times at 56 km and found that the females outperformed the males at 90 km. Regression analysis showed that the males outperformed the females at 5–42 km and that there were no gender differences in performance until an intercept of 66 km, after which the females had an increasing advantage.[84]

It is hoped that in the future there is an increased understanding of potential gender differences in metabolism and that specific recommendations for each of the genders can be made. Hopefully it will not take decades for this to come to fruition, as it did for people to realize that females could (and are probably even better suited to longer distances) complete a marathon.

REFERENCES

1. Sherman, W. M., Costill, D. L., Fink, W. J., and Miller, J. M., The effect of exercise-diet manipulation on muscle glycogen and its subsequent utilization during performance, *Int. J. Sports Med.*, 2:114, 1981.
2. Bergstrom, J. and Hultman. E., A study of the glycogen metabolism during exercise in man, *Scand. J. Clin. Lab. Invest.*, 19, 218, 1967.
3. Hultman, E., Studies on muscle metabolism of glycogen and active phosphate in man with special reference to exercise and diet, *Scand. J. Clin. Lab. Invest.*, 19, 94, 1967.
4. Karlsson, J. and Saltin, B., Diet, muscle glycogen, and endurance performance, *J. Appl. Physiol.*, 31, 203, 1971.
5. Tarnopolsky, M. A., Atkinson, S. A., Phillips, S. M., and MacDougall, J. D., Carbohydrate loading and metabolism during exercise in men and women, *J. Appl. Physiol.*, 78, 1360, 1995.
6. Brooks, G.A., Fahey, T.D., and White, T.P., *Exercise Physiology: Human Bioenergetics and its Applications.* Macmillan Publishing Co., 1996.
7. Kendrick, Z. V., Steffen, C. A., Rumsey, W. L., and Goldberg, D. I., Effect of estradiol on tissue glycogen metabolism in exercised oophorectomized rats. *J. Appl. Physiol.*, 63, 492, 1987.
8. Kendrick, Z. V. and Ellis, G. S., Effect of estradiol on tissue glycogen metabolism and lipid availability in exercised male rats, *J. Appl. Physiol.*, 71, 1694, 1991.
9. Hatta, H., Atomi, Y., Shinohara, S., Yamamoto, Y., and Yamada, S., The effects of ovarian hormones on glucose and fatty acid oxidation during exercise in female ovariectomized rats, *Horm. Metabol. Res.*, 20, 609, 1988.
10. Wilmore, J. H., Wambsgans, K. C., Brenner, M., Broeder, C. E., Paijmans, I., Volpe, J. A., and Wilmore, K. M., Is there energy conservation in amenorrheic compared with eumenorrheic distance runners? *J. Appl. Physiol.*, 72, 15, 1992.
11. Marcus, R. C., Madvig, C. P., Minkoff, J., Goddard, M., Bayer, M., Martin, M., Gaudiani, L., Haskell, W., and Genant, H., Menstrual function and bone mass in elite women distance runners, *Ann. Inter. Med.*, 102, 158, 1985.
12. Hoyenga, K. B. and Hoyenga, K. T., Gender and energy balance: sex differences in adaptations for feast and famine, *Physio. Behav.*, 28, 545, 1982.
13. Drinkwater, B. L., Nilson, K., Chestnut, C. H. III, Bremner, W. J., Shainholtz, S., and Southworth, M. B., Bone mineral content of amenorrheic and eumenorrheic athletes, *N. Engl. J. Med.*, 311, 277, 1984.
14. Sparling, P. B., A Meta-Analysis of studies comparing maximal oxygen uptake in men and women. *Med. Sci. Ex. Sport*, 51, 542, 1980.
15. Cureton, K. J., Matching of male and female subjects using $\dot{V}O_{2\ max}$, *Research Quarterly for Exercise and Sport*, 52, 264, 1981.
16. Nicklas, B.J., Hackney, A.C., and Sharp, R.L., The menstrual cycle and exercise: Performance, muscle glycogen, and substrate responses. *Int. J. Sports Med.*, 10:264-269, 1989.
17. Lamont L. S., Lemon P. W., and Bruot B. C., Menstrual cycle and exercise effects on protein catabolism, *Medicine and Science in Sports and Exercise*, 19, 106, 1987.

18. Baer, J. T., Endocrine parameters in amenorrheic and eumenorrheic adolescent female runners, *Int. J. Sports Med.*, 14, 191, 1993.

19. Jensen, M. D., Martin, M. L., Cryer, P. E, and Roust, L. R., Effects of estrogen on free fatty acid metabolism in humans, *Am. J. Physiol.*, 266, E914, 1994.

20. Ruby, B. C., Robergs, R. A., Waters, D. L., Bruge, M., Mermier, C., and Stolarczyk, L., Effects of estradiol on substrate turnover during exercise in amenorrheic females, *Med. Sci. Sports Exerc.*, 29, 1160, 1997.

21. Janssen, G.M.E. and ten Hoor, F., Sport and Health in a General Perspective, *Int. J. Sports Med.*, S3, S118, 1989.

22. Klein, S., Holland, O. B., and Wolfe, R. R., Importance of blood glucose concentration in regulating lipolysis during fasting in humans, *Am. J. Physiol.*, 258 (Endocrinol. Metab. 21), E32, 1990.

23. Phillips, S. M., Green, H. J., Tarnopolsky, M. A., Heigenhauser, G. J. R., Hill, R. E., and Grant, S. M., Effects of training duration on substrate turnover and oxidation during exercise. *J. Appl. Physiol.*, 81, 2182, 1996.

24. Holloszy, J. O., Dalsky, G. P., Nemeth, P. M., Hurley, B. F., Martin, W. H. III, and Hagberg, J. M., Utilization of fat as substrate during exercise: effect of training, in *Biochem. of Exercise* VI, Vol. 16, Saltin, B., (Eds.), Human Genetics, Champaign, IL, 1986.

25. Klein, S., Weber, J.-M., Coyle, E. F., and Wolfe, R. R., Effect of endurance training on glycerol kinetics during strenuous exercise in humans, *Metabolism*, 45, 357, 1996.

26. Haralambie, G. and Berg, A., Serum urea and amino nitrogen changes with exercise duration, *Eur. J. Appl. Physiol.*, 36, 39, 1976.

27. Romijn J. A., Coyle E. F., Sidossis S., Gastaldelli A., Horowitz J. F., Endert E., Wolfe R. R., Regulation of endogenous fat and carbohydrate metabolism in relation to exercise intensity and duration, *Am. J. Physiol.*, 265, E380, 1993.

28. Bergstrom, J. and Hultman, E. A study of the glycogen metabolism during exercise in man. *Scand. J. Clin Lab Invest.*, 19:218-228, 1967.

29. Gibala, M. J., Tarnopolsky, M. A., and Graham, T. E., Tricarboxylic acid cycle intermediates in human muscle at rest and during prolonged cycling, *Am. J. Physiol.*, 272(*Endocrinol Metab.35*):E239, 1997.

30. Jansson, E. and Kaijser, L., Substrate utilization and enzymes in skeletal muscle of extremely endurance-trained men, *J. Appl. Physiol.*, 62, 999, 1987.

31. Hurley, B. F., Nemeth, P. M., Martin, W. H. III, Hagberg, J. M., Dalsky, G. P., and Holloszy, J. O., Muscle triglyceride utilization during exercise: effect of training, *J. Appl. Physiol.*, 60, 562,1986.

32. Romjin, J. A., Klein, S., Coyle, E. F., Sidossis, S., and Wolfe, R. R., Strenuous endurance training increases lipolysis and triglyceride-fatty acid cycling at rest, *J. Appl. Physiol.*, 75, 108, 1993.

33. Tremblay, A., Simoneau, J.-A., and Bouchard, C., Impact of exercise intensity on body fatness and skeletal muscle metabolism, *Metabolism*, 43, 814, 1994.

34. Costill, D. L., Fink, W. J., Getchell, L. H., Ivy, J. L., and Witzman, F. A., Lipid metabolism in skeletal muscle of endurance-trained males and females. *J. Appl. Physiol.*, 47, 787, 1979.

35. Mole, P. A., Osgai, L. B., and Holloszy, J. O., Increase in levels of palmityl CoA synthetase, carnitine palmityltransferase, and palmityl CoA dehydrogenase, and in the capacity to oxidize fatty acids, *J. Clin. Inves.*, 50, 2323, 1971.

36. Poehlman, E. T., Gardner, A. W., Ariciero, P. J., Goran, M. I., and Calles-Escandon, J., Effects of endurance training on total fat oxidation in elderly persons, *J. Appl. Physiol.*, 76, 2281, 1994.

37. Seip, R. L., Angelopoulos, T. J., and Semenkovich, C. F., Exercise induces human lipoprotein lipase gene expression in skeletal muscle but not adipose tissue, *Am. J. Physiol. 268 (Endocrinol. Metab. 31)*, E$_2$29, 1995.

38. Roy, D. and Marette, A,. Exercise induces the translocation of GLUT 4 to transverse tubules from and intra-cellular pool in rat skeletal muscle. *Biochem. Biophys. Res. Comm.*, 223:147, 1996.

39. Hickner, R. C., Fisher, J. S., Hansen, P. A., Bracette, S. B., Mier, C. M., Turner, M. J., and Holloszy,J. O., Muscle glycogen accumulation after endurance exercise in trained and untrained individuals. *J. Appl. Physiol.*, 83:897, 1997.

40. Costill, D. L., Coyle, E., Dalsky, G., Evans, W., Fink, W., and Hoopes, D., Effects of elevated plasma FFA and insulin on muscle glycogen usage during exercise, *J. Appl. Physiol.*, 43, 695, 1977.

41. Dyck, D. J., Putman, C. T., Heigenhauser, G. J. F., Hultman, E., and Spriet, L. L., Regulation of fat-carbohydrate interaction in skeletal muscle during intense aerobic cycling, *Am. J. Physiol. 265 (Endocrinol. Metab. 28)*, E852, 1993.

42. Hargreaves, M., Kiens, B., and Richter, E. A., Effect of increased plasma free fatty acid concentrations on muscle metabolism in exercising men, *J. Appl. Physiol.*, 70, 194, 1991.

43. Coggan, A. R., Spina, R. J., Kohrt, W. M., and Holloszy, J. O., Effect of prolonged exercise on muscle citrate concentration before and after endurance training in men, *Am. J. Physiol.*, 264 *(Endocrinol. Metab.* 27), E215, 1993.

44. Dohm, G. L., Hecker, A. L., Brown, W. E., Klain, G. J., Puente, F. R., Askew, E. W., and Beecher, G. R. *Biochem. J.*, 164:705, 1977.

45. Henderson S. C., Black A. L., and Brooks G. A., Leucine turnover and oxidation in trained rats during exercise, *Am. J. Physiol.*, 249, E137, 1985.

46. Hood D. A. and Terjung R. L., Effect of endurance training on leucine metabolism in perfused rat skeletal muscle, *Am. J. Physiol.*, 253, E648, 1987.

46a. McKenzie, S., Phillips, S. M., Carter, S.L., Lowther, S., Gibala, M. J., and Tarnopolsky, M. A., Endurance exercise training attenuates leucine oxidation during exercise in humans. *FASEB J.*, 13(4), A81, 1999.

47. Helge, J. W., Wulff, B., and Kiens, B. Impact of a fat rich diet on endurance in man: Role of the dietary period. *Med. Sci. Sports Exerc.*, 30(3):456, 1998.

48. Forsberg, A. M., Nilsson, E., Werneman, J., Bergström, J., and Hultman, E., Muscle composition in relation to age and sex, *Clin. Sci.*, 81, 249, 1991.

49. Prince, F. P., Hikida, R. S., and Hagerman, F. C., Muscle fibre types in women athletes and non-athletes, *Pflügers Arch.*, 371, 161, 1977.

50. Tarnopolsky, M. A., Phillips, S. M., Gender Differences in intra-muscular triglyceride and β-3-hydroxyacl-CoA dehydrogenase activity, *Can. J. Appl. Phys.*, 20,51P, 1995.

51. Mandour, T., Kissebah, A. H., and Wynn, V., Mechanism of oestrogen and progesterone effects on lipid and carbohydrate metabolism: alteration in the insulin: glucagon molar ratio and hepatic enzyme activity, *Eur. J. Clin. Invest.*, 7, 181, 1977.

52. Ramirez, I., Estradiol-induced changes in lipoprotein lipase, eating, and body weight in rats, *Am. J. Physiol.*, 240 *(Endocrinol. Metab.* 3), E533, 1981.

53. Hamosh, M. and Hamosh, P., The effect of estrogen on the lipoprotein lipase activity of rat adipose tissue, *J. Clin. Invest.*, 55, 1132, 1975.

54. Gray, J. M. and Wade, G. N., Food intake, body weight, and adiposity in female rats: actions and interactions of progestins and antiestrogens, *Am. J. Physiol.*, 240:*(Endocrinol. Metab.* 3), E474, 1981

55. Wilson, D. E., Flowers, C. M., Carlile, S. I., and Udall, K. S., Estrogen treatment and gonadal function in the regulation of lipoprotein lipase, *Atherosclerosis*, 24, 491, 1976.

56. Ellis, G. S., Lanza-Jacoby, S., Gow, A., and Kendrick, Z. V., Effects of estradiol on lipoprotein lipase activity and lipid availability in exercised male rats, *J. Appl. Physiol.*, 77, 209, 1994.

57. Rebuffe-Scrive, M., Sex steroid hormones and adipose tissue metabolism in ovariectomized and adrenalectomized rats, *Acta Physiol. Scand.*, 129, 471, 1987.

58. Steingrimsdottir, L., Brasel, J., and Greenwood, M. R. C., *Am. J. Physiol.*, 239 *(Endocrinol. Metab.)*, E162, 1980.

59. Shirling, D., Ashby, J. P., and Baird, J. D., Effect of progesterone on lipid metabolism in the intact rat, *J. Endocrinol.*, 90, 285, 1981.

60. Hansen, F. M., Fahmy, N., and Nielsen, J. H., The influence of sexual hormones on lipogenesis and lipolysis in rat fat cells, *Acta Endocrinologica*, 95, 566, 1980.

61. Guerre-Millo, M., Leturque, A., Girard, J., and Lavau, M., Increased insulin sensitivity and responsiveness of glucose metabolism in adipocytes from female versus male rats, *J. Clin. Invest.*, 76, 109, 1985.

62. Nuutila, P., Knuuti, M. J., Mäki, M., Laine, H., Ruotsalainen, U., Teräs, M., Haaparanta, M., Solin, O., and Yki-Järvinen, H., Gender and insulin sensitivity in the heart and in skeletal muscles, *Diabetes*, 44, 31, 1995.

63. Richelsen, B., Increased α$_2$-but similar β-adrenergic receptor activities in subcutaneous gluteal adipocytes from females compared with males, *Eur. J. Clin. Invest.*, 16, 302, 1986.

64. Crampes, F., Riviere, D., Beauville, M., Marceron, M., and Garrigues, M., Lipolytic response of adipocytes to epinephrine in sedentary and exercise-trained subjects: sex-related differences, *Eur. J. Appl. Physiol.*, 59, 249, 1989.

65. Depres, J. P., Bouchard, C., Savard, R., Tremblay, A., Marcotte, M., and Therault, G., The effect of a 20-week endurance training program on adipose tissue morphology and lipolysis in men and women, *Metabolism*, 33(3), 235, 1984.

66. Ockner, R. K., Lysenko, N., Manning, J. A., and Monroe, S. E., Sex steroid modulation of fatty acid utilization and fatty acid binding protein concentration in rat liver, *J. Clin. Invest.*, 65, 1013, 1980.

67. Luxon, B. A. and Weisiger, R. A., Sex differences in intracellular fatty acid transport: role of cytoplasmic binding proteins, *Am. J. Physiol.*, 265 (*Gastrointest. Liver Physiol.* 28), G831, 1993.

68. van Breda, E., Keizer, H. A., York, M. M., Surtel, D. A. M., de Jong, Y., van derVusse, G. J., and Glatz, J. F. C., Modulation of fatty-acid-binding protein content of rat heart and skeletal muscle by endurance training and testosterone treatment, *Pflügers Arch.*, 421 (*European Journal of Physiology*), 274, 1992.

69. Jansson, G. M. E., Degenaar, P. P., Menheere, C. A., Habets, H. M. L., and Geurten, P., Plasma urea, creatinine, uric acid, albumin, and total protein concentrations before and after 15-, 25-, and 42-km contests, *Int. J. Sports Med.*, S132, 1989.

70. Gauthier, J. M., Thériault, R., Thériault, G., Gélinas, Y., and Simoneau, J.-A., Electrical stimulation-induced changes in skeletal muscle enzymes of men and women, *Med. Sci. Sports Exerc.*, 24, 1252, 1992.

71. Green, H. J., Fraser, I. G., and Ranney, D. A., Male and female differences in enzyme activities of energy metabolism in vastus lateralis muscle, *J. Neurol. Sci.*, 65, 323, 1984.

72. Simoneau, J.-A. and Bouchard, C., Human variation in skeletal muscle fiber-type proportion and enzyme activities, *Am. J. Physiol.*, 257 (*Endocrinol. Metab.*20), E567, 1989.

73. Friedmann, B. and Kindermann, W., Energy metabolism and regulatory hormones in women and men during endurance exercise, *Eur. J. Appl. Physiol.*, 59, 1, 1989.

74. Mendenhall, L.A., Sial, S., Coggan, A.R., and Klein, S., Gender differences in substrate metabolism during moderate intensity cycling, *Med. Sci. Sport. Exerc.*, 27, S213, 1995.

75. Ruby, B. C., Robergs, R. A., Waters, D. L., Bruge, M., Mermier, C., and Stolarczyk, L., Effects of estradiol on substrate turnover during exercise in amenorrheic females, *Med. Sci. Sports Exerc.*, 29, 1160, 1997.

76. Tarnopolsky, M. A., Ettinger, S., MacDonald, J. R., Roy, B. D., and MacKenzie, S., 17-β stradiol (E_2) does not affect muscle metabolism in males, *Med. Sci. Sports Exerc.*, 29(5):S93, 1997.

77. Walker, J. L., Heigenhauser, G. J. F., Huttman, E., and Spriet, L. L., Dietary carbohydrate muscle glycogen content and endurance performance in well-trained female athletes, *Physiologist*, 39:A10, 1996.

78. Tarnopolsky, M. A., Bosman, M., MacDonald, J. R., Vandeputte, D., Martin, J., and Roy, B.D., Post-exercise protein-carbohydrate and carbohydrate supplements increase muscle glycogen in men and women, *J. Appl. Physiol.*, 83: 1877, 1997.

79. Tarnopolsky, L. J., MacDougall, J. D., Atkinson, S. A., Tarnopolsky, M. A., and Sutton, J. R., Gender differences in substrate or endurance exercise, *J. Appl. Physiol.*, 68, 302, 1990.

80. Phillips, S. M., Atkinson, S. A., Tarnopolsky, M. A., and MacDougall, J. D., Gender differences in leucine kinetics and nitrogen balance in endurance athletes, *J. Appl. Physiol.*, 75(5), 2134, 1993.

81. Janssen, G. M. E., Degenaar, C. P., Menheerre, P. P. C. A., Habets, H. M. L., and Geurten, P., Plasma urea, creatinine, uric acid, albumin, and total protein concentrations before and after 15, 25, and 42 km contests, *Int. J. Sports Med.*, 10:S132, 1989.

82. Lariviere, F., Moussalli, R., and Garrel, D. R., Increased leucine flux and leucine oxidation during the luteal phase of the menstrual cycle in women, *Am. J. Phys.*, 267, E422, 1994.

83. Speechly, D. P., Taylor, S. R., and Rogers, G. G., Differences in ultra-endurance exercise in performance-matched male and female runners, *Med. Sci. Sports Exerc.*, 28, 359, 1996.

84. Bam, J., Noakes, T. D., Juritz, J., and Dennis, S. C., Could women outrun men in ultramarathon races? *Med. Sci. Sports Exerc.*, 29, 244, 1997.

CHAPTER 13

Nutritional Implications of Age Differences in Energy Metabolism

Nancy M. Lewis and Jean E. Guest

CONTENTS

0-8493-0755-4/00/$0.00+$.50
© 2000 by CRC Press LLC

13.1 INTRODUCTION

The human body hosts a dynamic physiologic process that begins with birth and ends with death. The time that encompasses these two events provides information and insight into the individual nature of this experience. Distinct time frames and their associated physiologic changes have been used to define the different stages of life. These definitions may vary, but the age associated physiologic changes that occur with each stage do not. Infancy, childhood, adolescence, and adulthood (young, middle, older, oldest) are commonly assigned definitions. This chapter explores the effects of adequate nutrition and physical exercise on body composition and energy metabolism across the life span.

13.2 BODY COMPOSITION

Changes in body composition are associated with aging. Decreases in basal metabolic rate (BMR) and physical activity with advancing age are presumed to be primarily responsible. Historically, changes in body composition have been accepted as natural and inevitable consequences of the aging process. A review of current literature supports a more modern view that body composition changes are not entirely inevitable, and they can be influenced in a positive manner with appropriate nutritional intake and physical activity. The fountain of youth does not exist, but a proactive approach to aging may delay or reverse changes that previously resulted in disability, and loss of independence.

13.2.1 Energy Expenditure By Age

Daily energy expenditure (EE) declines progressively throughout life. Energy requirements per body surface area are greatest at birth, remain high throughout the growth phases of infancy, childhood, and adolescence, then progressively diminish during adulthood. Each stage of life presents unique effects, and therefore requirements, on body composition and metabolism. EE in adults is determined by BMR, physical activity, and diet induced thermogenesis (DIT). These same factors apply to the pediatric population, but with one additional consideration: energy required for growth, which significantly increases EE.

The ideal method for determining BMR is direct or indirect calorimetry, which provides actual measured values.[1,2] However, these methods are not available in all settings. Where this is the case, the common method used to predict BMR in healthy individuals are prediction equations such as Harris-Benedict,[3] World Health Organization, Food and Agriculture Organization, United Nations University,[4] and Schofield.[5]

Firouzbakhsh et al.[6] assessed the reliability of prediction equations[3-5] for resting energy expenditure (REE) in the pediatric population. Indirect calorimetry measurements were performed on 92 males and 107 females ranging in age from 5 to 16 years. The prediction equations and indirect calorimetry measurements were compared. Their results indicated that the Schofield[5] and WHO/FAO/UNU[4] equations were reliable estimators of REE. However, these authors pointed out that the prediction equations include the erroneous assumption that the relationship between body composition and height and weight remain constant. They also suggested that Tanner[7] developmental stages should be considered when the equations are used for adolescents. Figure 13.1 provides selected characteristics associated with Tanner stages of sexual development.

Wong et al.[8] reported similar conclusions from their evaluation of ten prediction equations in 76 Caucasian and 42 African-American females aged 8 to 17 years. Nine out of ten prediction equations overestimated BMR by 60 ± 46 kcal per day (range 15 to 176 kcal per day). In six of the equations that controlled for age, weight, height, and sexual maturity, the overestimation was

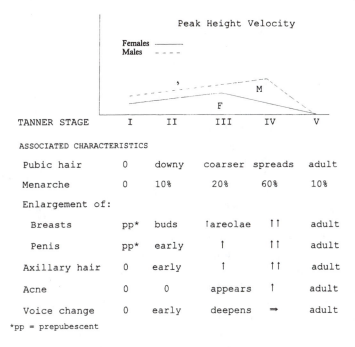

Figure 13.1 Characteristics associated with Tanner stages of sexual development.

significantly greater ($p < 0.05$) for African-Americans (77 ± 17 kcal per day) than Caucasians (25 ± 17 kcal per day). These authors suggest that ethnicity should also be considered.

A technique for determining EE in free living populations is the doubly labeled water method, which became available for use in adults in 1984.[9] This method utilizes water labeled with stable isotopes from both deuterium (^2H) and oxygen (^{18}O). EE is determined by calculating the difference in disappearance rates of the two isotopes after oral administration. Roberts and Young[10] validated the doubly-labeled water method in preterm infants in 1988, and Jones et al.[11] validated it in infants following abdominal surgery in 1987. However, Fomon[12] suggests several points to consider when this method is used in full-term healthy infants. First, the respiratory quotient (RQ) is more variable in infants, which allows for more error than in older individuals. Second, the physical exchange process of labeled and unlabeled molecules is unequal between pulmonary capillary blood and water vapor in the alveoli and through the skin. This is due to the differences in mass between hydrogen, deuterium, and ^{16}O and ^{18}O. Third, the possible sequestration of isotopes in body tissues may be interpreted as isotope loss due to the high fat (40% of energy) diet consumed by infants.

13.2.1.1 Pediatric

The focus of body composition and EE measurements in the pediatric population is assessment of normal growth as characterized by standardized growth charts.[13] Anthropometric data (height, weight, and head circumference in children ≤ 36 months of age) obtained by health maintenance providers are tracked over time. Adequacy of nutritional intake is judged by maintenance of normal growth patterns.[14] Aberrations in growth patterns indicate alterations in energy balance resulting in abnormal growth, but just as in the adult population the etiology may not be easily determined.

The relationship between total energy expenditure (TEE) and body composition in infants is complex. Energy requirements in the pediatric population have been based on the laws of thermodynamics where energy intake equals energy expended, plus energy stored. The ability to measure

EE in the pediatric population has been technically difficult. The doubly labeled water method allows for measurement of infants and children in free living conditions.

Wells et al.[15] investigated the relationship between body composition and EE using doubly labeled water in 92 full-term healthy infants aged 12 weeks. The difference between body weight and fat free mass (FFM) was used to calculate fat mass (FM). Age, gender, FFM, and total EE were entered into a multiple regression equation, with FM used as the dependent variable. Their results demonstrated that age was the only significant predictor of FM. These same researchers[16] further investigated the role of activity and EE in 34 full-term healthy infants aged 9 months and 12 months. They employed the same methodology as in their previous study,[15] with the addition of a behavioral activity diary (time spent feeding and time spent upset). Behavioral activity was used as an independent variable in the multiple regression analysis. Their results demonstrated no significant differences between the 9- and 12-month-old groups in body composition, total EE per kilogram of body weight, or behavioral measurements. Variance in TEE was explained by FFM (19.7%), body weight (18.7%), and behavioral activity (26.4%). Behavioral activity was inversely and significantly related to total EE. These authors concluded that behavioral activity should be considered along with body size to predict energy requirements in this age group.

Butte et al.[17] took another approach in their investigation into how age and body composition affect energy requirements, sedentary energy expenditure (SEE), and BMR. They examined 210 healthy participants, which included 101 infants (50 males and 51 females aged 3 months to 18 months), 82 females aged 9 to 16 years, and 27 adults (6 males and 21 females aged 20 to 46 years). EE, SEE, and BMR measurements were collected in a respiratory chamber for the children and adults while the infants were measured by indirect calorimetry (hood only or whole body chamber) and the doubly labeled water method. Statistical methods used to analyze the data were a linear regression without log transformation to determine the best model relating BMR and SEE to weight or FFM, multiple regression for independent effects, and t-test of homogeneity for differences between slopes. Their results indicate that SEE and BMR per unit of body size (kg) increased during infancy, declined in childhood, and leveled off in adulthood. These authors concluded that energy requirements from infancy to adulthood appear to be a power, not a linear, function of body weight and composition.

Goran et al.[18] investigated the physiologic determinants of REE in 113 healthy children aged 3.9 to 7.8 years. Measurements of body height, weight, skin-fold thicknesses, heart rate, physical activity (by questionnaire), REE (by indirect calorimetry), and FM and FFM (by bioelectrical impedance) were collected in 60 females (39 Caucasian and 21 Mohawk Indian) and 53 males (41 Caucasian and 12 Mohawk Indian). Regional body fat distribution was assessed by waist/hip ratio and skin-fold thicknesses expressed as a ratio of trunk skin folds (axilla, chest, and abdomen) to extremity skin folds (triceps, calf, and thigh). After statistical analysis, their results demonstrated a mean REE of 1054 ± 134 kcal per day (range 830 to 1480 kcal per day) with absolute REE in males being significantly higher than in females (1093 ± 138 kcal per day versus 1019 ± 121 kcal per day respectively, $p = 0.003$). Even after adjusting for FFM (which significantly correlated with REE), the REE in the males remained significantly higher than in the females (1071 ± 94 kcal per day versus 1039 ± 76 kcal per day, respectively, $p = 0.05$). FFM, gender, and FM were significant independent determinants of REE. Age, ethnicity, fat distribution, heart rate, and physical activity were not. These authors concluded that the same determinants (FFM, FM, and gender) that affect REE in adults are similar in children. They further concluded that just as REE is higher in adult males than adult females, the same is true in children.

Goran et al.[19] examined the relationship between FM, EE, and recreational activity in young children. Measurements for TEE by doubly labeled water method, FM and FFM by bioelectric resistance and skinfolds, and REE by indirect calorimetry were obtained in 101 children with a mean age of 5.3 ± 0.9 years. One year later, 68 of the children were re-examined when their mean age was 6.3 ± 0.9 years. Results of their study indicate that approximately 10% of the variance in FM in children was due to time devoted to recreational physical activity. Davies et al.[20] performed a similar study in 77 children aged 1.5 to 4.5 years. Their results demonstrate a significant association between high levels of body FM and low levels of physical activity. Maintaining appropriate weight for height during childhood and adolescence is important because they are associated with body composition in adulthood.[21]

Females — Rapid changes in EE and body composition are most dramatic during infancy and adolescence. Growth spurts result in increased EE with a concurrent increase in energy intake. The effect of gender is most noticeable during adolescence when the expression of these changes in EE and body composition results in an increased prevalence of obesity in females.[22] Goran et al.[23] examined 22 prepubertal children (11 males and 11 females) beginning at a mean age of 5.4 ± 0.9 years. Measurements for TEE, REE, physical activity-related EE, reported physical activity, FM, and FFM were obtained three times over a five-year period. Males and females demonstrated similar increases in body weight, FM, and FFM. Significant effects of time and gender in TEE were seen. Females increased EE from year 1 to year 2, but by year 5 they had a significant decrease. Reported physical activity in females remained comparable to males until there was a significant (50%) decrease observed between ages 8.5 and 9.5 years. Energy intake did not change during this period. These authors concluded that these results suggest the existence of an energy-conserving mechanism through reduced physical activity prior to puberty in females.

Body composition changes associated with puberty include increases in linear growth, body fat, and body fat percentage which begin in females between 10 and 12 years of age, and in males two years later.[24] The most significant difference in body composition change that occurs between females and males is the increase in body fat and percentage. This has been attributed to the effects of sex steroids on adipose tissue.[25] Cowell et al.[26] investigated body fat distribution patterns by utilizing anthropometric measurements (height, weight, and body mass index [BMI]) and dual energy X-ray absorptometry (DXA). These researchers examined 336 healthy children, adolescents, and young adults (169 males and 166 females) who had a mean age of 15.5 years (range 4 to 35 years). Their results demonstrated gender and age differences in total body fat, body fat percentage, and distribution pattern. Females after age 15 had a greater total body fat and body fat percentage (20% to 40%) than males ($\leq 20\%$). The distribution of this body fat was also significantly different between genders.

Expressing their data as trunk to leg fat ratio (the percentage of fat in the trunk divided by the percentage of fat in the leg) these researchers observed a steady linear increase with age in males, but not in females. Males younger than 13 had a significantly smaller trunk to leg fat ratio than females of the same age (mean 0.668 vs. 0.763, respectively, p = 0.004). However, after age 15, the trunk to leg fat ratio was significantly higher in males of all ages than in females (0.997 vs. 0.867, respectively, p = 0.0005).

Males — The report by Cowell et al.[26] discussed in the previous section suggests that changes in body fat distribution in males are temporally associated with puberty. Although body fat percentage does not increase significantly and consistently remains lower than that in females, the distribution pattern was that of accumulation in the trunk region rather than the lower limbs. Furthermore, the trunk to leg fat ratio was found to be independent of BMI expressed as a standard deviation score (used as a measurement of obesity) in males, whereas there was a weak association observed in females. These authors concluded that the tendency toward truncal fat accumulation in males was independent of adipose tissue mass, whereas in females it was associated.

13.2.1.2 Adult

In 1966, McGandy et al.[27] reported a statistically significant decline in mean total daily caloric intakes, BMR, and EE in males from ages 20 to 99 years. The age-dependent decrease in caloric intake was accounted for by decrements in BMR and EE required for physical activity. FFM or lean body mass (LBM) decreases approximately 15% between the third and eighth decade of life, contributing to a lower BMR in the elderly. Forbes and Reina[28] in 1970 reported an average loss of 12 kg of LBM in males, and 5 kg in females from age 25 to 70 years. Preservation of FFM and prevention of age-related skeletal muscle loss (sarcopenia) may help prevent the decrease in BMR that occurs with aging.

In addition to its role in energy metabolism, the age-related decline in skeletal muscle may be associated with reductions in bone density, insulin sensitivity, and aerobic capacity. For these reasons, strategies for preserving muscle mass and strength in aging individuals may be an important way to maintain functional independence and decrease the prevalence of many age-associated chronic diseases.

A study to assess FFM by use of total body potassium (TBK) was reported by Novak[29] in 1972. He assessed the body composition of more than 500 males and females between the ages of 18 and 85. His results demonstrated that body fat increased from 17.8% to 36.2% in men, and from 33% to 44.8% in women. Concomitantly, fat free and cellular mass decreased from 82.2% to 63.8% in aging males, and from 67% to 55.2% in aging females. More recently, Flynn et al.[30] in 1989 reported in an 18-year longitudinal study that the most rapid rate of TBK loss occurs between 41 and 60 years of age in males, and after age 60 in females.

Employing another technique, total body neutron activation, Cohn et al.[31] determined that FFM declined with muscle mass (MM) decrease, but with little change in less metabolically active FFM (i.e., cartilage, fibrous tissue, and skeletal tissue). This TBK drop was closely associated with a decline in total body calcium, suggesting a link between sarcopenia and osteopenia.

Loss in MM, particularly skeletal muscle, contributes to a loss of strength. Frontera et al.[32] examined muscle strength, age, and body composition in 200 healthy males and females 45 to 78 years of age. Muscle strength of the elbow and knee extensors and flexors was measured by an isokinetic dynamometer. FFM was estimated by hydrostatic weighing, and MM was determined by urinary creatinine excretion. FFM and MM were significantly lower in the older (mean age 65.5 years) than in the younger (mean age 49.2) males and females. The females had 42.2% to 62.8% of the absolute strength of the males. However, when strength was expressed per kilogram of MM, the gender differences diminished or disappeared. These researchers concluded that MM, not function or location, was responsible for age- and sex-related strength differences. Loss of muscle strength with advancing age may be the major determinant of functional disabilities in older individuals.

Alterations in body composition with aging[29] are not limited to FFM and MM. Body fat distribution also changes. Body fat, especially in the central regions of the body is associated with an increased risk for other health disorders, including atherosclerosis, hypertension, and type 2 (also known as Type II) diabetes, that occur with increasing frequency with aging.[33]

Kohrt et al.[34] reported on body composition in 74 young and 200 older sedentary males and females, and 59 young and 44 older endurance trained males and females with an age range of 18 to 72 years. Skinfold thicknesses were two to six-fold greater in upper, central body sites in both younger and older sedentary males and females than in their trained younger and older counterparts. Skinfold thicknesses at all sites (triceps, thigh, subscapula, pectoralis, umbilicus, suprailiac) were approximately 24% larger for the older than younger trained males, and 47% larger for the older than younger trained females. These authors suggested that people who exercise regularly appear to accumulate less adipose tissue in upper and central body regions as they get older and therefore reduce the risk for metabolic disorders associated with upper body obesity. Recognizing the need to maintain FFM and skeletal muscle strength while avoiding accumulation of central body fat throughout the aging process may lead to a stronger, healthier population.

Decreased caloric need is associated with a declining metabolic rate and activity level. The decline in energy needs with aging is the main factor associated with increased body fatness.[84] Tzankoff and Norris[35] reported that 24-hour creatinine excretion (an index of metabolically active, creatinine-producing skeletal muscle) was closely related to BMR at all ages in males.

Pannemans and Westerterp[36] reported on TEE and physical activity level in 26 males and females with a mean age of 69.5 years, and 29 males and females with a mean age of 28.8 years who were fed two isoenergetic diets for three weeks each in a cross-over design. The two diets provided 12% and 42%, or 21% and 33% of total energy intake from protein and fat, respectively. TEE was measured with the doubly labeled water technique. Gross energy intake or metabolizable energy (ME) was calculated by subtracting the energy content of the feces and urine from the energy content of the food consumed. Energy balance was then calculated by subtracting ME from TEE. BMR was calculated by an open-circuit, ventilated hood system. Physical activity was calculated as a physical activity index (PAI), where TEE was divided by BMR. The PAI for older males and females was a mean of 1.52 ± 0.20 and 1.66 ± 0.20 respectively, and 1.66 ± 0.15 and 1.67 ± 0.20 for younger males and females, respectively. When males and females were combined, the mean BMR values for the older and younger groups were 6.38 ± 0.56 MJ/d and 7.43 ± 0.95 MJ/d, respectively. Multiple regression analysis revealed that PAI and FFM combined explained 86% of the variance in BMR in older and younger males, and 80% in older and younger females. Maintaining FFM by balancing energy intake and output (with individualized physical activity and calorie intake) may significantly impact the decrease in BMR that occurs with aging. Other researchers have suggested that the remaining variance of 10%–15% is due to the thermic effect of feeding (TEF).[1]

Jette and Branch[37] surveyed 2654 males and females as part of the Framingham study. They reported 40% of females aged 55 to 64, approximately 45% aged 65 to 74, and 65% aged 75 to 84 years responded that they were unable to lift 4.5 kg (approximately 10 lb), and they experienced an inability to do heavy household work. Bassey et al.[38] reported a significant inverse relationship between isometric muscle strength of the plantar flexor of the foot and age, and a lower isometric strength in older females than in males. Declining muscle strength and functional ability with age is a public health concern as more individuals live longer.

Aerobically trained young females have a higher resting metabolic rate (RMR) than their sedentary counterparts.[39] Ryan and co-workers[40] conducted a study in 43 highly trained female athletes and 14 sedentary females aged 18 to 69 to assess body composition and EE. They report that although maximal oxygen consumption ($\dot{V}O_{2\,max}$) declined with age, athletes at all ages had a significantly higher $\dot{V}O_{2\,max}$ than nonathletes. Body weight and BMI did not differ among the younger and older athletes and young nonathletes, but older nonathletes had higher body weights and BMIs. There were no differences in FFM and percentage of body fat between the younger and older athletes. Despite comparable body fat (percent and weight in kilograms) in younger and older athletes, an increase in intra-abdominal adipose tissue (IAAT) was seen in older athletes. However, subcutaneous abdominal fat and sagittal diameter did not increase in the older athletes.

The Ryan et al. study[40] demonstrated that FFM as characterized by DXA and computed tomography (CT) can be maintained in older athletes. However, FFM is lower, while percentage of body fat, IAAT, and subcutaneous abdominal fat are higher in nonathletes than athletes regardless of age. RMR exhibited a significant cross-sectional decline from youngest to oldest athletes. RMR was similar among older athletes and nonathletes, while younger athletes had a significantly higher RMR than younger nonathletes. These authors concluded that intense chronic exercise in women athletes prevents FFM from declining with age. Older athletes have higher IAAT levels, even though their body fat levels were similar to younger athletes. Despite preservation of FFM in older athletes, RMR declines in women athletes with aging. Researchers are searching for an explanation for the drop in RMR with aging in the presence of maintenance of FFM. RMR can be influenced by menopausal status[41] and decline in $\dot{V}O_{2\,max}$[42] after age 50, which may explain the decreased RMR seen in the Ryan et al. study.[40]

RMR decreases in males approximately 1–2% per decade as men age from 20 to 75 years.[43] However, Poehlman et al.[44] in 1990 demonstrated that RMR was approximately 6% higher in physically active older men when compared to untrained older men. A similar effect was seen in a study conducted by Horber et al.[45] In this study, 42 healthy men were divided into three groups that ranged in age from 29–69 years. The first group consisted of young (31 ± 2.1 years) untrained men (no training in five years), the second group consisted of older (68.6 ± 1.2 years) untrained men (no training in five years), and the third group consisted of older (67.4 ± 1.2 years) trained men (joggers who participated in the Grand Prix of Berne had jogged at least 30 km per week for three years). Although RMR per kilogram of LBM decreased with increasing age, older trained men had RMR rates similar to young untrained men. Older untrained men had lower RMR rates than young untrained men. The attenuated decrease in RMR in older trained males in this study was positively correlated to plasma insulin-like growth factor-I (IGF-I). The effect of hormone alterations with aging may be influenced by regular physical training in males.

13.2.2 Hormone Supplementation

Growth hormone (GH) is a 190 amino acid protein that is synthesized and secreted by the anterior pituitary gland. One of its functions is to regulate skeletal and protein anabolism.[46] The role GH plays in body composition and energy metabolism varies throughout the life cycle. Circulating GH hormone levels increase during childhood and adolescence and decrease during adulthood. However, exercise can cause serum GH to rise at any age.[47]

13.2.2.1 Pediatric

GH deficiency (GHD) in children results in stunted linear growth, poor nitrogen retention, and increased fat mobilization and oxidation.[48,49] The primary focus of GH replacement treatment in GH-deficient children is restoration of normal growth and development.[50] The effect of GH replacement therapy (GHRT) on body composition, REE, and TEF was studied by Vaisman et al.[51] They examined ten prepubertal males with subnormal spontaneous GH secretion ages 6.2 to 9.5 years. Anthropometric data (heights, weights, and four-site subcutaneous skinfolds), TBK (by ^{40}K emission measurement), REE and TEF (by open-circuit indirect calorimetry), and seven-day food records (recorded prior to each study period) were collected before beginning daily injections of recombinant GH (0.2 IU/kg./d), and at two, four, and six months during the treatment period. Significant treatment effects were seen in height, weight, REE, TEF, TBK, percentage of body fat, and protein sparing (indirect calorimetry). However, after correcting for expected changes in body composition over time, their results demonstrated continued increases in height and weight, with a significant decrease in percentage of body fat. But by six months, all of the other effects plateaued or returned to pretreatment levels. Calorie and protein intakes increased during the treatment period but did not reach statistical significance. These authors concluded that significant body composition changes occurred and persisted with GHRT, but the energy metabolism changes were transient.

13.2.2.2 Adult

In addition to the decline in skeletal MM and strength with aging, another consequence of aging is decreased hormone levels. Therefore, in recent years replacement therapy for estrogen in females, and for GH in males has been investigated.

Females — Estrogen replacement therapy (ERT) for females is associated with increased risk for cancers such as uterine or breast.[52] These associated risk factors limit the population that may benefit from this therapy. The possibility that GH may positively affect whole body protein turnover, and therefore LBM, suggests a role for this anabolic hormone, which might prove to be a viable alternative to ERT in females for preventing sarcopenia.

Thompson et al.[53] studied the effect of recombinant human growth hormone (rhGH), and recombinant human insulin-like growth factor I (rhIGF-I) on body composition in 16 healthy females with a mean age of 71.9 ± 1.3 years. All study participants were within 20% of their ideal body weight, received a standardized diet designed for weight maintenance with a protein intake of $0.9 \text{ g} \cdot \text{kg body wt}^{-1} \cdot \text{day}^{-1}$, and were randomly assigned to one of three groups receiving rhGH (0.025 mg/kg) daily or rhIGF-I as either low-dose (0.015 mg/kg) or high-dose (0.06 mg/kg) twice per day, which were self-administered by subcutaneous injections over four weeks. Body composition by DXA and nitrogen balance were measured at baseline and at four weeks. Significant results included a decrease in FM in all groups and an increase in nitrogen retention and LBM in the rhGH and high-dose rhIGF-I groups. However, the high-dose rhIGF-I and rhGH groups experienced side effects, including headaches, lethargy, joint swelling/pain, and bloating. The low-dose rhIGF-I group did not experience these side effects.

Butterfield et al.[54] investigated the effect of rhGH and rhIGF-I on protein utilization in 14 healthy females aged 66 to 82 years. Four of the women were also receiving ERT. All participants were within 20% of their ideal body weight, received a diet with a mean caloric intake of 1904 ± 170 kcals per day with a protein intake of $0.9 \text{ g} \cdot \text{kg body wt}^{-1} \cdot \text{day}^{-1}$. They were randomly assigned to one of four treatment groups to receive self-administered subcutaneous injections of 0.025 mg rhGh/kg once daily or low (0.015 mg/kg), medium (0.03 mg/kg), and high (0.06 mg/kg) doses of rhIGF-I twice daily. Nitrogen balance, muscle protein synthesis, and whole body protein turnover were determined after a four-week treatment period. Their results indicate a significant increase in nitrogen balance in all treatment groups at week 1, but this decreased by 50% in the rhGH group at week 4. Protein synthesis and breakdown increased significantly in the rhGH group by 9% and 8%, respectively, low-dose rhIGF-I group by 4.5% and 4%, and high-dose group by 18% and 17%. Net protein synthesis increased significantly with rhGH (48%), mid-dose rhIGF-I (196%), and high-dose rhIGF-I (27%). Muscle protein synthesis increased significantly with rhGH (50%), mid-dose rhIGF-I (67%), and high-dose rhIGF-I (57%). These positive results indicate the ability of older females to respond to growth factor stimulation during short-term treatment.

Males — GH acts directly or indirectly by producing IGF-1 on a range of target tissues. GH injections have been shown to increase LBM and decrease percentage of body fat in healthy older men.[55] Reductions in total body and intra-abdominal fat, total and low-density lipoprotein cholesterol, and an increase in high-density lipoprotein cholesterol have been demonstrated in treated younger adults with GHD.[56] The beneficial effect on serum lipids seen in younger men has not been observed in older men.[57]

Poehlman and Copeland[58] studied IGF-I in 42 younger men aged 18 to 36 years and 26 older men aged 59 to 76 years. They reported that IGF-I was 33% lower in older men than in younger men, and it was inversely related to the percentage of body fat and indices of upper body fat distribution. IGF-I was positively related to $\dot{V}O_{2 \text{ max}}$ and leisure time physical activity, but it was not related to fat free weight or daily caloric intake. However, reductions in IGF-I levels have been associated with decreased caloric intakes by other researchers.[59,60] Additionally, macronutrient composition of the diet, especially protein, can impact the plasma concentration of IGF-I.[60,61]

The main benefit of GHRT in older men is increased tissue level effect (IGF-I axis), resulting in greater aerobic capacity for higher muscle function and thus greater strength. Vittone et al.[57] reported increased muscle strength after six weeks of treatment with single nightly injections of growth hormone-releasing hormone 1-29 (GHRH 1-29) in men aged 64 to 76 years. These researchers suggest that GHRH 1-29 alters baseline relationships between muscle strength and muscle bioenergetics consistent with a reduced need for anaerobic metabolism during exercise. Cuneo et al.[62] reported a 17% increase in $\dot{V}O_{2 \text{ max}}$ during a six-month, double-blind, placebo-controlled study in 18- to 55-year-old GH-deficient males treated with rhGH. These researchers suggest that the mechanisms for improvements in $\dot{V}O_{2 \text{ max}}$ and anaerobic threshold include increased LBM and MM, O_2 delivery, substrate flux, or a combination of these factors. In an earlier study, Cuneo et al.[63] reported increased LBM and skeletal muscle mass in these same subjects with rhGH treatment.

Younger GH-deficient adult males experience the same manifestations in body composition as the elderly in terms of decreased LBM, skeletal muscle mass, strength, $\dot{V}O_{2 \text{ max}}$, and an increase in body fat.[62] The implications of these studies on the daily functioning of aging individuals is to suggest that maintaining normal GH and IGF-I levels may attenuate some of the effects of aging on body composition, muscle strength, and performance of daily activities.

The importance of adequate caloric and nutrient intakes must also be stressed if the full potential of such treatment is to be realized. The use of human GH, rhGH, GHRH 1-29, or growth hormone-releasing hormone 1-44, as well as the optimal dosage(s) continues to be studied. Further research, including placebo-controlled trials, is needed to determine the optimal treatment for GHRT in males.

GHRT in males has not been shown to have any discernible adverse effects.[57] There have been reports of hyperglycemia associated with the administration of GH by some,[55,64] but not all,[65] researchers. However, this side effect appears to be dose-related.[64] A more recent report suggested a link between high levels of IGF-I and prostate cancer in males.[66]

13.3 ENERGY BALANCE

Daily EE and daily calorie intake determine energy balance in humans. EE is most accurately determined over a period of 24 hours or longer. The gold standard for this measurement is the use of a respiratory chamber in which indirect calorimetry, spontaneous physical activity, and TEF can be measured. This information can be combined with body composition (estimated by underwater weighing) to determine FFM.[1] However, because of their cost and size, respiratory chambers are usually accessible only to researchers located at major research centers. The practical need to accurately assess energy expenditure in free living individuals has led many researchers to the combined use of a doubly labeled water technique and indirect calorimetry to determine TEE and REE.[2]

13.3.1   Age Differences

Changes in body composition and functioning seen with time are attributed primarily to the aging process. Body composition and energy balance have a simple relationship. FM and FFM have a desirable ratio when energy intake and expenditure are balanced, and they have an undesirable ratio when they are not. Energy imbalance results in overnutrition (obesity) or undernutrition (wasting), which can be seen at any stage of life.

13.3.1.1 Pediatric

Healthy infants and toddlers do not selectively become under- or over-nourished. Body composition is determined by family history, feeding mode, and activity level.[67] Caregivers' actions influence energy balance more strongly in this age group than in healthy older children and adolescents. However, as toddlers grow into childhood and adolescence, the focus of current literature on energy balance is in the area of obesity prevention and treatment.

Goran et al.[68] investigated factors that contribute to total EE in 30 healthy children (16 males and 14 females) aged 4 to 6 years. Measurements for height, weight, heart rate, REE from indirect calorimetry, body composition by bioelectric impedance, and TEE over 14 days under free living conditions with the doubly labeled water method were collected. Activity EE was estimated from the difference between TEE and REE. REE in this study also included energy costs for DIT and spontaneous physical movement. FFM was calculated from bioelectric impedance data, and FM was derived from the differences between body weight and FFM. Their results demonstrate a significantly higher body fat percentage in females, TEE was approximately 25% lower than current recommendations for energy intake in 4- to 6-year-old children, and activity-related EE was estimated to be 17% ± 11% of total daily EE.

13.3.1.2 Adult

Roberts et al.[2] reported that BMR and physical activity accounted for 73% of the individual variation in TEE in young and old sedentary men. Meredith et al.[69] studied endurance-trained males between 20 and 60 years of age who consumed very high-calorie diets. They reported that the number of hours per week spent exercising and body fat levels were closely related regardless of age. The relationship between body composition, dietary intake, and physical activity appears to be maintained across the age continuum.

13.3.2 Gender and Age

Several researchers have studied the impact of gender and age on body composition, RMR, and EE. The reported studies provide mixed results.[70–72] Arciero et al.[73] studied 328 males and 194 females aged 17 to 81 years. Their purpose was to examine gender differences in RMR in healthy males and females spanning a broad range of age, body mass, and aerobic fitness levels. They reported that females have a 3% lower RMR than males. The lower RMR persisted in females after age comparison (premenopausal or postmenopausal) with men of similar ages. These researchers concluded that RMR is lower in females than males of similar age, but it is independent of differences in body composition and aerobic fitness.

Klausen et al.[74] examined 235 females and 78 males aged 15 to 64 years for gender and age effects on 24-hour EE, BMR, and SEE. They reported no significant difference in EE or BMR by gender. However, when adjustments for differences in body composition and activity level between younger men and women (20 to 29 years) and older men and women (50 to 65 years) were compared, there was a significantly lower BMR (4.6%) in the older group.

Vaughn et al.[75] studied 24-hour EE by use of a respiratory chamber. Their study included 17 males and 21 females aged 60 to 85 and 33 males and 31 females aged 18 to 30 years. They report a significantly lower (5%) BMR in older males and females than the younger males and females after adjusting for differences in body composition (FFM, fat mass) and gender.

Some authors[73,74] have offered observations regarding the various differences in results reported in the literature on BMR, gender, and age. Two areas suggested for consideration are sample size and methods for measuring of EE. The use of small sample sizes in some of the reported studies may have not been powerful enough to pick up small, but significant, differences (Type II error). The methods to measure EE vary from indirect methods that employ prediction equations to direct methods[1,2] where accuracy and technique may be confounding factors.

13.3.3 Ethnicity and Age

The Pima Indians of Arizona are a population prone to obesity and diabetes. As such, they have been the subject of numerous studies in these areas.[76,77] Rising et al.[78] collected longitudinal data from seven nondiabetic male Pima Indians at baseline and after seven years, and cross-sectional data from 131 Pima males. Results indicate an inverse correlation between BMR and age ($r = -0.21$, $p < 0.02$), while percentage of body fat was positively correlated with age ($r = 0.17$, $p < 0.05$). These results suggest an inherent risk factor for obesity such as a low BMR. If so, is it seen in the younger members of the population?

Fontvieille et al.[79] addressed this question in their study comparing Pima Indian children to Caucasian children. Body composition by bioelectric resistance and RMR by indirect calorimetry were measured in 43 Pima Indian children (22 males and 21 females with a mean age of 9.9 ± 1.1 years) and 42 Caucasian children (21 males and 21 females with a mean age of 9.7 ± 1.2 years). The Pima Indian children were taller, heavier and fatter and had a higher absolute RMR value than the Caucasian children. However, when differences in gender, body size, and composition were adjusted, the RMR values were similar, indicating no actual differences. These authors speculate that excess energy intake and/or low levels of physical activity may explain the obesity seen in these Pima Indian children.

13.4 SUBSTRATE OXIDATION

The impressive acceleration of growth seen in the first year of life as well as during puberty requires appropriate metabolic function. Adequate carbohydrate and fat oxidation provides a protein-sparing effect that promotes somatic growth. Metabolic dysfunction in the pediatric population results in associated diseases that are most commonly constitutional in origin.

Age-associated diseases seen with changes in body metabolism include type 2 diabetes, coronary artery disease, hypertension, osteoporosis, and obesity.[80] An appropriate nutritional and exercise program throughout life may affect body composition and metabolic function as much as any pharmocologic intervention. The primary outcomes would be improved health and increased independence, especially in older adults.

13.4.1   Age and Gender Effect

13.4.1.1 Pediatric

Le Stunff and Bougneres[81] investigated basal EE and lipid and glucose oxidation to determine the time course of metabolic dysfunctions in early-phase childhood obesity. They studied 31 (16 males and 15 females with a mean age of 11.9 ± 0.4 years) healthy children who had been obese[1] (mean $160 \pm 4\%$ of IBW) for 1 to 11.5 years, and they compared them with 14 (7 males and 7 females with a mean age of 11.9 ± 0.7 years) healthy non-obese (mean 95% of IBW), age-matched controls. Indirect calorimetry, fasting plasma glucose and free fatty acids, plasma insulin, FM (by skin fold thicknesses), and LBM (calculated by subtracting FM from total body weight) were collected. Dietary intake was regulated for three days prior to indirect calorimetry testing. All children received age-appropriate caloric intakes with carbohydrate contributing 50% of kilocalories. Their results demonstrate that the obese children oxidized twice as much lipid (56 ± 4 mg/min) as the non-obese controls (25 ± 5 mg/min, p = 0.0005). The increased lipid oxidation in the obese children was present in the early stages of obesity. Glucose oxidation decreased in the obese (93 ± 6 mg/min) as compared to the non-obese children (136 ± 6 mg/min, p = 0.0005). The diminished glucose oxidation was not present in early-phase obesity but appeared after approximately four years and worsened with obesity duration (r = 0.72, p < 0.0005). These results remained even after normalization for body surface area or LBM. Mean basal plasma insulin levels did not differ between obese and non-obese children, although there was a statistical tendency for increasing basal plasma insulin with obesity duration (r = 0.48, p < 0.01). These authors hypothesized that increased lipid oxidation is one of the dysfunctions present in early-phase obesity, and increased lipid oxidation may induce progressive decreases in glucose oxidation, resulting in insulin resistance, and increased fasting insulin secretion.

Molnar and Schutz[82] investigated the effect of body composition, body fat distribution, and puberty on fat oxidation in obese and non-obese prepubertal and adolescent children. They examined 235 healthy non-obese children (116 males and 119 females) and 159 obese children (93 males and 66 females) who ranged in age from 9.5 to 16.5 years. Age, gender, height, weight, triceps and subscapular skin-fold thicknesses, LBM (calculated by subtracting FM from body weight), RMR (by indirect calorimetry), and Tanner[7] stage were collected. Serum samples for plasma insulin and glucose concentrations were collected in a subset of 58 non-obese children and 94 obese children, and urinary nitrogen in 152 (76 non-obese and 76 obese) children selected by Tanner[7] stage. Their results indicate post-absorptive fat oxidation (absolute value and percentage of RMR) was significantly higher in obese children (76.7 ± 23.3 gm/24 hr; $42.3\% \pm 18.7\%$) than non-obese adolescents (40.0 ± 26.3 gm/24 hr; $28.7\% \pm 17.0\%$) even after adjustments for LBM. Fat oxidation corrected for body FM was significantly lower in females (mean of 48.3 ± 28.4 gm/24 hr) than males (mean of 59.7 ± 29.0 gm/24 hr). There was a significant increase in fat oxidation during puberty; however, it was explained mainly by changes in body composition. RMR, RQ, nonprotein RQ, and immunoreactive insulin levels were significantly increased in obese versus non-obese adolescents. These authors concluded that obese adolescents have a higher fat oxidative rate than their non-obese counterparts and that this could be explained by higher EE due to their increased metabolically active body mass.

Puberty is the stage of life during which numerous physiologic and metabolic changes occur. Among them are increased secretion of GH and IGF-I[83] and increased circulating insulin concentrations.[84] In addition to these hormonal changes, a prominent metabolic change is the evolution of transient insulin resistance.[85] Arslanian and Kalhan[86] examined the role of insulin resistance in protein metabolism during puberty. Whole body leucine kinetics were compared between 20 prepubertal Tanner[7] stage I (TI), and 21 pubertal Tanner[7] stage II to IV (TII-IV) healthy children and adolescents. One week prior to data collection, all children were prescribed a weight-maintaining diet containing 55% carbohydrate, 30% fat, and 15% protein. Body composition was determined by total body water $H_2^{18}O$-dilution method. Measurements of leucine flux, oxidation, and nonoxidative disposal were collected during primed constant infusion of [1-^{13}C] leucine tracer at baseline and during a stepwise hyperinsulinemic (10 and 40 mU · m^{-2} · min^{-1}) euglycemic clamp in combination with indirect calorimetry. Plasma glucose, insulin, and IGF-I levels are also measured.

Analysis of these data demonstrated no differences in fasting plasma glucose and insulin concentrations, gender, and nonoxidative leucine disposal (protein synthesis) between the TI and TII-IV groups. There was a significant decrease in whole body leucine flux (proteolysis) and oxidation at baseline in the TII-IV group versus the TI group. Leucine flux was also significantly decreased during the clamp in the TII-IV group versus the TI group. REE correlated positively with leucine turnover (r = 0.49, p = 0.001) and leucine oxidation (r = 0.73, p = 0.0009). IGF-I correlated negatively with whole body leucine flux (r = –0.41, p = 0.0004), oxidation (r = –0.27, p = 0.04), and nonoxidative disposal (r = –0.38, p = 0.007). These authors concluded that these data demonstrate decreased proteolysis and protein oxidation while protein synthesis remains unchanged. They also concluded that insulin action in inhibiting proteolysis was decreased and that increased IGF-I levels may contribute to decreased protein degradation during puberty when compared to prepuberty in children.

13.4.1.2 Adult

The assumption that aging causes a decline in substrate utilization concomitant to other metabolic alterations[87] and that substrate utilization may be positively affected by exercise[88] appears to have validity. Elderly individuals appear to exhibit a reduced capacity to oxidize stored lipid in response to short-term fasting and catecholamine stimulation.[87,88] The blunted lipolytic response to catacholamines seen in human fat cells with aging is due to decreased activation of hormone sensitive lipase.[87] Kohrt et al.[89] reported a blunted response to catacholamines in elderly persons perfoming exercise at the same relative intensity as young persons. The alteration in lipolytic response to exercise may affect fuel use and consequently carbohydrate and fat oxidation.[88,90]

Poehlman and co-workers[91] studied 18 healthy older males and females ranging in age from 65 to 67 years and demonstrated that endurance training increased fat oxidation. Norepinephrine appearance (NEapp) and FFM also increased. The increased NEapp in response to expected changes in body composition due to training explained 50% of the increase in fatty acid oxidation, while the increase in FFM explained 15%. The mechanism for regulating fat oxidation in older individuals appears to be influenced by Neapp (higher levels of beta-adrenergic stimulation), and FFM (shifting disposal of fatty acids from nonoxidative to oxidative pathways).

The relationship between decreased basal fat oxidation and aging may be due to a loss of FFM rather than age per se. Calles-Escandon and co-workers[92] studied 32 females aged 18 to 73 years and reported a negative correlation between age and fat oxidation, but they also reported a positive correlation between FFM and fat oxidation. Similar results were reported by Sial et al.[93] from a study in six older and six younger males and females during 60 minutes of moderate-intensity cycle ergometer exercise. Participants were matched for gender and LBM, and results were measured during exercise performed at the same absolute intensity in the older and younger males and females. The older group increased carbohydrate utilization by 35% while decreasing fat utilization by 25% to 35% when compared with the younger group. These authors attribute the shift in substrate utilization to a decrease in skeletal muscle in the older group.

13.4.2   Ethnic Differences By Age

The prevalence of obesity in Pima Indians (diabetic or non-diabetic) has stimulated interest in the examination of the numerous factors that contribute to this condition. Reduction in the ratio of fat to carbohydrate oxidation is one such factor. Rising et al.[78] reported a significantly increased 24-hour RQ over time in data from seven non-diabetic Pima Indian males aged 22 to 41 years studied longitudinally over a seven-year period. These data were analyzed with cross-sectional data from 131 Pima males aged 18 to 71 years. Results indicate that as age increased, there was a lower net ratio of fat to carbohydrate oxidation. RQ increased from 0.084 to 0.86 from the youngest to the oldest.

Zurlo et al.[94] studied 152 non-diabetic Pima Indians using indirect calorimetry, gender, body composition, and energy balance to assess the ratio of carbohydrate to fat oxidation. The most significant factor was familial affiliation. A low ratio of fat to carbohydrate oxidation was associated with subsequent weight gain independent of low EE.

13.5 RECOMMENDATIONS

13.5.1   Nutritional

The most recent complete edition of Recommended Dietary Allowances (RDA) published in 1989 by the National Research Council (NRC)[95] is currently under revision. These standards are the primary reference points for the evaluation and prescription of nutritional intake in the United States. The WHO/FAO/UNU[4] publishes nutritional recommendations intended to serve as guidelines for populations of all nations.

13.5.1.1 Energy

Historically, the NRC has used a factorial method to estimate energy requirements using TEE in healthy individuals assumed to be in energy balance. Additional energy requirements are provided for lactating women and growing infants and children.[95] However, they do not provide recommendations for older individuals (older than 51 years). Nor do they account for differences in body composition or activity levels. The energy needs of physically active individuals, regardless of age, may be significantly different than their sedentary counterparts.

Pediatric — Fontvielle et al.[96] investigated the relationship between current daily energy requirement recommendations, TEE, and physical activity in 28 healthy, free living 5-year-old children (13 females and 15 males). TEE was measured with the doubly labeled water method (during a seven-day period), RMR by indirect calorimetry, and physical activity by PAI (reported by primary caregiver). Their results demonstrate a significantly higher RMR (5%) with a significantly lower

TEE (24%) than predicted by current FAO/WHO/UNU[4] energy recommendations of 90 kcal/kg/d. The value suggested by their results was 70 kcal/kg/d. FFM and body weight were significantly related to TEE and RMR in children. The energy cost of physical activity accounted for 16% ± 7% of TEE. There was a positive correlation observed between PAI, TEE, and RMR (r = 0.52, p < 0.01) and the energy cost of physical activity (r = 0.56, p < 0.005).

Past-year sport-leisure activity also correlated with differences between measured and predicted values with FFM, FM, and gender (r = 0.40, p < 0.05). Males exhibited a correlation between physical activity with TEE/RMR ratio (r = 0.064, p < 0.05) and the energy cost of physical activity (r = 0.63, p < 0.05). There was also a correlation between past-year sport-leisure activity with the energy cost of physical activity and with TEE that was not found in females. These authors concluded that current FAO/WHO/UNU[4] energy requirements overestimate actual needs in 5-year-old children. Furthermore, they suggested that lower-than-expected physical activity in children may be responsible. EE from physical activities may vary significantly from sports-and-leisure-type exercise to less-strenuous activities involved in daily living, such as watching television. Table 13.1 provides current estimates of time spent in physical activity by children.

Table 13.1 Current Estimates of Time Spent in Leisure and Daily Physical Activity by Children (hr/d)

	Fontvielle	Goran
Past year sport-leisure activities	1.87	1.77
Daily physical activities	6.35	4.25
Watching television	3.00	3.90

Adapted from Fontvielle, A. M., Harper, I. T., Ferraro, R. T., Spraul, M., and Ravussin, E., Daily energy expenditure by five-year-old children, measured by doubly labeled water, *J. Pediatr.*, 123, 200, 1993, and Goran, M. I., Hunter, G., Nagy, T. R., and Johnson, R., Physical activity related energy expenditure and fat mass in young children, *Int. J. Obes.*, 21, 171, 1997.

Adult — Roberts et al.[97] investigated the energy requirements in 15 healthy young males (mean age 24.2 ± 0.5 years) and 9 healthy older males (mean age 70.3 ± 2.2 years). Their ten-day metabolic balance study determined TEE by the doubly labeled water technique, REE by indirect calorimetry, ME intake by adiabatic bomb calorimetry aliquot analysis of prepared diets, and body composition by total body water ($H_2^{18}O$) dilution in free living individuals. Their results indicate both the younger and older males had significantly higher values for ME intake and TEE than the current RDA for energy. They concluded that the current RDA for energy may underestimate usual energy needs in both younger and older males.

The same laboratory conducted a similar study in healthy younger and older females. Sawaya et al.[98] studied ten normal-weight younger females (mean age 25.2 ± 1.1 years) and ten normal-weight older females (mean age 74.0 ± 1.4 years). Their nine-day experiment measured TEE by the doubly labeled water technique, body composition by hydrodensitometry, and REE by indirect calorimetry. Their results indicate a significant underprediction of energy requirements by the RDAs for the younger females but not for the older females.

The issue of accurately predicting energy requirements in older males and females has been investigated by other authors. Calloway et al.[99] studied six healthy males aged 63 to 77 years over seven weeks in a metabolic unit. Their study assessed energy intake, BMR, body composition, and EE. These authors reported minimum maintenance energy requirements to be 1.5 × BMR in healthy older males. This requirement agrees with the current RDA activity factor (1.5 × BMR) identified for males and females over 50 years of age.[95]

Goran et al.[100] studied 13 older males and females with an age range of 56 to 78 years. They measured TEE by the doubly labeled water technique, RMR by respiratory gas analysis, FFM by underwater weighing, energy intake by a three-day food diary, and leisure time activity (LTA) by structured interviews. They reported a range of TEE from 1856 to 3200 kcal per day or 1.25 to 2.11 times RMR (range 1227 to 1930 kcal per day). TEE was best predicted by $\dot{V}O_{2 \, max}$ and LTA. These authors concluded that TEE varies greatly between healthy older adults due to variations in physical activity and under-reported energy intakes. Interestingly, males under-reported energy intakes by 12% , while females under-reported by 31%.

Flynn et al.[101] followed 144 males over a 20-year period from 1969 to 1989. Routine determinations of body composition by whole body counting, TBK, serum lipid profiles, blood pressure, and four-day diet records were collected. They reported decreases in height, LBM (percentage of body fat increased), TBK, and energy intakes over time. A mean weight increase was observed between ages 41 to 50 years, after which it plateaued and decreased later in life. Intake of all nutrients decreased significantly longitudinally and with time. In this study, energy intake decreased equally from carbohydrate, protein, and total fat sources.

Similar results were reported by Garry et al.[102] from a longitudinal survey conducted from 1980 to 1989. This study included 157 males and females with a mean age of 70 years in 1980. These researchers report significantly decreased intakes of energy, protein, and fat in males over time. The females demonstrated a significantly decreased fat intake with an increased carbohydrate intake over time. The gender differences in carbohydrate and fat intake were attributed to female responsiveness to voluntary fat reduction from national education programs rather than a true dimorphism due to gender.

Energy needs are based on RMR 60% to 70% of TEE.[4] The remaining 30% to 40% is attributed to body composition, physical activity, spontaneous physical activity, and TEF. Although males and females age differently, RMR and FFM decrease in both up to age 80. Data in individuals over age 80 years is incomplete. The question of whether RMR decreases due to decreased FFM or vice versa is not clear.[103,104] What effect these changes have on energy intake continues to be examined.

The changes reported in energy metabolism with aging confirm the need for age- and gender-specific recommendations. This area of research needs to be expanded to include studies examining energy requirements for individuals over 80 years of age. There is a paucity of information in this area.

13.5.1.2 Protein

The established recommended protein intake for healthy adult males and females is 0.8 g · kg.$^{-1}$ · d^{-1}.[95] These recommendations are based on nitrogen balance studies, which are the standard method for establishing total protein (nitrogen) requirements. The World Heath Organziation[4,95] also uses this method. The current protein recommendations for older adults were extrapolated from nitrogen balance studies conducted in healthy young males. Insufficient data in elderly subjects has been cited to justify this decision.[4,95] However, newer tracer studies are available to evaluate protein requirements.

Gersovitz et al.[105] conducted a nitrogen balance study in seven males (mean age 75 ± 4 years) and eight females (mean age 78 ± 9 years). An experimental diet containing 0.8 g egg protein · Kg.$^{-1}$ · d^{-1} was fed as the sole source of protein. The contribution toward total caloric intake from carbohydrate protein, and fat were 46%, 10%, and 44%, respectively. Body weight and TBK were monitored. Despite adequate energy intake, 43% of males and 50% of females were not in nitrogen balance during the final five days of the 30-day study. These authors concluded that in males and females over 70 years of age, the current protein recommendation is not adequate for nitrogen balance.

Campbell et al.[106] randomly assigned 12 males and females aged 56 to 80 years to consume either a diet of 0.8 ± 0.01 or 1.62 ± 0.02 g protein · kg.$^{-1}$ · d^{-1} for 11 days. Their results of nitrogen balance studies were a negative balance for the lower protein intake and a posititve balance for the higher level. These authors estimate a 1.0 to 1.25 g · Kg.$^{-1}$ · d^{-1} of high quality protein as a safe intake recommendation.

Maintenance of positive nitrogen balance is a significant marker for good health as individuals age. Additionally, the role of whole body protein turnover in this state of equilibrium is becoming more evident as studies in protein metabolism become more sophisticated.

Pannemans et al.[107] examined the effect of two levels of protein intake on nitrogen balance and whole body protein turnover in males (n = 17) and females (n = 11) with different activity levels. The mean age for males was 74 ± 12 years and for females 69 ± 9 years. A cross-over study design was used with two protein levels that were fed for three weeks each with a three-week washout period in between. Both diets were isocaloric. Diet A contained 12% of total calories from protein, or a mean of 0.9 g/kg body weight, and diet B contained 21%, or a mean of 1.5 g/kg of body weight. Body composition, PAI, BMR, nitrogen balance, and whole body protein turnover by [^{15}N]glycine were measured during each diet period. Their results indicate a positive nitrogen balance was maintained with both diets, protein turnover was significantly increased with diet B, and protein turnover during both diet periods was significantly higher in males than females when body composition was considered. These authors speculate that the significance of lower protein turnover in older females may be hormonal, but further studies are needed.

Morais et al.[108] tested the hypothesis that FFM alterations associated with aging affect whole body protein turnover. These researchers compared healthy older males (n = 8) and females (n = 8) whose mean age was 72.6 years with healthy younger males (n = 8) and females (n = 7) whose mean age was 28.4 years. Dietary intake was based on the older group's usual diet, with the younger group receiving comparable levels of energy and protein. Energy intakes ranged from 1.36 to 1.82 × RMR in the older group, while the younger group received a mean of 1.7 × RMR. Protein intakes were a mean of 1.24 g · kg.$^{-1}$ · d^{-1} and 1.27 g · kg.$^{-1}$ · d^{-1} in the older and younger groups, respectively. Body composition (bioelectrical impedance), RMR (ventilated hood method), nitrogen balance, skeletal muscle protein breakdown (urinary 3-methylhistidine), and protein turnover (oral [^{15}N]glycine) rates were collected. Their results indicate rates of whole body protein kinetics were not significantly affected by age when FFM was considered. Older females have significantly lower muscle protein catabolism. Whole body protein breakdown was lower in the older group (mean 24.05%) than the younger group (35.35%). These authors concluded that the lower rates of flux, synthesis, and breakdown seen in older males and females was due to body composition changes associated with aging.

13.5.2 Exercise

The Centers for Disease Control and Prevention and the American College of Sports Medicine report 78% of all Americans are inadequately active or completely sedentary.[109] Physical inactivity or "bed rest" was considered standard medical practice in treating illnesses or disabilities. It was also accepted as a natural consequence of aging in older individuals. Current medical recommendations endorse physical activity for enhancement of cardiovascular function, body composition, and maintenance of musco-skeletal strength and mass necessary for good health.[110,111] Decline in physical performance occurs with aging, but functional capacity can be maintained with physical conditioning.[112]

Sherman et al.[113] reported their findings from the Framingham Heart Study in females aged 75 years or older. The females who remained physically active were more independent and lived longer than their sedentary counterparts. In addition to physical well being, psychosocial benefits can be demonstrated. Bozoian and McAuley[114] reported their study in 33 females (mean age 86.4 years) who completed a ten-week program of either flexibility or strength exercises. The strength exercise group significantly improved their upper body strength and their ability to perform activities of daily living. Both exercise groups increased in positive effect and decreased in negative effect, but the strength group was significantly more satisfied with life than the flexibility group.

The focus of any exercise program should be to build (in children) and maintain (in adults) MM, strength, and bone density. Individualized exercise prescription to determine mode, frequency, and intensity should be utilized to achieve maximal benefit.

13.5.2.1 Endurance

Pediatric — Aerobic fitness is considered the best indicator of an individual's capacity to perform exercise involving oxidative mechanisms. Cardiovascular, pulmonary, and hematologic systems coordinate the delivery of oxygen during muscular performance. The rate of use or uptake of oxygen expressed as $\dot{V}O_{2\,max}$ is recognized as the foremost index of aerobic fitness. Armstrong et al.[115] investigated the conventional wisdom of using $\dot{V}O_2$ plateau as the standard for establishing $\dot{V}O_{2\,max}$ during progressive, incremental exercise testing in children. They studied healthy females (n = 18) and males (n = 7) with a mean age of 9.9 ± 0.4 years by conducting three progressively intense (grade and speed increased) treadmill tests to exhaustion. Each treadmill test was separated by one week. Age, gender, height, weight, body mass, $\dot{V}O_2$, heart rate, respiratory exchange ratio, blood lactate, minute ventilation, and respiratory frequency were collected at each test. Their results demonstrate mean peak $\dot{V}O_2$ values in tests two and three (supramaximal tests), which did not significantly differ from values in test one despite significantly higher indicators (minute ventilation, respiratory frequency, heart rate, respiratory exchange ratio, and blood lactate) of increased anaerobic contribution. Only 38.9% of the females and 35.3% of the males demonstrated a $\dot{V}O_2$ plateau ($\leq$ 2ml · kg^{-1} · min^{-1}); however, there were no significant differences between those who plateaued and those who did not. These authors concluded that $\dot{V}O_{2\,max}$ in children may not involve a $\dot{V}O_2$ plateau.

Other authors[116,117] agree that $\dot{V}O_{2\,max}$ may be less valid an indicator of cardiopulmonary function, endurance capacity, and response to training in children and adolescents than in adults. $\dot{V}O_{2\,max}$ capacity increases at similar rates in males and females up to age 12. It continues to increase in males up to age 18 and plateaus in females at around age 14.[117]

The National Institutes for Health[118] recommended that all children (and adults) set a long-term goal to accumulate at least 30 minutes or more of moderate-intensity physical activity on all, preferably most, days of the week.

Adult — The effects of endurance training on the cardiovascular system and water compartments was the focus of a study conducted by Pickering et al.[119] The mean age of ten sedentary, but otherwise healthy, males and females was 62 ± 2 years. Supervised training was performed on cycle ergometer three times per week with progressive intensity (50% to 85% $\dot{V}O_{2\,max}$). Measurements of exercise capacity, body composition, water compartment volumes, $\dot{V}O_{2\,max}$, and echocardiography were performed before training, after two months, at four months when training ended, and four months after training stopped. Their results demonstrate a 16% increase in $\dot{V}O_{2\,max}$ and an 11% increase in induced plasma volume expansion (indicates improved cardiac contractility function). No changes were seen in FFM, body composition, body weight, or other body water compartment volumes. However, after four months of detraining (resumption of sedentary life styles) the improvements noted above were totally lost.

Coggan et al.[112] measured muscle metabolic response with ^{31}P magnetic resonance spectroscopy and measured muscle mass with ^{1}H magnetic resonance imaging in younger (21 to 33 years) and older (58 to 68 years) trained and untrained males. Endurance training was associated with significantly increased (60% to 100%) muscle citrate synthase (CS) activity in both younger and older trained males compared with their untrained counterparts. Despite this response to endurance training, CS activity in both older groups was 20% lower than in corresponding younger groups. Smaller MM and lower muscle respiratory capacity were associated with the decreased muscle metabolism demonstrated by the older groups. These authors concluded that endurance training does improve metabolic responses to exercise in older males, but it cannot totally prevent age-related changes or decreased MM that occurs with aging.

Meredith et al.[120] studied the effects of endurance training at 70% $\dot{V}O_{2\,max}$ in ten older (65.1 ± 2.9 years) and ten younger (23.6 ± 1.8 years) males and females. Measurements of body compostition, MM, $\dot{V}O_{2\,max}$, and RMR were completed before and after training. Their results demonstrated that the older group had more adipose tissue and less MM than the younger group and training had no significant effect on weight or body composition in either group. The initial peak $\dot{V}O_2$ was lower in the older group, but after training the absolute increase of 5.5 ml to 6.0 ml · kg^{-1} · min^{-1} was similar in both groups. Significant increases were observed in glycogen stores (28%) and muscle O_2 consumption (128%) after training in the older group. The increase in muscle oxidative capacity was greater in the older group than in the younger group, which these authors suggested may indicate peripheral adaptions to aerobic exercise training in older individuals.

Kohrt et al.[121] examined the effect of endurance training on body composition and fat distribution in 47 males and 46 females aged 60 to 70 years of age. Body composition (by hydrodensitometry) and fat distribution (by skinfolds and circumference measures) were compared before and after training. The supervised endurance exercise consisted primarily of walking or jogging although some participants used rowing and cycle ergometers. Training sessions were a mean of 46 ± 5 minutes per day, 4.0 ± 0.6 days per week at 80% ± 5% of maximum heart rate, and they were carried out for nine to 12 months. Body weight, percentage of body fat, and FM decreased significantly in males and females. The males decreased a mean of 3.4 ± 4.4 kg. in body weight and females lost a mean of 1.6 ± 3.8 kg. FFM did not significantly change in either males or females. Reductions in skinfold thickness and circumference measures at the central body (trunk) area were significantly greater than at other sites (extremities). These authors concluded that endurance training can favorably affect central body composition by reducing abdominal fat distribution, thus reducing the risk for diseases associated with this type of body habitus.

The American College of Sports Medicine[122] recommendations for developing and maintaining cardiorespiratory fitness, body composition, muscular strength and endurance, and flexibility in healthy adults are summarized in Table 13.2.

Table 13.2 Exercise Recommendations for Healthy Adults

Recommendation	Amount
Frequency	3–5 days per week
Intensity	55*/65%–90% of maximum heart rate or 40*/50%–85% $VO_{2\,max}$
Duration	20–60 min continous aerobic activity; adjust for intensity of activity, i.e., shorter time periods for higher intensity and longer time periods for moderate to lower intensity
Mode	any activity that uses large muscle groups, can be maintained continuously, and is rhythmical and aerobic in nature

* Applicable to very unfit individuals

Adapted from American College of Sports Medicine, The recommended quantity and quality of exercise for developing and maintaining cardiorespiratory and muscular fitness, and flexibility in healthy adults, *Med. Sci. Sports Exerc.*, 30, 975, 1998.

13.5.2.2 Resistance

Pediatric — The safety and effectiveness of weight training in prepubescent children has been controversial. The American Academy of Pediatrics (AAP)[123] policy statement on weight training and weight lifting in 1983 suggested a minimal benefit was received from weight training in prepubescent athletes, while maximal benefit was obtained by the postpubertal athlete.

Vrijens[124] reported no strength gains in a study where 10- to 17-year-old males participated in an eight-week strength training program (1 set, 8–12 repetitions, 3 times/week). Docherty et al.[125] reported results of no strength gains for 12-year-old hockey and soccer players who trained following their competitive season. However, more recently in 1990 the AAP[126] provided definitions to differentiate weight training, weight lifting, and body building along with recommendations for weight training in pediatric athletes. The AAP[126] supports supervised weight training (by well-trained adults), but not maximal competitive weightlifting, power lifting, or body building in children prior to Tanner[7] Stage V.

Recommendations for weight training programs in children based on Kraemer et al.[127] and the American Orthopaedic Society for Sports Medicine[128] are summarized in Table 13.3.

Table 13.3 Recommendations for Weight Training in Children

Recommendation	Amount
Frequency	2–3 times per week
Intensity	low (12–15 RM*)
	moderate (10–12 RM)
	high (8–10 RM)
Duration	low intensity — 2–6 weeks
	moderate intensity — 8–24 weeks
	high intensity — ongoing
Mode	low intensity — 1–2 sets with 2–3 minutes of rest between sets
	moderate intensity — 2–3 sets with 2 minutes of rest between sets
	high intensity — 3–4 sets with 2 minutes of rest between sets

* repetition maximum

Adapted from Kraemer, W. J., Fry, A. C., Frykman, P. N., Conroy, B., and Hoffman, J., Resistance training and youth, *Ped. Exer. Sci.*, 1, 336, 1989, and American Orthopaediatric Society for Sports Medicine, *Proceedings of the Conference on Strength Training and the Prepubescent*, Cahill, B. R., Ed., American Orthopaediatric Society for Sports Medicine, 1988.

Adult — Klitgaard et al.[129] examined maximal isometric torque and MM (by CT scan) in older males (mean age 69 years) who had been strength training (three times per week at 70% to 90% of their one repetition maximum) for the previous 12 to 17 years. These strength-trained males were age-matched with runners and swimmers. Controls were younger males. The older strength-trained males had significantly greater upper arm and mid-thigh strength and mass than the endurance-trained, age-matched subjects. The older strength-trained males had similar muscle cross-sectional areas and strength to the younger controls.

McCartney et al.[130] studied 119 healthy older adults in a 42-week study comparing the effects of progressive weight-lifting training on dynamic muscle strength, peak power output, progressive treadmill walking and stair climbing, knee extensor cross-sectional areas, and bone mineral density and content. Participants were randomized into either exercise or control groups and were matched for age and gender. The exercise group trained two times per week. Controls were offered a low-intensity walking program two times per week, which was not heavily utilized, and were instructed to pursue normal activities of daily living. Their results indicate significant increases in the exercise group as compared to the control group in one repetition maximum (1RM) strength, peak power output, progressive treadmill walking, and knee extensor cross-sectional areas. No changes were seen in stair climbing or bone mineral density and content between the two groups. These authors conclude that resistance training does increase dynamic muscle strength, muscle size, and functional capacity.

Chandler et al.[131] studied the effect of lower extremity strength training in 100 frail community-dwelling males and females with a mean age of 77.6 ± 7.6 years. The study design was a prospective controlled clinical trial with baseline and postintervention measures of lower extremity strength, physical performance (balance, walking, and chair rise), and disability (physical functioning). Participants were randomly assigned to either the exercise or control groups. The exercise group received ten weeks of lower extremity resistance training three times per week in their homes, which was supervised by a physical therapist. Their results demonstrate a significant strength gain for mobility skills (sitting balance and reach, transfer, rising from a chair, standing balance, picking up an object from the floor, walking, turning, stopping suddenly, stepping over a shoe box, and stair climbing). Chair rise performance was significant only in the more impaired subjects. Strength gain was associated with increased gait speed and falls efficacy (perception of ability to avoid falls), but not with balance, endurance, or disability measures. The lack of significant improvement in balance and endurance was attributed to the short duration and low intensity of the exercise in this study. These authors concluded that the importance of demonstrating strength gains with strength training in this population is to document the concept that strength training is a viable intervention for health status improvements in the elderly.

Fiatarone et al.[132] explored the use of high-intensity strength training in ten nonagenarians (mean age 90.2 ± 1.1 years). All the participants were residents of a long-term care facility where they were classified as needing minimal to moderate assistance with activities of daily living. Anthropometric assessment indicated that four of the ten participants were undernourished (72%–88% of ideal body weight). An eight-week program of progressive resistance training consisting of concentric and ecentric muscle contraction performed three times per week was completed by nine of the participants (one male dropped out after four weeks due to stress on an inguinal hernia repair site). Dietary intake assessment indicated a mean energy intake of 29.1 ± 2.2 kcal/kg/d and a mean protein intake of $1.3 ± 0.1g \cdot kg^{-1} \cdot d^{-1}$. Strength gains were highly significant with a mean of 174% ± 31% (n = 9). Mid-thigh muscle area increased significantly in seven subjects, with a mean of 11.7% ± 5.0% for total area, 14.5% ± 7.8% for quadriceps, and 10.6% ± 9.1% for hamstrings and adductors. There was no significant change in subcutaneous or intramuscular fat areas nor did strength gains correlate with increased muscle size by CT scan. After four weeks of detraining, 1RM testing was repeated in seven of the nine subjects who completed training. There was a significant loss of 37% of maximum strength observed. Although strength training can increase strength significancy even in nonagenarians, there is also a significant loss of gained strength upon detraining. Therefore, to maintain strength gains, strength training must be ongoing.

The American College of Sports Medicine[122] recommends resistance training as part of adult fitness programs. The strength training should be of a moderate intensity that is sufficient to develop and maintain FFM. A recommended minimum is one set of 8 to 12 repetitions of 8 to 10 exercises that condition the major muscle groups two to three days per week.

13.6 CONCLUSION

Quality of life is enhanced by good physical health. Children and adolescents should experience appropriate growth, early to middle-aged adults should maintain an active life style, and older adults should enjoy the ability to perform the functions of daily living which allow independence. The effect of adequate nutritional intake and maintenance of appropriate body composition strongly influences these desired outcomes.

Energy metabolism is a strong modulator on body composition, therefore, MM, FFM, and FM. Preservation of FFM and avoidance of age-related accumulation of adipose tissue may attenuate the declines in muscle function, skeletal integrity, and overall strength that occur with aging. Obesity-related diseases commonly seen with aging are not inevitable. The positive role of exercise, both endurance and resistance training, on body composition and, therefore, energy metabolism is important in achieving optimal physiological functioning and good health. The ability and motivation to integrate an exercise program based on current recommendations in conjunction with an adequate nutritional intake should result in increased well being and quality of life.

REFERENCES

1. Ravussin, E., Lillioja, S., Anderson, T. E., Christin, L., and Bogardus, C., Determinants of 24-hour energy expenditure in man: methods and results using a respiratory chamber, *J. Clin. Invest.*, 78, 1568, 1986.

2. Roberts, S. B., Fuss, P., Heyman, M. B., and Young, V. R., Influence of age on energy requirements, *Am. J. Clin. Nutr.*, 62, 1053S, 1995.

3. Harris, J. and Benedict, F., *A biometric study of basal metabolism in man*, Washington, D.C., Carnegie Institute of Washington, 279, 1919.

4. World Health Organization, Food and Agriculture Organization, United Nations University, Energy and protein requirements, *WHO Tech. Rep. Ser.*, 724, 1985.

5. Schofield, W. N., Predicting basal metabolic rate, new standards and review of previous work, *Hum. Nutr. Clinc. Nutr.*, 39C, 5, 1985.

6. Firouzbakhsh, S., Mathis, R. K., Dorchester, W. L., Oseas, R. S., Groncy, P. K., Grant, K. E., and Finklestein, J. Z., Measured resting energy expenditure in children, *J. Pediatr. Gastroenterol. Nutr.*, 16, 136, 1993.

7. Tanner, J. M., *Growth at Adolescence*, 2nd ed., Blackwell Scientific, Oxford, 1962.

8. Wong, W. W., Butte, N. F., Hergenroeder, A. C., Hill, R. B., Stuff, J. E., and Smith, E. O., Are basal metabolic rate prediction equations appropriate for female children and adolescents?, *J. Appl. Physiol.*, 81, 2407, 1996.

9. Schoeller, D. A. and Webb, P., Five-day comparison of the doubly labeled water method with repiratory gas exchange, *Am. J. Clin. Nutr.*, 40, 153, 1984.

10. Roberts, S. B. and Young, V. R., Energy cost of fat and protein depostion in the human infant, *Am. J. Clin. Nutr.*, 48, 951, 1988.

11. Jones, P. J. H., Winthrop, A. L., Schoeller, D. A., Swyer, P. R., Smith, J., Filler, R. M., and Heim, T., Validation of doubly labeled water for assessing energy expenditure in infants, *Pediatr. Res.*, 21, 242, 1987.

12. Fomon, S. J., *Nutrition of Normal Infants*, Mosby, St. Louis, MO, 1993, 104.

13. Hamill, P. V. V., Drizd, T. A., Johnson, C. L., Reed, R. B., Roche, A. F., and Moore, W. M., Physical growth: National Center for Health Statistics percentiles, *Am. J. Clin. Nutr.*, 32, 607, 1979.

14. Fomon, S. J., *Infant Nutrition*, 2nd ed., W. B. Saunders, Philadelphia, 1974, pp. 34–63.

15. Wells, J. C. K., Cole, T. J., and Davies, P. S. W., Total energy expenditures and body composition in early infancy, *Arch. Dis. Child.*, 75, 423, 1996.

16. Wells, J. C. K., Hinds, A., and Davies, P. S. W., Free-living energy expenditures and behaviour in late infancy, *Arch. Dis. Child.*, 76, 490, 1997.

17. Butte, N. F., Moon, J. K., Wong, W. W., Hopkinson, J. M., and Smith, E. O., Energy requirements from infancy to adulthood, *Am. J. Clin. Nutr.*, 62S, 1047S, 1995.

18. Goran, M. I., Kaskoun, M., and Johnson, R., Determinants of resting energy expenditure in young children, *J. Pediatr.*, 125, 362, 1994.

19. Goran, M. I., Hunter, G., Nagy, T. R., and Johnson, R., Physical activity-related energy expenditure and fat mass in young children, *Int. J. Obes.*, 21, 171, 1997.

20. Davies, P. S. W., Gregory, J., and White, A., Physical activity and body fatness in pre-school children, *Int. J. Obes.*, 19, 6, 1995.

21. Harsher, D. W. and Bray, G. A., Body composition and childhood obesity, in *Obesity Endocrinology Metabolism Clinic North America*, Bray, G. A., Ed., W. B. Saunders, Philadelphia, 1996, pp. 871-876.

22. Figueroa-Colon, R., Lee, J., Aldridge, R., and Alexander, L., Obesity is prevalent and progressive in Birmingham school children, *Int. J. Obes.*, 18, 26, 1994.

22. Figueroa-Colon, R., Lee, J., Aldridge, R., and Alexander, L., Obesity is prevalent and progressive in Birmingham school children, *Int. J. Obes.*, 18, 26, 1994.

23. Goran, M. I., Gower, B. A., Nagy, T. R., and Johnson, R. K., Developmental changes in energy expenditure and physical activity in children: evidence for a decline in physical activity in girls before puberty, *Pediatrics*, 101, 887, 1998.

24. Committee on Nutrition, American Academy of Pediatrics, *Pediatric Nutrition Handbook*, 4th ed., Kleinman, R.E., Ed., American Academy of Pediatrics, Elk Grove Village, IL, 141,1998.

25. Bjorntorp, P., Growth hormone, insulin-like growth factor-I and lipid metabolism: interactions with sex steroids, *Horm. Res.*, 46, 188, 1996.

26. Cowell, C. T., Briody, J., Lloyd-Jones, S., Smith, C., Moore, B., and Howman-Giles R., Fat distribution in children and adolescents–the influence of sex and hormones, *Horm. Res.*, 48, S93, 1997.

27. McGandy, R. B., Barrows, C. H. Jr., Spanias, A., Meredith, A., Stone, J.L., and Norris, B. A., Nutrient intakes and energy expenditure in men of different ages, *J. Gerontol.*, 21, 581, 1966.

28. Forbes, G. B., and Reina, J. C., Adult lean body mass declines with age: some longitudinal observations, *Metabolism*, 19, 653, 1970.

29. Novak, L. P., Aging, total body potassium, fat-free mass, and cell mass in males and females between 18 and 85 years, *J. Gerontol.*, 27,438, 1972.

30. Flynn, M. A., Nolph, G. B., Baker, A. S., Martin, W. M., Krause, G., Total body potassium in aging humans: a longitudinal study, *Am. J. Clin. Nutr.*, 50, 713, 1989.

31. Cohn, S. H., Vartsky, D., Yasumura, S., and Vaswani, A. N., Indexes of body cell mass: nitrogen versus potassium, *Am. J. Physiol.*, 244, E305, 1983.

32. Frontera, W. R., Hughes, V. A., and Evans W.J., A cross-sectional study of upper and lower extremity muscle strength in 45–78 year old men and women, *J. Appl. Physiol.*, 71, 644, 1991.

33. Depres, J. P., Moorjani, S., Lupien, P. J., Tremblay, A., Nadeau, A., Bouchard, C., Regional distribution of body fat, plasma lipoproteins, and cardiovascular disease, *Arteriosclerosis*, 10, 497, 1990.

34. Kohrt, W. M., Malley, M. T., Dalsky, G. P., and Hollowszy, J. O., Body composition of healthy sedentary and trained, younger and older men and women, *Med. Sci. Sports Exerc.*, 24, 832, 1992.

35. Tzankoff, S. P., and Norris, A. H., Effect of muscle mass decrease on age-related BMR changes, *J. Appl. Physiol*, 45, 536, 1977.

36. Pannemans, D. L. E., and Westerterp, K. R., Energy expenditure, physical activity and basal metabolic rate of elderly subjects, *Br. J. Nutr.*, 73, 571, 1994.

37. Jette, A. M., and Branch, L. G., The Framingham disability study II: physical disability among the aging, *Am. J. Public Health*, 71, 1211, 1981.

38. Bassey, E. J., Bendall, M. J., and Pearson, M., Muscle strength in the triceps surae and objectively measured customary walking activity in men and women over 65 years of age, *Clin. Sci.* 74, 85, 1988.

39. Ballor, D. L., and Poehlman, E. T., Resting metabolic rate and coronary-heart-disease risk factors in aerobically and resistance trained women, *Am. J. Clin. Nutr.*, 56, 968, 1992.

40. Ryan, A. S., Nicklas, B.J. ,and Dariush, E., A cross-sectional study on body composition and energy expenditure in women athletes during aging, *Am. J. Physiol.*, 271, E916, 1996.

41. Poehlman, E. T., Toth, M. J., and Gardner, A. W., Changes in energy balance and body composition at menopause: a controlled longitudinal study, *Ann. Intern. Med.*, 123, 673, 1995.

42. Drinkwater, B. L., Horvath, S. M., and Wells, C. L., Aerobic power of females, ages 10 to 68, *J. Gerontol.*, 30, 385,1975.

43. Keys, A., Taylor, H. L., and Grande, F., Basal metabolism and age of adult man, *Metabolism*, 22, 579, 1973.

44. Poehlman, E.T., McAuliffe, T. L., Van Houten, D.R., and Danforth, E. Jr., Influence of age and endurance training on metabolic rate and hormones in healthy men, *Am. J. Physiol.*, 259, E66, 1990.

45. Horber, F. F., Kohler, S. A., Lippuner, K., and Jaeger, P., Effect of regular physical training on age-associated alteration of body composition in men, *Eur. J. Clin. Invest.*, 26, 279, 1996.

46. Kashiwagi, A., Bogardus, C., Lilloja, S., Huecksteadt, T. P., Brady, D., Verso, M. A., and Foley, J. E., *In vitro* insensitivity of glucose transport and antilipolysis to insulin due to receptor and postreceptor abnormalities in obese Pima Indians with normal glucose tolerance, *Metabolism*, 33, 772, 1984.

47. Roth, J., Glick, S. M., Yalow, R. S., and Berson, S. A., Secretion of human growth hormone: physiologic and experimental modification, *Metabolism*, 12, 577, 1963.

48. Henneman, D. H., and Henneman, P. H., Effects of human growth hormone on levels of blood and urinary carbohydrate and fat metabolites in man, *J. Clin. Invest.*, 39,1239,1960.

49. Manson, J. McK., and Wilmore, D. W., Positive nitrogen balance with human growth hormone and hypocaloric intravenous feeding, *Surgery*, 100, 188, 1986.

50. Kaplan, S. A., Growth and growth hormone: disorders of the anterior pituitary, in *Clinical Pediatric and Adolescent Endocrinology*, Kaplan, S. A., Ed., W. B. Saunders, Philadelphia, 1982, 25.

51. Vaisman, N., Zadik, Z., Akivias, A., Voet, H., Katz, I., Yair, S., and Ashkenazi, A., Changes in body composition, resting energy expenditure, and thermic effect of food in short children on growth hormone therapy, *Metabolism*, 43, 1543, 1994.

52. Hankinson, S. E., Willett, W. C., Colditz, G. A., Hunter, D. J., Michaud, D. S., Deroo, B., Rosner, B., Speizer, F. E., and Pollak, M., Circulating concentrations of insulin-like growth factor-I and risk of breast cancer, *Lancet*, 351, 1393, 1998.

53. Thompson, J. L., Butterfield, G. E., Marcus, R., Hintz, R. L., Van Loan, M., Ghiron, L., and Hoffman, A. R., The effects of recombinant human insulin-like growth factor-I and growth hormone on body composition in elderly women, *J. Clin. Enocrinol. Metab.*, 80, 1845, 1995.

54. Butterfield G. E., Thompson, J., Rennie, M. J., Marcus, R., Hintz, R. L., and Hoffman, A. R., Effect of rhGH and rhIGF-I treatment on protein utilization in elderly women, *Am. J. Physiol.*, 272, E94, 1997.

55. Rudman, D., Feller, A. G., Nagraj, H. S., Gergans, G.A., Lalitha, P. Y., Goldberg, A. F., Schlenker, R. A., Cohn, L., Rudman, I. W., and Mattson, D. E., Effect of human growth hormone in men over 60 years old, *New Engl. J. Med.*, 323, 1, 1990.

56. Bengtsson, B., Staffan, E., Lonn, L., Kvist, H., Stokland, A., Lindstedt, G., Bosaeus, I., Tolli, J., Sjostrom, L., and Isaksson, G. P., Treatment of adults with growth hormone deficiency with recombinant human growth hormone, *J. Clin. Endocrinol. Metab.*, 76, 309, 1993.

57. Vittone, J., Blackman, M. R., Busby-Whitehead, J., Tasiao, K. J., Stewart, K. J., Tobin, J., Stevens, T., Bellantoni, M.R., Rogers, M.A., Baumann, G., Roth, J., Harman, S. M., and Spencer, R.G.S., Effects of single nightly injections of growth hormone-releasing hormone (GHRH 1-29) in healthy elderly men, *Metabolism*, 46, 89, 1997.

58. Poehlman, E.T., and Copeland, K.C., Influence of physical activity on insulin-like growth factor-I in healthy younger and older men, *J. Clin. Endocrinol. Metab.*, 71, 1468, 1990.

59. Isley, W. L., Underwood, L. E., and Clemmons, D.R., Changes in plasma somatomedin-C in response to ingestion of diets with variable protein and energy content, *J. Parent. Enteral. Nutr.*, 8, 407, 1984.

60. Clemmons, D. R., Klibinski, A., and Underwood, L. E., Reduction of plasma immunoreactive somatomedin C during fasting in humans, *J. Clin. Endocrinol. Metab.*, 53, 1247, 1981.

61. Isely, W. L., Underwood, L. E., and Clemmons, D. R., Dietary components that regulate serum somatomedin-C concentrations in humans, *J. Clin. Invest.*, 71, 175, 1983.

62. Cuneo, R. C., Salomon, F., Wiles, C.M., Hesp, R., and Sonksen, P. H., Growth hormone treatment in growth hormone-deficient adults: effects on exercise performance, *J. Appl., Physiol.*, 70, 695, 1991.

63. Cuneo, R. C., Salomon, F., Wiles, C. M., Hesp, R., and Sonksen, P. H., Growth hormone treatment in growth hormone-deficient adults. I. effects on muscle mass and strength, *J. Appl. Physiol.*, 70, 688, 1991.

64. Marcus, R., Butterfield,G., Holloway, L., Gilliland, D. J., Hintz, R. L., and Sherman, B. M., Effects of short administration of recombinant human growth hormone to elderly people, *J. Clin. Endocrinol. Metab.*, 70, 519, 1990.

65. Kaiser, F. E., Silver, A. J., and Morely, J. E., The effect of recombinant human growth hormone on malnourished older individuals, *J. Am. Geriatr. Soc.* 39, 235, 1991.

66. Chan, J. M., Stampfer, M. J., Giovannucci, E., Gann, P. H., Ma, J., Wilkinson, P., Hennekens, C. H., and Pollak, M., Plasma insulin-like growth factor-1 and prostate cancer risk: a prospective study, *Science*, 279, 563, 1998.

67. Butte, N. F., Moon, J. K., Wong, W. W., Ferlic, L., Smith E. O., Klein, P.D., and Garza, C., Energy expenditure and deposition of breast-fed and formula-fed infants during early infancy, *Pediatr. Res.*, 28, 631, 1990.

68. Goran, M. I., Carpenter, W. H., and Poehlman, E. T., Total energy expenditure in 4- to 6-year-old children, *Am. J. Physiol.*, 264, E706, 1993.

69. Meredith, C. N., Zackin, M. J., Frontera, W. R., and Evans, W. J., Dietary protein requirements and body protein metabolism in endurance-trained men, *J. Appl. Physiol.*, 66, 2850, 1989.

70. Ferraro, R., Lillioja, S., Fontevielle, A. M., Rising, R., Bodardus, C., and Ravussin, E., Lower sedentary metabolic rate in women compared to men, *J. Clin. Invest.,* 90, 1, 1992.

71. Fukagawa, N. K., Bandini, L. G., and Young, J. B., Effect of age on body composition and resting metabolic rate, *Am. J. Appl. Physiol.,* 259, E233, 1990.

72. Poehlman, E. T., Melby, C. L., and Badylak, S. F., Relation of age and physical status on metabolic rate in younger and older healthy men, *J. Gerontol.,* 46, B54, 1991.

73. Arciero, P. J., Goran, M. I., and Poehlman, E. T., Resting metabolic rate is lower in women than in men, *J. Appl. Physiol.,* 76, 2514, 1993.

74. Klausen, B., Toubro, S., and Astrup, A., Age and sex effects on energy expenditure, *Am. J. Clin., Nutr.,* 65, 895, 1997.

75. Vaughn, L., Zurlo, F., and Ravussin, E., Aging and energy expenditure, *Am. J. Clin. Nutr.,* 53, 821, 1991.

76. Foley, J.E., Mechanisms of impaired insulin action in isolated adipocytes from obese and diabetic subjects, *Diabetes Metab. Rev.,* 4, 487, 1988.

77. Kashiwagi, A., Bogardus, C., Lilioja, S., Huecksteadt, T. P., Brady, D., Verso, M. A., and Foley, J. E., Invitro insensitivity of glucose transport and antilipolysis to insulin due to receptor and postreceptor abnormalities in obese Pima Indians with normal glucose tolerance, *Metabolism,* 33, 772, 1984.

78. Rising, R., Tataranni, P. A., Snitker, S., and Ravussin, E., Decreased ratio of fat to carbohydrate oxidation with increasing age in Pima Indians, *J. Am. Coll. Nutr.,* 15, 309, 1996.

79. Fontvieille, A. M., Dwyer, J., and Ravussin, E., Resting metabolic rate and body composition of Pima Indian and Caucasian children, *Int. J. Obes.,* 16, 535, 1992.

80. Evans, W. J., Exercise, nutrition, and aging, *Clin. Geriatr. Med.,* 11, 725, 1995.

81. Le Stunff, C., and Bougneres, P., Time course of increased lipid and decreased glucose oxidation during early phase of childhood obesity, *Diabetes,* 42, 1010, 1993.

82. Molnar, D., and Schutz, Y., Fat oxidation in nonobese and obese adolescents: effect of body composition and pubertal development, *J. Pediatr.,* 132, 98, 1998.

83. Juul, A, Bang, P., Hertel, M. T., Main, K., Dalgaard, P., Jorgensen, K., Muller, J., Hall, K., and Skakkebaek, M. E., Serum insulin-like growth factor-I in 1430 healthy children, adolescents, and adults: relation to age, sex, stage of puberty, testicular size, and body mass index, *J. Clin. Endocrinol. Metab.,* 78, 744, 1994.

84. Caprio, S., Plewe, G., Diamond, M. P., Simonson, D. C., Boulware, F. D., Sherwin, R. S., and Tamberlane, W. V., Increased insulin secretion in puberty: a compensatory response to reductions in insulin sensitivity, *J. Pediatr.,* 114, 963, 1989.

85. Arslanian, S. A., and Kalhan, S. C., Correlations between fatty acids and glucose metabolism potential explanation of insulin resistance of puberty, *Diabetes,* 43, 908, 1994.

86. Arslanian, S. A., and Kalhan, S. C., Protein turnover during puberty in normal children, *Am. J. Physiol.,* 270, E79, 1996.

87. Lonnqvist, F., Nyberg, B., Wahrenberg, H., and Arner, P., Catacholamine-induced lipolysis in adipose tissue of the elderly, *J. Clin. Invest.,* 85, 1614, 1990.

88. Terjung, R. L. V. H., Lipid metabolism during exercise, *Diabetes Metab. Rev.,* 2, 33, 1986.

89. Kohrt, W. M., Spina, R. J., Ehsani, A. A., Cryer, P. E., and Holloszy, J. O., Effects of age adiposity, and fitness level on plasma catacholamine responses to standing and exercise, *J. Appl. Physiol.,* 75, 1828, 1993.

90. Holloszy, J. O., and Coyle, E. F., Adaptions of skeletal muscle to endurance exercise and their metabolic consequences, *J. Appl. Physiol.,* 56, 831, 1984.

91. Poehlman, E. T., Gardner, A. W., Arciero, P. J., Goran, M. I., and Calles-Escandon, J., Effects of endurance training on total fat oxidation in elderly persons, *J. Appl. Physiol.,* 76, 2281, 1994.

92. Calles-Escandon, J., Archiero, P. J., Gardner, A. W., Bauman, C., and Poehlman, E. T., Basal fat oxidation decreases with aging in women, *J. Appl. Physiol.,* 78, 266, 1995.

93. Sial, S., Coggan, A. R., Carroll, R., Goodwin, J., and Klein, S., Fat and carbohydrate metabolism during exercise in elderly and young subjects, *Am. J. Physiol.,* 271, E983, 1996.

94. Zurlo, F., Lillioja, S., Esposito-Del Puente, Nyomba, B. L., Raz, I., Saad, F. M., Swinburn, B. A., Knowler, W. C., Bogardus, C., and Ravussin, E., Low ratio of fat to carbohydrate oxidation as predictor of weight gain: study of 24-h RQ, *Am. J. Physiol.,* 259, E650, 1990.

95. National Research Council, Recommended Dietary Allowances, 10th ed., National Academy of Sciences, Washington, D.C., 1989.

96. Fontvielle, A. M., Harper, I. T., Ferraro, R. T., Spraul, M., and Ravussin, E., Daily energy expenditure by five-year-old children, measured by doubly labeled water, *J. Pediatr.*, 123, 200, 1993.

97. Roberts, S. B., Young, V. R., Fuss, P Heyman, M. B., Fiatarone, M., Dallal, G. E., Cortiella, J., and Evans, W. J., What are the dietary energy needs of elderly adults?, *Int. J. Obes.*, 16, 969, 1992.

98. Sawaya, A. L., Saltzman, E., Fuss, P., Young, V. R., and Roberts, S., Dietary energy requirements of young and older women determined by using the doubly labeled water method, *Am. J. Clin. Nutr.*, 62, 338, 1995.

99. Calloway, D. H., and Zanni, E., Energy requirements and energy expenditure of elderly men, *Am. J. Clin. Nutr.*, 33, 2088, 1980.

100. Goran, M. I., and Poehlman, E. T., Total energy expenditure and energy requirements in healthy elderly people, *Metabolism*, 41, 744, 1992.

101. Flynn, M. A., Nolph, G. B., Baker, S., and Krause, G., Aging in humans: a continuous 20-year study of physiologic and dietary parameters, *J. Am. Coll. Nutr.*, 11, 660, 1992.

102. Garry, P. J., Hunt, W. C., Koehler, K. M., VanderJagt, D. J., and Vellas, B. J., Longitudinal study of dietary intakes and plasma lipids in healthy elderly men and women, *Am. J. Clin. Nutr.*, 55, 682M, 1992.

103. Poehlman, E. T., Goran, M., I., Gardner, A. W., Ades, P. A., Arciero, P. J., Katzman-Books, S. M., Montgomery, S. M., Toth, M. J., and Sutherland, P. T., Determinants of decline in resting metabolic rate in aging females, *Am. J. Physiol.*, 264, E450, 1993.

104. Poehlman, E. T., Berke, E. M., Joseph, J. R., Gardner, A. W., Katzman-Books, S. M., and Goran, M. I., Influence of aerobic capacity, body composition, and thyroid hormones on the age-related decline in resting metabolic rate, *Metab. Clin. Exp.*, 41, 915, 1992.

105. Gersovitz, M., Motil, K., Munro, H. N., Scrimshaw, N. S., and Young, V.R., Human protein requirements: assessment of adequacy of the current recommended dietary allowance for dietary protein in elderly men and women, *Am. J. Clin. Nutr.*, 35, 6, 1982.

106. Campbell, W. W., Crim, M. C., Dallal, G. E., Young, V. R., and Evans, W. J., Increased protein requirements in elderly people: new data and retrospective reassessments, *Am. J. Clin. Nutr.*, 60, 501, 1994.

107. Pannemans, D. L. E., Halliday, D., and Westerterp, K. R., Whole-body protein turnover in elderly men and women: responses to two protein intakes, *Am. J. Clin. Nutr.*, 61, 33, 1995.

108. Morais, J. A., Gougeon, R., Pencharz, P. B., Jones, P. J. H., Ross, R., and Marliss, E. B., Whole-body protein turnover in the healthy elderly, *Am. J. Clin. Nutr.*, 66, 880, 1997.

109. Pate, R. R., Pratt, M., Blair, S. N., Haskell, W. L., Macera, C. A., Bouchard, C., Buschner, D., Ettinger W., Heath G. W., and King, A. C., Physical activity and public health: a recommendation from the Centers for Disease Control and Prevention and the American College of Sports Medicine, *J. Am. Med. Assoc.*, 273, 402, 1995.

110. National Institutes of Health Consensus Statement: Physical activity and health, 13, 1, 1995.

111. Shepard, R. J., Aging, physical activity, and health, *Human Kinetics*, Champain, IL, 1997.

112. Coggan, A. R., Abduljalil, A. M., Swanson, S. C., Earle, M. S., Farris J. W., Mendenhall, L. A., and Robitaille P., Muscle metabolism during exercise in young and older untrained and enduranced-trained men, *J. Appl. Physiol.*, 75, 2125, 1993.

113. Sherman, S. E., DíAgostino, R. B., Cobb, J. L., and Kannel, W. B., Does exercise reduce mortality rate in the elderly? Experience from the Framingham Heart Study, *Am. Heart J.*, 128, 965, 1994.

114. Bozoian, S. and McAuley, E., Strength training effects on subjective well-being and physical function in the elderly, *Med. Sci. Sports Exerc.*, 26, S156, 1994.

115. Armstrong, N., Welsman, J., and Winsley, R., Is peak $\dot{V}O_2$ a maximal index of children's aerobic fitness?, *Int. J. Sports Med.*, 17, 356, 1996.

116. Rowland, T. W., Oxygen uptake and endurance fitness in children: a developmental perspective, *Ped. Exer. Sci.*, 1, 313, 1989.

117. Bar-Or, O., Metabolic response to acute exercise, in *Pediatric Sports Medicine*, Katz, M., and Carpentier, R. S., Eds., Springer-Verlag, New York, 1983, pp.3-4.

118. National Institutes of Health Consensus Conference, Physical activity and cardiovascular health, *J. Am. Med. Assoc.*, 276, 241, 1996.

119. Pickering, G. P., Fellmann, N., Morio, B., Ritz, P., Amonchot, A., Vermorel, M., and Coudert, J., Effects of endurance training on the cardiovascular system and water compartments in elderly subjects, *J. Appl. Physiol.*, 83, 1300, 1997.

120. Meredith, C. N., Frontera, W. R., Fisher, E. C., Hughes, V. A., Herland, J. C., Edwards, J., and Evans, W. J., Peripheral effects of endurance training in young and old subjects, *J. Appl. Physiol.*, 66, 2844, 1989.

121. Kohrt, W. M., Obert, K. A., and Holloszy, J. O., Exercise training improves fat distribution patterns in 60- to 70-year-old men and women, *J. Gerontol.*, 47, M99, 1992.

122. American College of Sports Medicine, The recommended quantity and quality of exercise for developing and maintaining cardiorespiratory and muscular fitness, and flexibility in healthy adults, *Med. Sci. Sports Exerc.*, 30, 975, 1998.

123. American Academy of Pediatrics, Policy statement on weight training and weight lifting: information for the pediatrician, *Phys. Sports Med.*, 11, 157, 1983.

124. Vrijens, J., Muscle strength development in the pre- and post-pubescent age, *Med. Sport*, 11, 152, 1978.

125. Docherty, D., Wenger, H. A., Collis, M. L., and Quinney, H. A., The effects of variable speed resistance training on strength development in prepubertal boys, *J. Hum. Mov. Stud.*, 13, 377, 1987.

126. American Academy of Pediatrics, Strength training, weight and power lifting, and body building by children and adolescents, *Pediatrics*, 86, 801, 1990.

127. Kraemer, W. J., fry, A. C., Frykman, P. N., Conroy, B., and Hoffman, J., Resistance training and youth, *Ped. Exer. Sci.*, 1, 336, 1989.

128. American Orthopaediatric Society for Sports Medicine, *Proceedings of the Conference on Strength Training and the Prepubescent*, Cahill, B. R., Ed., American Orthopaediatric Society for Sports Medicine, 1988.

129. Klitgaard, H. Mantoni, M., Schiaffino, S., Ausoni, S., Gorza, L., Lauren-Winter, C., Schnohr, P., and Saltin, B., Function, morphology and protein expression of aging skeletal muscle: a cross-sectional study of elderly men with different training backgrounds, *Acta. Physiol. Scand.*, 140, 41, 1990.

130. McCartney, N., Hicks, A. L., Martin, J., and Webber, C. E., Long-term resistance training in the elderly: effects on dynamic strength, exercise capacity, muscle, and bone, *J. Gerontol.*, 50A, B97, 1995.

131. Chandler, J. M., Duncan, P. W., Kochersberger, G., and Studenski, S., Is lower extremity strength gain associated with improvement in physical performance and disability in the frail, community-dwelling elder? *Arch. Phys. Med. Rehabil.*, 79, 24, 1998.

132. Fiatarone, M. A., Marks, E. C., Ryan, N. D., Meredith, C. N., Lipsitz, L. A., Evans, W. J., High-intensity strength training in nonagenarians: effects on skeletal muscle, *J. Am. Med. Assoc.*, 263, 3029, 1990.

CHAPTER 14

Body Weight Regulation and Energy Needs: Weight Loss

Janice L. Thompson and Melinda M. Manore

CONTENTS

14.1 INTRODUCTION

Weight loss among many athletes is a common goal. For certain sports, such as wrestling, distance running, gymnastics, and dance, a low body weight is considered a necessity for ensuring successful performance. In addition to performance pressures, athletes are also susceptible to societal pressures to be thin. This is especially true among many female athletes, and this drive for thinness can become obsessive, leading to disordered eating behaviors and potential health consequences. It has been reported that dieting is pervasive in our society, with approximately 40% of adult U.S. women attempting to lose weight.[1,2] Even more alarming is that 44% of high school-aged females (grades 9 through 12) reported trying to lose weight.[2]

When is it appropriate for an athlete to lose weight? There are situations in which weight loss in an athlete may be warranted. Some athletes may gain body fat in the off-season, and their performance is enhanced when they lose the excess body fat. However, there are also many circumstances in which the athlete or coaching staff may have unrealistic goals and expectations regarding body weight and performance. If weight loss appears necessary, what is the safest way to encourage weight loss in an athlete? The information presented in this chapter attempts to answer these questions. A review of energy balance, fuel oxidation, and the relationship of these factors to weight loss is included, as are discussions of safe and pathogenic weight loss strategies and health concerns that are consistently associated with weight loss among athletes. Weight loss in the athlete needs to be approached with care, prudence, and realistic expectations for all involved in the process.

14.2 MANIPULATION OF ENERGY BALANCE TO INDUCE WEIGHT LOSS

Weight loss is generally brought about by an imbalance between energy intake and energy expenditure. Energy intake can be intentionally reduced below the level of energy expenditure, or energy intake can remain stable while energy expenditure exceeds the level of energy intake. While manipulating energy balance appears simplistic, there are several factors that affect an individual's ability to lose weight. These factors include changes in the components of the energy balance equation and the manipulation of fuel oxidation through alterations in nutrient composition.

14.2.1   Energy Balance Equation

The energy balance equation states that body weight is maintained if energy intake equals energy expenditure. Energy intake is composed of all foods consumed, and the three components of total daily energy expenditure (TDEE) are the resting metabolic rate (RMR), thermic effect of food (TEF), and the energy expenditure due to physical activity. The RMR represents the energy expended to support all resting metabolic functions (e.g., maintaining body temperature, ventilation, cellular electrical activity, etc.). The TEF represents the energy expended as a result of digestion, absorption, transport, and storage of foods consumed. The energy cost of physical activity accounts for all activities done above resting level, including very low-level activities and high-intensity exercise bouts.

RMR has been reported to account for 60–75% of TDEE, and TEF and energy cost of physical activity account for 6–10% and 15–34% of TDEE, respectively.[3,4] Increasing total energy expenditure to result in weight loss can be accomplished by manipulating one or more of these three components.

14.2.2   Manipulation of the Components of Energy Balance Equation

Although it has long been claimed that exercise increases RMR, the effects of exercise on RMR are equivocal. Some cross-sectional studies comparing athletes to untrained subjects have found athletes to have significantly higher RMR values,[5,6] while Broeder et al.[7] found no difference in RMR among untrained and trained individuals. Results of training studies show that some individuals experience an increase in RMR with training,[8,9] while others do not.[10] It is likely that many factors affect one's metabolic response to exercise, including genetics and the type, intensity, and duration of exercise training. These factors may contribute to the inconsistencies in these data.

RMR is known to have a genetic component, with approximately 40% of the variability in RMR explained by genetics in twins and pairs of parents and children after adjusting for the influences of age, gender, and fat-free mass.[11] The type of training employed could impact the RMR. The strongest predictor of RMR is fat-free mass, with approximately 80% of the variance in RMR accounted for by fat-free mass (Figure 14.1).[3] It would seem that increasing one's fat-free mass through resistance training would increase fat-free mass and, in turn, increase RMR. Resistance training has been shown to increase fat-free mass,[12,13] but RMR did not increase with a 12-week resistance training program that resulted in a gain of fat-free mass of 1 kg.[13] Interestingly, Bosselaers et al.[14] found that body builders had a significantly higher absolute 24-hour energy expenditure than inactive controls, but this difference disappeared when adjustments were made for differences in fat-free mass among the two groups. Exercise has been found to prevent some of the decline in RMR that occurs with energy restriction,[15] but it appears to be protective only when energy restriction is not severe.[16]

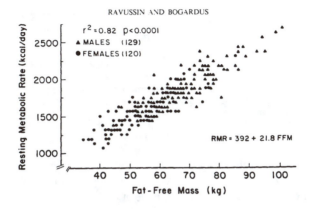

Figure 14.1 Relationship between resting metabolic rate and fat-free body mass in 249 nondiabetic Pima Indians (59 hidden observations). Note that 82% of the variance in resting metabolic rate can be attributed to the differences in fat-free body mass (r^2 = .82) and that the relationship is similar in men and women.

Exercise intensity and duration also impact RMR and TDEE. Fat is the predominant fuel source during endurance-type exercise of low- to moderate-intensity.[17] As exercise intensity increases above 60–70% of $\dot{V}O_{2\,max}$, carbohydrate contributes proportionately more energy than fat (Figure 14.2).[18] In addition, most individuals can perform low- to moderate-intensity exercise for a longer duration than high-intensity exercise, resulting in greater energy expenditure over time. These findings have led to the recommendation that weight loss is best achieved by performing moderate-intensity endurance-type exercise for 45–60 minutes.

A recent study by Tremblay et al.[19] challenges these recommendations. Individuals participating in high-intensity bicycling training were shown to have a greater reduction in skinfold thickness than individuals who performed moderate-intensity, continuous bicycling training. The high-intensity training reduced body fat more despite the fact that the energy cost of the high-intensity training was less than half of moderate-intensity training. The authors concluded that high-intensity training may significantly increase loss of body fat by affecting an increase in beta-oxidation enzyme activity. This study could have important implications for athletes trying to lose weight. As many athletes are fit and can perform high-intensity training on a regular basis, this type of training combined with moderate dietary restriction could result in desirable body fat changes.

In addition to its potential impact on RMR, exercise can also increase TDEE through an increase in energy expenditure above RMR during a brief period following the exercise bout. This increase in energy expenditure is referred to as excess post-exercise oxygen consumption (EPOC). Bahr et al. found that 80 minutes of exercise at 70% $\dot{V}O_{2\,max}$ significantly increased EPOC by 15%, as did performing three bouts of exercise at 108% $\dot{V}O_{2\,max}$ for two minutes per bout.[20] This elevation in EPOC occurred as long as four to 12 hours following exercise. Weight lifting has also been found to increase EPOC. Melby et al. found EPOC was elevated 5 to 10% above RMR

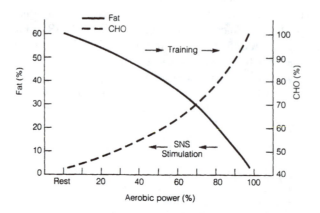

Figure 14.2 The balance of carbohydrate and lipid use during exercise is explained by the "cross-over concept." At low- to moderate-intensity exercise, carbohydrates and lipids both play major roles as energy substrates. However, when relative aerobic power output reaches 60–65%, carbohydrates (CHO) become increasingly important and lipids become less important. Because of the cross-over phenomenon, in most athletic activities, glycogen stores provide the greatest fuel for exercise. Lipids become important energy sources during recovery. SNS refers to the sympathetic nervous system and the metabolic effects of epinephrine and norepinephrine.

when measured the morning following resistance exercise.[21] Burleson et al. reported that EPOC was elevated at 30 and 90 minutes following weight training exercise that was performed for 27 minutes.[22] In this same study, treadmill running done at the same intensity and duration as weight training did not elevate EPOC. From these studies, it appears that endurance exercise of longer duration or exercise performed at higher intensities may be sufficient to increase EPOC, which would subsequently elevate TDEE.

The composition of the diet influences the TEF. Flatt reported that the thermogenic effects of carbohydrate (or glucose), protein, and fat are 5 to 10%, 20 to 30%, and 3 to 5% of the total energy consumed, respectively.[23] This means that little energy is needed to metabolize and store fat, while processing and storing protein and carbohydrate is less energy-efficient. The magnitude of TEF also depends on the total daily energy intake. As TEF accounts for 6 to 10% of the energy intake,[4] an individual with a daily energy intake of 2500 kcal per day would have a TEF of 150 to 250 kcal per day. To increase TEF, one would need to increase energy intake (which could result in positive balance and weight gain) or alter the nutrient composition of the diet. Because TEF accounts for a relatively small proportion of TDEE, attempts to alter TEF will have little significant impact on weight loss.

The third component of TDEE is the energy expended from performing physical activity. This component accounts for energy expended above RMR. The TDEE can be increased by performing exercises that cost more energy (e.g., jogging, running, cycling, etc.) and by spending less time doing low-level activities (e.g., sleeping less, walking instead of driving, exercising while watching television, etc.). Because the energy expended doing physical activities is the most variable of the three components of energy expenditure, it is the one most easily manipulated to result in weight loss. Increasing this component in some athletes is not practical, as they may already be exercising a great deal. In fact, it is common for many endurance athletes to expend 1000 to 2000 kcal per day while engaging in sport-related activities. Thompson et al. found that the RMR of a group of elite male endurance athletes accounted for only 38–47% of TDEE (as opposed to 60–75% in less active people) due to their high levels of training.[24] Thus, the present activity level of the athlete attempting to lose weight needs to be assessed before recommendations regarding physical activity can be made.

14.3 DIET COMPOSITION AND FUEL UTILIZATION

The ability of an individual to lose body weight and change body composition is influenced not only by alterations in energy intake and energy expenditure, but also by the oxidation rates of the nutrients that are consumed. It is now known that under normal physiological conditions, carbohydrate, protein, and alcohol are not readily converted to triglycerides or stored as adipose tissue.[25,26] This is due to an increased oxidation rate in response to intakes of carbohydrate, protein, and alcohol.

When carbohydrates are consumed, glycogen storage and glucose oxidation are increased, and fat oxidation is decreased (Figure 14.3).[27] The glucose that is not stored is utilized for energy.[27,28] As the carbohydrate that is eaten is utilized, little, if any, excess carbohydrate will be stored as body fat. Protein intake is also accompanied by an increase in protein oxidation, and any excess amino acids are deaminated and the carbon skeletons can be used to meet energy demands.[27] Alcohol is considered a priority fuel in that it is the primary fuel oxidized upon its consumption. Excess alcohol is not stored as fat. Although excess carbohydrate, protein, and alcohol are not directly stored as fat, they can indirectly contribute to body fat storage by providing alternative sources of fuel for oxidation. Thus, the excess energy remaining will be from the dietary fat consumed, and this excess energy is stored as adipose tissue.

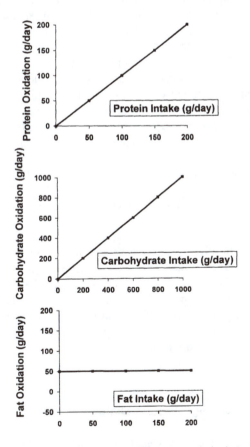

Figure 14.3 Relationship between intake and oxidation of protein, carbohydrate (CHO), and fat in 21 weight stable men (n = 11) and women (n = 10) after seven days of consuming a diet that contained 62% of energy from carbohydrate, 26% of energy from fat, and 12% of energy from protein.

The effect of inadequate energy or carbohydrate intake has a unique impact on protein balance, and it is a key concern for athletes attempting to lose weight. Inadequate intakes of carbohydrate or energy will result in a negative protein balance.[29] Thus, a higher protein/kcal ratio is required to maintain protein balance when energy or carbohydrate intake is insufficient. To prevent loss of fat-free mass, it is important that both carbohydrate and protein are eaten in adequate quantities to maximize protein sparing in the athlete attempting to lose body fat.

Fat balance differs from protein and carbohydrate balance in that the oxidation of fat does not increase proportionately with the increase in fat intake (Figure 14.3). The failure to oxidize dietary fat results in the excess energy consumed as dietary fat being stored in the adipose tissue. The variable responses to carbohydrate, protein, alcohol, and fat intake emphasizes the importance of nutrient composition when designing weight-loss programs for athletes.

14.3.1 High-Carbohydrate, Low-Fat Diets

According to the energy balance equation, weight loss will occur when energy intake is lower than energy expenditure. However, the composition of the diet can play an important role in the composition of the weight lost and in providing the energy necessary for exercise training. A common recommendation for weight loss is the consumption of a high-carbohydrate, low-fat diet. The previous discussion of fuel oxidation sheds light on how this type of diet can result in the loss of body fat. The consumption of excess energy results in fat storage due to the sparing of dietary fat, as it is the fuel least likely to be oxidized in proportion to its intake. Because excess carbohydrate is not readily stored as body fat, a high-carbohydrate, low-fat diet is less likely to result in body fat accumulation.

A high-carbohydrate, low-fat diet is defined as providing 60–65%, 20–25%, and 10–20% of total energy from carbohydrates, fat, and protein, respectively. Weight loss has been accomplished with this type of diet even when dieters are given *ad-libitum* access to food. The weight loss that accompanies *ad-libitum* food intake may be beneficial to athletes who maintain heavy training schedules while trying to lose body fat. Two primary mechanisms have been identified to explain weight loss despite *ad-libitum* food intake on high-carbohydrate diets. These mechanisms are as follows:

- Significantly less energy is consumed with a high-carbohydrate diet due to its higher fiber and lower fat content.[30-32]
- One feels less hungry when consuming a high-carbohydrate diet due to the increased bulk of the foods eaten.[30]

High-carbohydrate, low-fat diets that would benefit athletes include food plans comprised of an abundance of complex carbohydrate foods such as whole grains, fruits, and vegetables. It is very easy to consume a high-carbohydrate, low-fat diet by eating a diet high in simple carbohydrates. Simple carbohydrate foods include sugared beverages, hard candy, fruit juice, and low- or non-fat crackers and cookies. Although these types of food provide glucose, they do not supply many other nutrients (such as vitamins and minerals), and they easily lead one to consume excess energy. Although the excess simple carbohydrates will not likely be stored as fat, any dietary fat included in the plan that is not utilized for energy will be stored in the adipose, and body fat and weight gain will result.

14.3.2 Low-Carbohydrate, High-Protein Diets

A constant presence in the arena of weight loss plans is the low-carbohydrate, high-protein diet. Although packaged under a variety of names and marketing strategies, this type of diet is composed of foods that contain less than 45% of total energy intake from carbohydrate, more than 20% of total energy intake from protein, and the balance of energy derived from fat. There are two mechanisms proposed to support the use of the high-protein-type diet:

- Weight loss is faster than the loss achieved using higher carbohydrate plans.
- Reducing dietary carbohydrate will prevent the excessive production of insulin (or insulin "surges") that result from eating a high-carbohydrate meal; lower levels of insulin leads to reduced fat storage and improved glucose regulation.

The rate of weight loss is reported to be accelerated using very-low-energy, high-protein, low-carbohydrate diet plans.[33] In contrast, Golay et al. found no difference in the amount of weight lost using isocaloric (1000 kcal per day) diets containing either low carbohydrate (15% of energy from carbohydrate, 32% of energy from protein, and 53% of energy from fat) or higher carbohydrate (45% of energy from carbohydrate, 29% of energy from protein, and 26% of energy from fat).[34] One major disadvantage of applying a low-carbohydrate diet plan to the lifestyle of an athlete is that the body uses its carbohydrate stores for energy for all activities throughout the day. This will result in glycogen depletion, leaving the athlete with limited or no capability to perform high-intensity activities. Another disadvantage of a low-carbohydrate diet plan is that body weight decreases more rapidly due to the increased diuresis, or loss of body water, that accompanies the oxidation of stored carbohydrate. Although the weight loss goals are achieved, these diets leave one feeling lethargic, short-tempered, dehydrated, and unable to perform much physical activity. Carbohydrate is the most critical fuel for athletic performance, and consuming inadequate amounts of carbohydrate will hinder the athlete's ability to train and perform optimally, and it could lead to fluid and electrolyte imbalances that can be harmful.

Recent claims regarding the risks of consuming a high-carbohydrate diet include concerns about the regulation of glucose and insulin metabolism and the storage of excess carbohydrate as body fat. As insulin signals the cells to store glucose, amino acids, and fat, and dietary carbohydrate results in the secretion of insulin, dietary carbohydrate is claimed to be dangerous if consumed in large proportions, and it is blamed for insulin insensitivity, mood swings, and increased body fat. It is important to understand that much of the studies published on glucose/insulin regulation, weight loss, and responses to various diets included obese subjects, and individuals with Type II diabetes or other glucose regulation problems. These individuals are not the metabolic peers of highly trained athletes. Athletes have been reported to have improved glucose tolerance and insulin sensitivity,[35,36] and athletes could respond quite differently to the dietary regimens imposed upon obese, diabetic individuals. However, Tegelmen et al. found that hockey players who normally consumed a low-carbohydrate (45% of energy), high-fat (42% of energy) diet experienced a reduction in fasting insulin and insulin resistance when they consumed a higher-carbohydrate diet (52–58% of energy from carbohydrate, 25–30% of energy from fat, and 17–19% of energy from protein).[36] These findings show that although exercise training can improve glucose metabolism, dietary intake also plays a significant role in glucose and insulin regulation.

To insure glycogen repletion, it has been suggested that male athletes and larger female athletes try to consume at least 500 g (or 2000 kcal) of carbohydrate per day (8 to 10 g of carbohydrate per kg body weight). Smaller athletes, or athletes consuming lower energy intakes, should try to consume 6 to 8 g of carbohydrate per kg body weight to support training and competition.[17,37] These goals are not possible to achieve if one reduces both total energy and the amount of dietary carbohydrate consumed.

14.4 OPTIMAL BODY WEIGHT AND COMPOSITION FOR EXERCISE PERFORMANCE

There are numerous studies that show a negative relationship between body fat and performance.[38–41] Although body weight can affect performance in sports that require moving the body horizontally or vertically through space, the composition of the body, or amount of body fat, appears to be a more significant predictor of performance than body weight.[42,43] Examples of sports where lower body fat is advantageous include distance running, diving, gymnastics, wrestling, and figure skating. There is also a visual component to many sports, such as gymnastics and body building, which requires a lean physique for successful performance. There are many instances where fat mass, in adequate amounts, is advantageous. Examples include contact sports, where the application and absorption of force and momentum are critical components, and long-distance swimming, where fat mass assists with maintaining buoyancy and body temperature.[44]

Although all athletes need to be fit and prepared for competition, not all individuals should be classified into the same body weight category. Unfortunately many abuses of weight standards occur, and extreme dieting behaviors can lead to poor performance, illness, disordered eating behaviors, menstrual dysfunction in female athletes, and in extreme cases, death. How can healthy and responsible weight recommendations be made for athletes? In reality, weight standards for groups of athletes are not appropriate and should not be applied if at all possible. There are some sports, such as gymnastics, where physical appearance is critical to performance and closely linked with the maintenance of a relatively low body weight. Thus, it is important to assist these athletes with combining a competitive body weight with healthy eating practices.

The most effective strategy for assessing appropriate weight loss is to measure the body composition of the athlete, and if body fat levels are higher than is considered optimal, weight loss can be responsibly guided by reducing body fat and maintaining fat-free mass. A detailed description of the procedure to assist an athlete with healthy and responsible weight loss is provided later in this chapter (see Section 14.5). Assessment of body composition is helpful in determining both the levels of body fat and fat-free mass. Body composition is not error-free, however, and the results should be applied appropriately. Even with the best assessment methods used (e.g., hydrostatic weighing or dual-energy X-ray absorptiometry), the error in estimating percentage body fat ranges from 1 to 3%.[45] Using other methods increases this range of error. Using skinfold or bioelectrical impedence measures very carefully and applying the correct prediction equations will at best result in a prediction error of 3% body fat.[45,46] This means that if percentage of body fat is measured at 16%, actual percentage of body fat may be as low as 13% or as high as 19%. Because many individuals who assess body composition in athletes are not adequately trained, the prediction error will be even greater.

As with body weight standards, there are many abuses of values derived using measures of body composition. The following is an example of inappropriate use of skinfold measures in an athlete. A female distance runner has her body composition assessed using skinfold calipers. Her percentage of body fat is calculated to be 15% body fat. The team standard for body fat is 14%, and this athlete is instructed to lose approximately 10 pounds (4.5 kg) in an attempt to reduce her body fat to desirable levels. As just reviewed, even under the best circumstances of measurement this athlete's percentage body fat may be as low as 12% or as high as 18%. Thus, this athlete may already have a percentage of body fat within desirable ranges, and weight loss is not necessary. In addition, the goal for weight loss is based on an arbitrary decision and is not based on an athlete's existing body fat stores or performance ability. Lohman suggests that the minimal levels of percentage body fat that are compatible with health are 12% body fat for women and 5% body fat for men.[45] The scenario just presented is common, especially among collegiate athletic teams. In this type of situation, it is important not only to have realistic and healthy percentage body fat goals but to also measure body composition using another, preferably more accurate, method to get a clearer picture of whether this athlete has a percentage body fat that falls within desirable ranges.

Unfortunately, there are numerous situations in which starting lineups, scholarship status, and punitive exercise measures are determined solely upon an athlete's percentage of body fat. Athletes can also be devastated by the results of these tests, and they may be driven to extreme measures to reach a goal that may not be realistic. It is critical that the athlete, coach, and family of the athlete are aware of the limitations of body composition assessments to gain a realistic attitude toward ways to improve performance and avoid focusing on reducing body weight and body fat entirely as factors to enhance performance.

Table 14.1 illustrates ranges of percentage body fat for some sports.[47-68] This figure is not provided as a standard for all athletes to follow, but to give an example of the ranges of percentage

**Table 14.1 Ranges of Percentage Body Fat
for Athletes From a Variety of Sports**

Sport	Males	Females
Basketball	8–11	18–29
Volleyball	—[a]	21–27
Swimming	14[b]	16–24
Distance Running	10–11	14–20
Gymnastics	—[a]	13–23
Soccer	9–16	26[b]
Cycling	9–15	—[a]
Wrestling	9–11	—[a]
Combined Endurance Training	8–10	16–23

[a] Denotes no values reported.

[b] Denotes one published value.

body fat for athletes participating in various sports. Wilmore[69] and Berning and Steen[70] have also provided ranges for percentage fat among various sports. Referring to these values can assist an athlete and coach with setting realistic goals for percentage of body fat. If weight loss is indicated, it is important to maintain as much fat-free mass as possible. This can be accomplished by setting realistic body weight and body fat goals based upon the existing fat-free mass. The new goal weight can be calculated using the following formula:[69]

$$\text{Goal Weight} = \frac{\text{Fat-free mass}}{1 - \text{desired \% body fat}}$$

For example, a male basketball player has been measured at 230 pounds (104.5 kg) and 17% body fat. The goal for this player is to reduce body fat to a range of 10 to 13%. His current fat-free mass is 191 pounds (86.8 kg). Applying the range of desired percentage body fat values, this athlete's goal weight range is 212 to 220 pounds (96.4 to 100 kg). This calculation assumes that the athlete will lose predominantly fat mass, and maintain fat-free mass. Applying this equation to the previously discussed scenario with the female athlete, and assuming she weighs 115 pounds, or 52.3 kg, to reduce her percentage body fat from 15% to 13%, she would need to lose only 2 to 3 pounds (or 0.9 to 1.4 kg), not the 10 pounds (4.5 kg) recommended.

14.5 WEIGHT LOSS STRATEGIES

There are many strategies one can employ to lose weight. Although there are a variety of healthy plans an athlete can follow for weight loss, there also is an abundance of strategies available that can be harmful and potentially deadly for the athlete. A review of both safe and pathogenic weight loss strategies is provided in this section.

14.5.1 Safe Strategies

Successful and safe weight loss depends upon many factors. One critical factor is designing a program that will meet an athlete's needs. Because training and performance depend on sound nutrition, designing a program that addresses individual habits, food preferences, health needs, and training schedules will help ensure that the athlete will meet weight loss and performance goals.

Table 14.2 outlines the steps to follow when designing a weight loss plan for an athlete.[71,72] Although the athlete and coaching staff can use this information to design a weight loss program, it

Table 14.2. Steps to Follow When Designing a Weight Loss Plan for an Athlete

1.   Assess body composition using the most accurate method(s) available. Be sure that trained technicians are employed to determine body composition. Avoid using methods that show poor validity (e.g., Futrex 5000). Calculate a reasonable goal weight range for the athlete using the following equation:

$$\text{Goal weight} = \frac{\text{fat-free mass}}{1 - \text{desired \% body fat}}$$

2.   Assess current dietary intake using diet records.[1] Include information regarding dietary habits and time and places where food is consumed. Determine situations that may trigger the athlete to overeat.

3.   Determine the athlete's current activity level using activity records or published questionnaires.[1] Analyze the athlete's activity patterns. Are they optimal for inducing weight loss? If not, determine any adjustments that need to be made in daily activity patterns to increase total daily energy expenditure.

4.   Estimate energy balance by subtracting energy expenditure from energy intake. Energy restriction should equal approximately 500 kcal per day less than the current energy needed to maintain body weight. *Note: it is common for individuals to under-report energy intake (Black et al., 1993; Schoeller, 1995), and overweight individuals are more likely to report eating a lower energy intake than would be expected from activity levels (Edwards et al., 1993). If the energy intake of the athlete appears to be low, use either the energy expenditure estimate from the activity records or the mid-point value between reported energy intake and energy expenditure as the energy intake goal for weight loss.

5.   The diet plan should be designed so that it contains the percentage of total energy from carbohydrate, fat, and protein as 60–65%, 20–25%, and 10–20%, respectively. Larger male and female athletes should try to consume 500 g (or 8 to 10 g per kg body weight) of carbohydrate per day. For smaller male and female athletes, it is recommended that 6 to 8 g of carbohydrate per kg body weight be consumed. Protein needs of athletes are higher than the general population, and protein intake should be 1.5 to 2 g per kg body weight per day. Low-fat protein sources should be eaten, including lean meats, beans, soy products, and non-fat dairy products.

6.   All athletes on a reduced-energy diet plan should take a multivitamin and mineral supplement. Women may also need to take an additional calcium supplement. Iron supplementation can benefit those at risk for iron deficiency and anemia; taking iron supplements should be done under the supervision of a physician or a trained health professional.

7.   Encourage regular fluid intake. The minimum suggested water intake for sedentary people is 64 fluid ounces per day. Athletes, depending on training schedules and environmental conditions, may need to consume at least twice this amount. Use sport drinks when appropriate to provide adequate energy to train regularly, especially in hot environments.

8.   Encourage athletes to eat numerous, smaller meals throughout the day to reduce feelings of hunger.

9.   Encourage the athlete to maintain healthy dietary practices. Stress the importance of maintaining training and performance while achieving gradual weight loss of 1 to 2 pounds (or 0.5 to 0.9 kg) per week.

[1] For details on using diet and activity records to estimate energy balance, refer to Thompson and Manore, 1998.

is most beneficial to seek assistance from an individual trained in sports nutrition. Many universities have full- and part-time faculty who can assist athletes with meeting their weight loss goals, and there are registered dietitians working in the community who specialize in sports nutrition. If possible, weight loss should be accomplished during the off-season, as losing weight during the season can negatively impact training and performance. The ideal rate of weight loss is 1 to 2 pounds (0.5 to 0.9 kg) per week, as faster weight loss can lead to loss of fat-free mass.[69] Measuring the body composition, current dietary intake, and typical activity level of an athlete is necessary to determine the energy and macronutrient needs of the athletes. As discussed in Section 14.3, prescribing a high-carbohydrate diet for an athlete will help ensure adequate carbohydrate for training and glycogen repletion and will allow an athlete to eat numerous small meals, so hunger is less of a problem. It is also important to ensure that an athlete eats adequate protein, as protein requirements increase during situations of energy restriction. It is always a good idea for the athlete to take a general multivitamin/mineral supplement. This is especially critical for athletes who consume less than 2000 kcal per day.

14.5.2 Pathogenic Strategies

Pathogenic weight loss strategies include any behaviors or actions that are potentially harmful to the athlete. These strategies include restrained eating, binging and purging, skipping meals, excessive exercise, and dehydration. Although participating in these behaviors can lead to weight loss, athletes need to be educated about the risks of these types of behaviors.

Restrained eating can also be referred to as chronic dieting. It is common to find that restrained eaters are of normal body weight but desire to lose 5 to 10 pounds (2.3 to 4.5 kg).[73] As these individuals regularly restrict food intake, they are at increased risk for poor nutrient intakes. Restrained eaters do not have a clinical eating disorder such as bulimia nervosa or anorexia nervosa, but they may suffer from a sub-clinical eating disorder. Beals and Manore reported that female athletes with sub-clinical eating disorders reported having lower energy, protein, and fat intakes, while energy expenditure (assessed from activity records) was similar.[74]

Binging and purging are behaviors practiced by athletes participating in various sports and includes individuals with sub-clinical eating disorders and those diagnosed with bulimia nervosa. Weight-class athletes who participate in rapid weight-loss practices, such as wrestlers and boxers, also employ this practice to meet their assigned weight categories.[75] Binging includes consuming large quantities of food at one time, followed by purging using practices such as self-induced vomiting, laxatives, diuretics, and excessive exercise. Binging and purging are extremely dangerous practices and can lead to clinical eating disorders, tooth decay, poor performance, dehydration, and death due to fluid and electrolyte imbalances.[76,77]

Skipping meals can lead to overeating at subsequent meals and can also lead to more severe food restriction patterns. Adequate fuel is critical to maintain athletic practice and performance, and skipping meals will limit access to necessary nutrients. Excessive exercise is a form of purging and is commonly used by individuals to attempt to prevent storage of any excess energy that may be consumed. Our experiences have shown that many college females keep a meticulous count of kilocalories consumed over the day and use exercise as a means to punish self-proclaimed "bad" eating behaviors. Athletes should not deprive themselves of favorite foods or use excessive exercise as a punitive measure. To maintain health and performance capabilities, athletes need to eat healthy diets containing a variety of foods, and the exercise performed should be done to enhance fitness, health, and performance.[73]

Dehydration is a practice commonly used for rapid weight loss in athletes needing to "make weight." Wrestlers are athletes who dehydrate themselves by exercising intensely in hot environments while wearing vapor-impermeable suits. They may also combine this activity with fluid restriction, the use of diuretics and laxatives, and vomiting.[75] This practice is extremely dangerous and has been forbidden by the NCAA.[78] Despite attempts to prevent the use of dehydration to achieve rapid weight loss, these practices are still used by high school and collegiate-level wrestlers. Fogelholm reported that the effects of dehydration and rapid weight loss on exercise performance include a decrease in endurance exercise capacity, impaired anaerobic performance, and reduced muscular strength.[75] In extreme cases, death can result;[79] this consequence will be discussed in more detail in the following section.

14.6 HEALTH CONCERNS RELATED TO WEIGHT LOSS

Numerous health problems can result if weight loss is not approached using safe and healthy strategies. Some of the most common health concerns that can result from practicing pathogenic weight loss strategies are eating disorders, macro- and micronutrient imbalances, and inadequate fluid intakes. Each concern can negatively impact the health and performance of athletes. Although many athletes and coaches may view these problems as acute and having no long-term impact on health, the following evidence suggests that these concerns can seriously threaten the long-term health of an athlete.

14.6.1   Disordered Eating

Disordered eating behaviors, including clinical disorders such as anorexia nervosa and bulimia nervosa, are prevalent among athletes. Participation in disordered eating behaviors among athletes in aesthetic and weight-dependent sports (e.g., gymnastics, dance, distance running, and figure skating) are reported to be significantly higher than in the general population.[80] The prevalence of disordered eating in elite or world-class females athletes is reported to be as high as 50%.[81] Disordered eating is also prevalent among young female swimmers.[82] As previously mentioned, persistent dietary restriction can lead to binge eating, which can increase the risk of exhibiting a clinical eating disorder. These facts stress the importance of encouraging gradual weight loss among athletes who need to lose weight and discouraging the use of pathogenic weight loss strategies.

One negative health consequence related to disordered eating is menstrual dysfunction in female athletes. Menstrual dysfunction, which includes amenorrhea, oligomenorrhea, and sub-clinical ovulatory disturbances, also occurs in many female athletes who do not have an eating disorder. Physical and psychological stress, low energy intakes, low percentage of body fat, and intense training have been implicated in contributing to menstrual disturbances in female athletes.[83] An athlete's hormonal status, energy stores, and the severity of energy restriction interact to play a significant role in the onset of menstrual dysfunction. Figure 14.4 highlights a model illustrating the interaction of energy drain, or negative energy balance, with the aforementioned physiological factors in the development of menstrual dysfunction in female athletes.[83] The

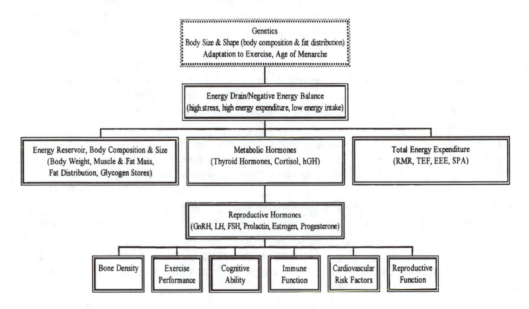

Figure 14.4 Model to illustrate the influence of energy drain on the development of menstrual dysfunction in active women and the potential health and performance outcomes due to low reproductive hormones and high cortisol levels. HGH = human growth hormone, GnRH = gonadotropin-releasing hormone, LH = luteinizing hormone, FSH = follicle-stimulating hormone, RMR = resting metabolic rate, TEF = thermic effect of food, EEE = exercise energy expenditure, SPA = spontaneous physical activity.

potential health problems associated with menstrual dysfunction also are identified and include decreased bone mineral density, impaired reproductive function, and increased risk for cardio-vascular disease.

14.6.2 Nutrient Imbalances

Energy restriction and dieting in athletes can pose difficulties when one is attempting to consume adequate levels of macro- and micronutrients. Many female athletes report consuming energy and nutrient intakes that are below 75% of the RDA.[84,85] Carbohydrate, iron, calcium, B-vitamins, folate, iron, and zinc are nutrients particularly affected by energy restriction among athletes. All of these nutrients are critical for optimal health and performance. Chronic under-consumption of these nutrients can lead to glycogen depletion, decreased oxygen-carrying capac-ity, increased incidence of bone fractures, and higher injury rates due to fatigue and impaired cell growth and repair. With these concerns in mind, athletes reducing body weight will benefit from taking a complete multivitamin and mineral supplement. Female athletes may also need to take supplemental calcium.

14.6.3 Inadequate Fluid Intakes

Fluid losses during exercise training can be quite large, and athletes must replenish fluids to maintain health and performance. Achieving rapid weight loss using dehydration and other patho-genic purging strategies can adversely affect thermoregulation, renal and cardiovascular function, nerve conduction, and electrolyte balance.[86–88] For more information regarding the effects of rapid weight loss on performance, refer to the review by Fogelholm.[75]

Wrestlers are a group of athletes known to regularly participate in dehydration to achieve rapid weight loss. Reductions in body weight of 4 to 8% over 12 to 96 hours have been reported.[89–91] The American College of Sports Medicine recommends that athletes should not compete at a body weight that places a wrestler at less than 5% body fat, and this weight is referred to as the minimum wrestling weight (MWW).[92] It is unclear how much body weight and percentage of body fat influence performance in wrestling. Horswill et al. found no relationship between first round success in a collegiate wrestling tournament and body weight;[93] in contrast, Wroble and Moxley reported that high school wrestlers who performed at a weight lower than MWW were the most successful in state-qualifying tournaments.[94]

The recent deaths of three collegiate wrestlers emphasize the risk of using dehydration to achieve rapid weight loss.[79] All three wrestlers used similar rapid weight-loss strategies over 3 to 12 hours, including restricted food and fluid intake and excessive exercise in hot environments while wearing vapor-impermeable suits. Preliminary reports suggest that death resulted from hyperthermia, which was induced by the use of pathogenic strategies. Reported weight loss for collegiate wrestlers is 16 pounds, or 10% of total pre-season body weight, and the three wrestlers who died lost an average of 30 pounds, or 15% of total pre-season weight.[79] It is obvious from these findings that practicing dehydration during periods of extreme weight loss can be fatal. Thus, strategies for maintaining regular fluid intake should be an integral part of a safe weight loss plan.

14.7 CONCLUSIONS AND RECOMMENDATIONS

It is apparent that a plethora of weight-loss strategies are available to athletes. The key to successful weight loss includes providing a diet plan that allows for maintenance of training, health, and performance. Pathogenic weight loss strategies, although used frequently by some athletes, should be avoided at all times. Table 14.3 reviews recommendations for healthy weight loss among

Table 14.3. Recommendations for Healthy Weight Loss for Athletes

1. The athlete should work with a coach, athletic trainer, team physician, and dietitian to determine if weight loss is necessary.
2. Realistic goals for weight loss should be determined. If possible, athletes should avoid weight loss during the season. If weight loss during the season is necessary, athletes must be closely monitored to ensure energy and nutrient intake is adequate to support health, training, and competition.
3. Athletes should be encouraged to eat a variety of foods. The focus should be on eating whole grains and five fruits and vegetables per day; this will help with optimizing fiber and nutrient intake from foods and should reduce hunger.
4. The athlete's diet should be designed to encourage healthy eating behaviors, such as reducing excess fat and saturated fat, avoiding foods that are high in calories, and eating only when hungry.
5. Breakfast should always be eaten, even if it is a small piece of fruit or bread. Athletes should avoid skipping meals, and carry food with them throughout the day to provide energy when needed.
6. The overweight athlete should avoid consuming alcoholic beverages and other forms of "empty" calories. Drinking alcohol will lead to increased fat storage, as dietary fat is less likely to be oxidized when alcohol is available for fuel.

athletes. It is hoped that athletes, coaches, and sport medicine professionals will use the information in this chapter to guide reasonable and healthy weight loss.

REFERENCES

1. Horm, J. and Anderson, K., Who in American is trying to lose weight?, *Ann. Intern. Med.*, 119, 672, 1993.
2. Serdula, M. K., Collins, M. E., Williamson, D. F., Anda, R. F., Pamuk, E., and Byers, T. E., Weight control practices of U.S. adolescents and adults, *Ann. Intern. Med.*, 119, 667, 1993.
3. Ravussin, E. and Bogardus, C., Relationship of genetics, age, and physical fitness to daily energy expenditure and fuel utilization, *Am. J. Clin. Nutr.*, 49, 968, 1989.
4. Poehlman, E. T., A review: exercise and its influence on resting energy metabolism in man, *Med. Sci. Sports Exer.*, 21, 515, 1989.
5. Poehlman, E. T., Melby, C. L., and Badylak, S. F., Resting metabolic rate and postprandial thermogenesis in highly trained and untrained males, *Am. J. Clin. Nutr.*, 47, 793, 1988.
6. Poehlman, E. T., Melby, C. L., Badylak, S. F., and Calles, J., Aerobic fitness and resting energy expenditure in young adult males, *Metabolism*, 38, 85, 1989.
7. Broeder, C. E., Burrhus, K. A., Svanevik, L. S., and Wilmore, J. H., The effects of aerobic fitness on resting metabolic rate, *Am. J. Clin. Nutr.*, 55, 795, 1992.
8. Tremblay, A., Fontaine, E., Poehlman, E. T., Mitchell, D., Perron, L., and Bouchard, C., The effect of exercise-training on resting metabolic rate in lean and moderately obese individuals, *Int. J. Obesity*, 10, 511, 1986.
9. Campbell, W. W., Crim, M. C., Young, V. R., and Evans, W. J., Increased energy requirements and changes in body composition with resistance training in older adults, *Am. J. Clin. Nutr.*, 60, 167, 1994.
10. Broeder, C. E., Burrhus, K. A., Svanevik, L. S., and Wilmore, J. H., The effects of either high-intensity resistance or endurance training on resting metabolic rate, *Am. J. Clin. Nutr.*, 55, 802, 1992.
11. Bouchard, C., Tremblay, A., Nadeau, A., Després, J. P., Thériault, G., Boulay, M. R., Lortie, B., Lablanc, C., and Fournier, G., Genetic effect in resting and exercise metabolic rates, *Metabolism*, 38, 364, 1989.
12. Ballor, D. L., Katch, V. L., Becque, M. D., and Marks, C. R., Resistance weight training during caloric restriction enhances lean body weight maintenance, *Am. J. Clin. Nutr.*, 47, 19, 1988.
13. Van Etten, L. M. L. A., Westerterp, K. R., and Verstappen, F. T. J., Effect of weight-training on energy expenditure and substrate utilization during sleep, *Med. Sci. Sports Exer.*, 27, 188, 1995.
14. Bosselaers, I., Buemann, B., Victor, O. J., and Astrup, A., Twenty-four-hour energy expenditure and substrate utilization in body builders, *Am. J. Clin. Nutr.*, 59, 10, 1994.

15. Thompson, J. L., Manore, M. M., and Thomas, J. R., Effects of diet and diet-plus-exercise programs on resting metabolic rate: a meta-analysis, *Int. J. Sport Nutr.*, 6, 41, 1996.

16. Donnelly, J. E., Jacobsen, D. J., Jakiei, J. M., and Whatley, J. E., Very low calorie diet with concurrent versus delayed and sequential exercise, *Int. J. Obesity*, 18, 469, 1994.

17. Coyle, E. F., Substrate utilization during exercise in active people, *Am. J. Clin. Nutr.*, 61(suppl), 968S, 1995.

18. Brooks, G. A., Fahey, T. D., and White, T. P., *Exercise Physiology: Human Bioenergetics and Its Applications*, Mayfield Publishing Company, Mountain View, CA, 1996, 117.

19. Tremblay, A., Simoneau, J., and Bouchard, C., Impact of exercise intensity on body fatness and skeletal muscle metabolism, *Metabolism*, 43, 814, 1994.

20. Bahr, R., Ingnes, I., Vaage, O., Sejersted, O. M., and Newsholme, E. A., Effect of duration of exercise on excess postexercise O_2 consumption, *J. Appl. Physiol.*, 62, 485, 1987.

21. Melby, C., Scholl, C., Edwards, G., and Bullough, R., Effect of acute resistance exercise on post-exercise energy expenditure and resting metabolic rate, *J. Appl. Physiol.*, 75, 1847, 1993.

22. Burleson, M. A., Jr., O'Bryant, H. S., Stone, M. H., Collins, M. A., and Triplett-McBride, T., Effect of weight training exercise and treadmill exercise on post-exercise oxygen consumption, *Med. Sci. Sports Exer.*, 30, 518, 1998.

23. Flatt, J. P., The biochemistry of energy expenditure, in *Obesity*, Bjorntorp, P. and Brodoff, B.N., Eds., Lippincott Co., Philadelphia, 1992, chap. 8.

24. Thompson, J., Manore, M. M., and Skinner, J. S., Resting metabolic rate and thermic effect of a meal in low- and adequate-energy intake male endurance athletes, *Int. J. Sport Nutr.*, 3, 194, 1993.

25. Swinburn, B. and Ravussin, E., Energy balance or fat balance?, *Am. J. Clin. Nutr.*, 57(suppl), 766S, 1993.

26. Abbott, W. G. H., Howard, B. V., Christin, L., Freymond, D., Lillioja, S., Boyce, V. L., Anderson, T. E., Bogardus, C., and Ravussin, E., Short-term energy balance: relationship with protein, carbohydrate, and fat balances, *Am. J. Physiol.*, 255, E332, 1988.

27. Thomas, C. D., Peters, J. C., Reed, G. W., Abumrad, N. N., Sun, M., and Hill, J. O. Nutrient balance and energy expenditure during ad libitum feeding of high-fat and high-carbohydrate diets in humans, *Am. J. Clin. Nutr.*, 55, 934, 1992.

28. Schutz, Y., Flatt, J. P., and Jéquier, E., Failure of dietary fat intake to promote fat oxidation: a factor favoring the development of obesity, *Am. J. Clin. Nutr.*, 50, 307, 1989.

29. Krempf, M., Hoerr, R. A., Pelletier, V. A., Marks, L. A., Gleason, R., and Young, V. R., An isotopic study of the effect of dietary carbohydrate on the metabolic fate of dietary leucine and phenylalanine, *Am. J. Clin. Nutr.*, 57, 161, 1993.

30. Duncan, K. H., Bacon, J. A., and Weinsier, R. L., The effects of high and low energy density diets on satiety, energy intake, and eating time of obese and nonobese subjects, *Am. J. Clin. Nutr.*, 37, 763, 1983.

31. Lissner, L., Levitsky, D. A., Strupp, B. J., Kalkwarf, H. J., and Roe, D. A., Dietary fat and the regulation of energy intake in human subjects, *Am. J. Clin. Nutr.*, 46, 886, 1987.

32. Tremblay, A., Plourde, G., Deprés, J. P., and Bouchard, C., Impact of dietary fat content and fat oxidation on energy intake in humans, *Am. J. Clin. Nutr.*, 49, 799, 1989.

33. Blackburn, G.L., Lynch, M. E., and Wong, S. L., The very-low-calorie diet: a weight-reduction technique, in *Handbook of Eating Disorders: Physiology, Psychology, and Treatment of Obesity, Anorexia, and Bulimia*, Brownell, K. D., and Foreyt, J. P., Eds., Basic Books, New York, 1986, chap. 10.

34. Golay, A., Allaz, A-F., Morel, Y., de Tonnac, N., Tankova, S., and Reaven, G., Similar weight loss with low- or high-carbohydrate diets, *Am. J. Clin. Nutr.*, 63, 174, 1996.

35. Ebeline, P., Bourey, R., Koranyi, L., Tuominen, J. A., Groop, L. C., Henriksson, J., Mueckler, M., SoviJarvi, A., and Koivisto, V. A., Mechanism of enhanced insulin sensitivity in athletes. Increased blood flow, muscle glucose transport protein (GLUT-4) concentration, and glycogen synthase activity, *J. Clin. Invest.*, 92, 1623, 1993.

36. Tegelman, R., Åberg, T., Eklöf, R., Pousette, Å., Carlström, K., and Berglund, L., Influence of a diet regimen on glucose homeostasis and serum lipid levels in male elite athletes, *Metabolism*, 45, 435, 1996.

37. O'Keeffe, K. A., Keith, R. E., Wilson, G. D., and Blessing, D. L., Dietary carbohydrate intake and endurance exercise performance in trained female cyclists, *Nutrition Research*, 9, 819, 1989.

38. Leedy, H. E., Ismail, A. H., Kessler, W. V., and Christian, J. E., Relationships between physical performance items and body composition, *Research Quarterly*, 36, 158, 1965.

39. Katch, F. I., McArdle, W. D., Czula, R., and Pechar, G. S., Maximal oxygen uptake, endurance running performance, and body composition in college women, *Research Quarterly*, 44, 301, 1973.

40. Cureton, K. J. and Sparling, P. B., Distance running performance and metabolic responses to running in men and women with excess weight experimentally equated, *Med. Sci. Sports Exer.*, 12, 288, 1980.

41. Pate, R. R., Barnes, C., and Miller, W., A physiological comparison of performance-matched female and male distance runners. *Research Quart. Exer. Sport*, 56, 245, 1985.

42. Malina, R. M., Physique and body composition: effects on perfomance and effects on training, semistarvation, and overtraining, in *Eating, Body Weight, and Performance in Athletes*, Brownell, K. D., Rodin, J., and Wilmore, J. H., Eds., Lea & Febiger, Philadelphia, 1992, pp. 94-114.

43. Pate, R. R., Slentz, C. A., and Katz, D. P., Relationships between skinfold thickness and performance of health related fitness test items, *Research Quart. Exer. Sport*, 60, 183, 1989.

44. Sinning, W. E., Body composition and athletic performance, in *Limits of Human Performance*, Clarke, D. H. and Eckert, H. M., Eds., Human Kinetics, Champaign, IL, 1985, pp. 45-56.

45. Lohman, T. G., *Advances in Body Composition Assessment*, Human Kinetics, Champaign, IL, 1992, 7.

46. Lukaski, H. C., Methods for the assessment of human body composition: traditional and new, *Am. J. Clin. Nutr.*, 46, 537, 1987.

47. Johnson, G. O., Nebelsick-Gullett, L. J., Thorland, W. G., and Housh, T. J., The effect of a competitive season on the body composition of university female athletes, *J. Sports Med. Phys. Fit.*, 29, 314, 1989.

48. Nichols, D. L., Sanborn, C. F., Bonnick, S. L., Gench, B., and DiMarco, N., Relationship of regional body composition to bone mineral density in college females, *Med. Sci. Sports Exer.*, 27, 178, 1995.

49. Mokha, R. and Sidhu, L. S., Body fat in various sportive groups, *J. Sports Med.*, 27, 376, 1987.

50. Nowak, R. K., Knudsen, K. S., and Schulz, L. O., Body composition and nutrient intakes of college men and women basketball players, *J. Am. Dietetic Assoc.*, 88, 575, 1988.

51. Bale, P., Anthropometric, body composition and performance variables of young elite female basketball players, *J. Sports Med. Phys. Fit.*, 31, 173, 1991.

52. Siders, W. A., Bolonchuk, W. W., and Lukaski, H. C., Effects of participation in a collegiate sport season on body composition, *J. Sports Med. Phys. Fit.*, 31, 571, 1991.

53. Bolonchu, W. W., Lukaski, H. C., and Siders, W. A., The structural, functional, and nutritional adaptation of college basketball players over a season, *J. Sports Med. Phys. Fit.*, 31, 165, 1991.

54. Meleski, B. W. and Malina, R. M., Changes in body composition and physique of elite university-level female swimmers during a competitive season, *J. Sports Sci.*, 3, 33, 1985.

55. Roby, F. B., Buono, M. J., Constable, S. H., Lowdon, B. J., and Tsao, W. Y., Physiological characteristics of champion synchronized swimmers, *Physic. Sportsmed.*, 11, 136, 1983.

56. Phillips, S. M., Atkinson, S. A., Tarnopolsky, M. A., and MacDougall, J. D., Gender differences in leucine kinetics and nitrogen balance in endurance athletes, *J. Appl. Physiol.*, 75, 2134, 1993.

57. Luc'a, A., Chicharro, J. L., Pérez, M., Serratose, L., Bandrés, F., and Legido, J. C., Reproductive function in male endurance athletes: sperm analysis and hormonal profile, *J. Appl. Physiol.*, 81, 2627, 1996.

58. Fogelholm, G. M., Kukkonen-Harjola, T. K., Taipale, S. A., Sievänen, H. T., Oja, P., and Vuori, I. M., Resting metabolic rate and energy intake in female gymnasts, figure-skaters and soccer players, *Int. J. Sports Med.*, 16, 551, 1995.

59. Moffatt, R. J., Surina, B., Golden, B., and Ayres, N., Body composition and physiological characteristics of female high school gymnasts, *Research Quart. Exer. Sport*, 55, 80, 1984.

60. Vercruyssen, M. and Shelton, L., Intraseason changes in the body composition of collegiate female gymnasts, *J. Sports Sci.*, 6, 205, 1988.

61. Kirkendall, D. T., The applied sport science of soccer, *Physic. Sportsmed.*, 13, 53, 1985.

62. Maughan, R. J., Energy and macronutrient intakes of professional football (soccer) players, *Brit. J. Sports Med.*, 31, 45, 1997.

63. Giada, F., Vigna, G. B., Vitale, E., Baldo-Enzi, G., Bertaglia, M., Crecca, R., and Fellin, R., Effect of age on the response of blood lipids, body composition, and aerobic power to physical conditioning and deconditioning, *Metabolism*, 44, 161, 1995.

64. Enns, M. P., Drewnowski, A., and Grinker, J. A., Body composition, body size estimation, and attitudes towards eating in male college athletes, *Psychosomatic Medicine*, 49, 56, 1987.

65. Song, T. M. K. and Cipriano, N., Effects of seasonal training on physical and physiological function on elite varsity wrestlers, *J. Sports Med.*, 24, 123, 1984.

66. Laughlin, G. A., and Yen, S. S. C., Nutritional and endocrine-metabolic aberrations in amenorrheic athletes, *J. Clin. Endocrin. Metabol.*, 81, 4301, 1996.

67. Ryan, A. S., Nicklas, B. J., and Elahi, D., A cross-sectional study on body composition and energy expenditure in women athletes during aging, *Am. J. Physiol.*, 271, E916, 1996.

68. Meredith, C. N., Zackin, M. J., Frontera, W. R., and Evans, W. J., Dietary protein requirements and body protein metabolism in endurance-trained men, *J. Appl. Physiol.*, 66, 2850, 1989.

69. Wilmore, J. H., Body weight standards and athletic performance, in *Eating, Body Weight and Performance in Athletes. Disorders of Modern Society*, Brownell, K.D., Rodin, J., and Wilmore, J.H., Eds., Lea & Febiger, Philadelphia, 1992, chap. 20.

70. Berning, J. S. and Steen , S. N., *Sports Nutrition for the 90's. The Health Professional's Handbook*, 1st edition, Aspen Publishers Inc., Gaithersburg, MD, 1991, p. 265.

71. Thompson, J. L. and Manore, M. M., Energy balance, in *Nutrition for Sports and Exercise*, Berning, J.R. and Steen, S.N., Eds., Aspen Publishers Inc., Gaithersburg, MD, 1998, 167–186.

72. Manore, M. M. and Ryan, M., Nutrient intake assessment, in *Sports Nutrition: A Guide for the Professional Working with Active People*, 2nd edition, Benardot, D.., Ed., American Dietetic Association, Chicago, 1993, p. 52.

73. Manore, M. M., Running on empty. *ACSM's Health Fit. J.*, 2, 24, 1998.

74. Beals, K .A. and Manore, M. M., Nutritional status of female athletes with subclinical eating disorders, *J. Am. Dietetic Assoc.*, 98, 419, 1998.

75. Fogelholm, M., Effects of bodyweight reduction on sports performance, *Sports Medicine*, 18, 249, 1994.

76. Eichner, E. R., General health issues of low body weight and undereating in athletes, in *Eating, Body Weight and Performance in Athletes: Disorders of Modern Society*, Brownell, K., Rodin, J., and Wilmore, J., Eds., Lea & Febiger, Phildelphia, 1992, pp. 191-201.

77. Pomeroy, C. and Mitchell, J. Medical complications and management of eating disorders, *Psychiatry Annals*, 19, 488, 1989.

78. National Collegiate Athletic Association, *NCAA Sports Medicine Handbook*, 9th edition, National Collegiate Athletic Association, Overland Park, Kansas, 1997.

79. Division of Nutrition and Physical Activity, Hyperthermia and dehydration-related deaths associated with intentional rapid weight loss in three collegiate wrestlers—North Carolina, Wisconsin, and Michigan, *Morbidity and Mortality Weekly*, 47, 105, 1998.

80. Rosen, L. W., McKeag, D. B., Hough, D. O., and Curley, V., Pathogenic weight control behavior in female athletes, *Physic. Sportsmed.*, 14, 79, 1986.

81. Houtkooper, L. B., Exercise and eating disorders, in *Perspectives in Exercise Science and Sports Medicine. Exercise, Nutrition, and Control of Body Weight*, Lamb, D. and Murray, Eds., Cooper Publishing Group, City, 1998.

82. Dummer, G. M., Rosen, L. W., Heusner, W. W., Roberts, P. J., and Counsilman, J. E., Pathogenic weight-control behaviors of young competitive swimmers, *Physic. Sportsmed.*, 15, 75, 1987.

83. Dueck, C. A., Manore, M. M., and Matt, K .S., Role of energy balance in athletic menstrual dysfunction, *Int. J. Sport Nutr.*, 6, 165, 1996.

84. Benardot, D. , Schwarz, M., and Heller, D. W., Nutrient intake in young, highly competitive gymnasts, *J. Am. Dietetic Assoc.*, 89, 401, 1989.

85. Benson, J., Gillien, D. M., Bourdet, K., and Loosli, A. R., Inadequate nutrition and chronic calorie restriction in adolescent ballerinas, *Physic. Sportsmed.*, 13, 79, 1985.

86. Horswill, C. A., Applied physiology of amateur wrestling, *Sports Medicine*, 14, 114, 1992.

87. Steen, S. N. and Brownell, K. D., Patterns of weight loss and regain in wrestlers: has the tradition changed? *Med. Sci. Sports Exer.*, 22, 762, 1990.

88. Sawka, M. N., Young, A. J., Francesconi, R. P., Muza, S. R., and Pandolf, K. B., Thermoregulatory and blood responses during exercise at graded hypohydration levels, *J. Appl. Physiol.*, 59, 1394, 1985.

89. Webster, S., Rutt, R., and Weltmen, A., Physiological effects of a weight loss regimen practiced by college wrestlers, *Med. Sci. Sports Exer.*, 22, 229, 1990.

90. Zambraski, E. J., Foster, D. T., Gross, P. M., and Tipton, C. M., Iowa wrestling study: weight loss and urinary profiles of collegiate wrestlers, *Med. Sci. Sports Exer.*, 8, 105, 1976.

91. Klinzing, J. E. and Karpowicz, W., The effect of rapid weight loss and rehydration on a wrestling performance test, *J. Sports Med. Phys. Fit.*, 26, 149, 1986.

92. Thorland, W. G., Tipton, C. M., Lohman, T. G., Bowers, R. W., Housh, T. J., Johnson, G. O., Kelly, J. M., Oppliger, R. A., and Tcheng, T. K., Midwest wrestling study: prediction of minimal weight for high school wrestlers, *Med. Sci. Sports Exer.*, 23, 1102, 1991.

93. Horswill, C. A., Scott, J. R., Dick, R. W., and Hayes, J., Influence of rapid weight gain after the weigh-in on success in collegiate wrestlers, *Med. Sci. Sports Exer.*, 26, 1290, 1994.

94. Wroble, R. R. and Moxley, D. P., Weight loss patterns and success rates in high school wrestlers, *Med. Sci. Sports Exer.*, 30, 625, 1998.

CHAPTER **15**

Body Weight Regulation and Energy Needs: Weight Gain

Jenna Anding

CONTENTS

15.1 INTRODUCTION

Adverse health consequences are not strictly limited to the obese. Individuals who are significantly underweight, defined as a body mass index (weight in kilograms/height in meters[2]) less than 20,[1] could be a sign of undernutrition. In males, being underweight can negatively impact performance and increase their risk of sustaining injury.[2] Underweight females are prone to poor performance and increased injuries, but they also experience amenorrhea and bone demineralization, which increases their risk for developing osteoporosis.[2] For some individuals, heredity plays a defining role in their leanness. For others, medical, economic, and psychological factors contribute to being underweight. For underweight individuals, a comprehensive physical exam should be conducted to rule out any underlying illness that may be impairing nutrient intake and metabolism. Psychological, social, and economic factors related to eating disorders and poverty, should also be examined and addressed as needed.

This chapter focuses on athletes who have a need to gain weight or "bulk up" for reasons unrelated to medical illnesses, eating disorders, or economic hardships. More specifically, this chapter addresses the nutritional and physiological needs of athletes who desire to gain weight to improve their physical appearance or enhance their athletic performance. For these individuals, the challenge is to increase their body weight by building lean body mass, not by adding additional pounds of adipose tissue. This will require the athlete to adopt a lifestyle that includes not only a healthy diet but also exercise — more specifically resistance training.

15.2 NUTRITIONAL CONSIDERATIONS FOR INCREASING LEAN BODY TISSUE

15.2.1 Energy

Energy intake plays a significant role in the athlete's ability to gain lean body tissue just as it does in the athlete who is trying to lose body fat. Theoretically, the overweight athlete must induce a negative energy balance of 3500 kcal, either by reducing caloric intake or increasing energy expenditure, to lose 1 pound of body fat. For the athlete trying to gain weight, it might seem logical that if one reversed the energy balance, the opposite would occur. Unfortunately, this is not the case if the athlete is trying to gain muscle.

An estimated 70% of muscle is water.[3] Approximately one-fifth of the tissue is protein, with carbohydrate, fat, and minerals comprising the remaining 8%. Based on this composition, one pound of muscle equals an estimated 700 to 800 kcals.[3] However, to synthesize one pound of muscle, the energy requirements greatly exceed 800 kcal. The National Research Council[4] suggests that five additional kilocalories are required to nourish the growth and development of 1 g of muscle. Because one pound of muscle equals 454 grams, individuals striving to increase their lean muscle mass must increase their energy intake by an estimated 2500 kcal (10,500 kilojoules).[4] Manjarrez and Birrer[5] and Pearson[6] have suggested that a slow rate of weight gain is more likely to result in an increase in lean muscle than adipose tissue. Therefore, it is recommended that the athlete increase his/her caloric intake by 700 to 1000 kcal per day to promote a maximum weight gain of 0.7 kg per week.[7]

15.2.2 Macronutrients

Adding extra kilocalories to one's daily intake might seem effortless for non-athletes. For many athletes, however, ingesting enough energy to promote lean body tissue synthesis can be challenging because their energy requirements are typically higher in comparison to their non-athletic counterparts.[3] Moreover, the muscle-gaining athlete must be selective with respect to the foods selected because food choices play an integral role in the success an athlete has in muscle synthesis.

15.2.2.1 Protein

Athletes generally believe protein is one of the most important dietary factors that impact one's gain lean body tissue.[8] According to Lemon, this belief has been debated in the literature as early as the 1840s when von Liebig[9,10] hypothesized that the primary fuel utilized during times of physical activity was protein. Subsequent research recanted that hypothesis[4,11,12] but more recent research[13–16] appears to be leaning in favor of the hypothesis that athletes have higher protein requirements than non-athletes. This may be due to a better understanding of protein intake and its effect on nitrogen balance and muscle synthesis particularly during times of resistance/strength training. Recommendations for protein intake range from 0.8 grams/kg body weight/day to 2.0 grams/kg body weight/day.[4,10,17] The recommendation of 0.8 grams/kg body weight/day reflects the Food and Nutrition Board's Recommended Dietary Allowances (RDA).[4] However, researchers have made the argument that the RDAs reflect energy and nutrient needs of average adults, most of who are sedentary.[17]

Lemon has recommended a protein intake that represents 12 to 15% of total energy intake.[17–19] Because an athlete's energy requirements are higher than non-athletes, this would obviously result in an increase in the grams of protein consumed per kilogram of body weight. More specifically, protein recommendations for strength/resistance training athletes range from 1.2 to 1.8 grams/kg body weight/day.[10,17] Recommendations for protein among endurance athletes are slightly lower, ranging from 1.2 to 1.4 grams/kg body weight/day.[10] Because research suggests that the protein requirements for athletes are generally higher during the initial two to three weeks of resistance training,[19] beginning athletes might want to consider consuming at the high end of the recommended range for protein during the beginning stages of training. Most athletes can meet the recommended level of protein by eating a balanced diet.

It is well known that athletes often exceed the recommended levels of protein in part from the usage of specialized supplements. There has been a concern among dieticians and nutritionists that excessive protein intakes might have adverse physiological consequences, including a compromise in renal function[20] and an increase in urinary calcium excretion.[21] Excessive protein intake, especially if derived from high-fat animal products, may place an individual at risk for the development of cardiovascular disease[2] and may be counterproductive to the athlete who is trying to control his/her percentage body fat. Lemon[19] has counteracted these concerns by noting that the previously reported connection between high-protein intake and renal disease was based on a study with patients who already had existing renal disease. Furthermore, it has been argued that the demonstrated calcium losses have been with purified proteins, which were inadequate in phosphate. By increasing the phosphate intake in a manner that would naturally reflect the consumption of protein from food sources, the urinary losses of calcium could be prevented.[23] Still, there is no scientific basis to support the promotion of diets that exceed more than 2.0 g of protein/kilogram body weight/day.[10]

In recent years, individual amino acids have received a great amount of attention with respect to their proposed effects on muscle tissue generation. Numerous amino acid supplements sold in gyms and health food stores, including those with arginine and ornithine, claim to enhance muscle growth and development by promoting the secretion of human growth hormone.[22,23] Research studies supporting these claims, however, are inconclusive. Elam[24] supplemented inactive males daily with 1 g of both arginine and ornithine or a placebo, five days a week for a five-week period. During this period, subjects were instructed to follow a prescribed resistance training regimen, which was completed three times a week. Body mass index, percentage body fat, and composite body girth were measured prior to and at the end of the study. Subjects receiving the amino acid supplements demonstrated an average reduction in body fat by 8.45%, which was significantly higher than the 1.6% reduction reported by the control group. Although diet was not a variable addressed in this study and serum levels of human growth hormone were not examined, the authors concluded that these amino acids promoted more positive anthropometric changes than would have be seen from resistance training alone.

Elam and colleagues[25] reported similar results one year later when they supplemented sedentary males with either 1 g each of ornithine and arginine or a placebo and evaluated body composition and total strength after five weeks of resistance training. Serum levels of human growth hormone were not measured. Instead, urinary hydroxyproline, an indirect measure of the body's ability to recover from stress, was measured.[25] This post-test study did not examine or control dietary intake except during the 24-hour period in which the urinary hydroxyproline was measured. Subjects in the experimental group demonstrated significantly higher lean body mass and total strength and significantly lower levels of urinary hydroxyproline in comparison to the placebo group. In addition, the urinary hydroxyproline was much lower among subjects in the experimental group, leading the authors to conclude that these subjects were able to recover from the resistance training and generate more significant results with their resistance training because of the amino acid supplementation.

Elam's hypothesis that arginine and ornithine promote an increase in human growth hormone secretion have been supported by Bucci et al. who reported an increase in serum growth hormone among trained athletes 90 minutes after ingesting 170 mg of ornithine per kilogram of body weight.[26] Isidori et al. also demonstrated that a combination of arginine and lysine (1200 mg each) could stimulate growth hormone release levels in humans. However, when supplemented individually, the effect on growth hormone release was much lower.[27] Other studies[28–32] have not substantiated the claim that these amino acids stimulate an increase in growth hormone.

In addition to its proposed ability to promote human growth hormone release, ornithine is also being touted as a stimulant for insulin secretion.[33] Bucci et al.[34] studied the effect of varying degrees of ornithine supplementation on insulin release among trained body builders (three females and nine males). Subjects were administered an oral dose of 40, 100, and 170 mg of ornithine per kilogram of body weight on three mornings, one week apart, following an overnight fast. Regardless of the dosage, oral ornithine supplementation failed to induce an increase in insulin secretion and at the highest dose caused gastrointestinal distress among subjects. Other researchers have reported similar findings with respect to ornithine's inability to promote insulin release.[35,36]

Because the data does not clearly support the use of amino acid supplements, athletes would be wise to use these supplements with great caution, if at all. As previously noted, excessive amounts of ornithine can result in gastrointestinal distress.[34] Furthermore, excessive intakes of individual amino acids may impair the absorption of other vital amino acids[37] and have been reported to generate toxic consequences.[37–39]

15.2.2.2 Carbohydrate

If caloric intake becomes inadequate, dietary protein is sacrificed to meet the required energy needs of the body. To prevent this from occurring, athletes are encouraged to consume the majority of their energy requirements from carbohydrates.

Athletes who alter their diet and exercise regimen to promote muscle synthesis should try to consume approximately 60 to 65% of their energy from carbohydrate.[2] According to Snyder and Naik,[2] consuming adequate carbohydrates can help promote an increase in insulin levels, which is believed to aid in muscle synthesis, especially when combined by an increased protein intake. Furthermore, Volek et al.[40] have suggested that consuming a diet composed of 15% protein and 60% carbohydrate (a 1:4 ratio) can increase resting levels of testosterone, another anabolic hormone known to stimulate muscle synthesis.

15.2.2.3 Fat

Dietary fat contains approximately 9 kcal per gram, providing twice the amount of energy contributed from carbohydrates (4 kcal per gram). The effects of high-fat diets (reaching up to 90% of the energy from fat) on athletic performance have been studied on short- and long-term levels without any conclusive results. Notwithstanding, if an athlete consumes 15% of his energy from protein and 60% of his energy from carbohydrate, then only 25% of the energy remaining can come from fat. This level falls within several recommendations calling for athletes to limit their dietary fat to 20% to 30% of total energy.[41] Although there is limited research that suggests that higher-fat diets might improve athletic performance among endurance athletes,[42] the efficacy of high-fat diets for weight-training athletes have not been clearly demonstrated and therefore not recommended at this time.

15.2.3 Vitamins

Vitamins play important roles in energy metabolism as well as red blood cell production and connective tissue repair. Antioxidants, including vitamin C, beta carotene, and vitamin E provide protective benefits from free radicals and lipid peroxidation.[6,43,44] B-vitamins, which include thiamin, riboflavin, niacin, vitamin B6, and pantothenic acid, play vital roles in the metabolism of energy, which is why the recommended intakes are partly based on energy intake. Because weight-gaining athletes have higher energy intakes than non-athletes, it has been argued that the current recommended dietary intakes might not be adequate for athletes.[43] However, this is generally not a concern for the athlete who consumes a varied diet. Likewise, there is no conclusive research to suggest that athletes will be able to enhance their muscle building potential by consuming megadoses of selected vitamins.[43,45] A multivitamin/mineral supplement that provides no more than 100% of the RDA is a practice accepted by most registered dietitians, especially when the athlete consumes a restrictive diet or presents with multiple food intolerances or aversions. A multivitamin/mineral supplement, however, is no substitute for a well-balanced diet and exercise.

15.2.4 Minerals and Trace Elements

Few minerals have been studied for their ability to promote lean tissue development. Yet as with the vitamins, mineral supplements with the promise of increased muscle development are abundant.

Early reports regarding the potential of boron to increase serum testosterone levels helped launch this mineral into the spotlight among weight-training athletes.[45] The report was later discounted[3] and a subsequent study by Ferrando and Green[46] demonstrated not only a lack of testosterone increase but also a lack of improvement in strength and lean body mass as a result of boron supplementation. Although not currently recognized as an essential nutrient for humans, a recommended range of acceptable intake between 500 to 1000 micrograms has been suggested.[47] Meeting this level should not be difficult because it can easily be obtained through the consumption of plant foods, with high amounts of the mineral reported in dried fruits and nuts.[47] Given boron's unproven anabolic abilities, further supplementation is not advised.

Chromium is an essential trace element that has been shown to potentiate the action of insulin.[48] It is often combined with picolinate and other compounds to increase its bioavailability.[49] Research suggests that most Americans fail to consume diets that contain the estimated safe and adequate daily dietary intake (ESADDI), which ranges from 50 micrograms to 200 micrograms.[4] Inadequate intakes combined with early research suggesting that chromium increased muscle mass and reduces body fat[50,51] have probably contributed to its popularity among body builders and athletes desiring to gain muscle. Unfortunately, subsequent and more well-controlled studies have disputed these claims.[52–54] Although insulin resistance may occur when a chromium deficiency is present, there are not enough well-controlled research studies to support the widely promoted anabolic properties of this mineral. Weight-gaining athletes are advised to consume food high in chromium, including mushrooms, asparagus, brewer's yeast, and prunes.[55] Consuming a supplement that contains no more than 200 micrograms of chromium may be beneficial if food preferences or dietary practices prohibit the inclusion of chromium-rich foods.[55] Ingesting more than the ESADDI is not advised, however, because of the concern that excessive supplementation may impair the absorption of other vital minerals, including iron.[53]

Magnesium is an essential mineral known for its role in more than 300 enzymes and for its involvement in all metabolic processes that involve adenosine triphosphate (ATP). Muscle contraction is also linked to magnesium.[3,4] The RDA for magnesium among adult males and females is 350 mg and 280 mg, respectively.[4] Although Americans are believed to consume diets inadequate in magnesium, deficiencies have not been reported.[4] Still, the link between magnesium and muscle contraction is intriguing and several researchers have investigated magnesium's effects on lean muscle mass and strength. Brilla and Haley[56] supplemented 26 untrained male subjects with either 8 mg/kg/body weight/day magnesium or a placebo while the subjects underwent strength training for seven weeks. Although both groups reported gains in quadriceps muscle torque, the gains were significantly higher among the experimental group in comparison to the control.[56] Studies by

Terblance et al.[57] and McDonald and Keen,[58] however, did not find any benefit of magnesium supplementation.

Vanadium is another trace mineral in which essentiality in humans has not been determined. The mineral is believed to enhance the action of insulin, although the exact mechanism is not known.[49] Because of its possibility to act in an anabolic manner, vanadium is often promoted as a muscle builder when supplemented in the diet as vanadyl, vanadate, or vanadyl sulfate. In clinical trials, non-insulin-dependent diabetics supplemented with vanadyl sulfate have shown improvements in glucose control and decreased hepatic insulin resistance.[59,60] In weight-training subjects supplemented orally with 0.5 mg/kg body weight/day of vanadyl sulfate for 12 weeks, Fawcett et al.[61] reported that the mineral was ineffective in promoting an increase in muscle tissue. The subjects did demonstrate a significant increase in selected performance parameters, leading the authors to postulate the possibility that vanadium enhances performance, particularly during the first month of use. No other human studies to date have examined the mineral's effectiveness on muscle synthesis, although the popularity of this mineral remains strong. Nielsen has suggested that consuming 10 micrograms per day should be sufficient to meet any proposed physiological requirement.[62] Ingesting vanadium in amounts as high as 18 mg per day might result in adverse outcomes, includinggastrointestinal disturbances, diarrhea, and a reduction in food intake.[62] Using this mineral to obtain its proposed anabolic effects does not appear to be prudent at this time.

15.3 RESISTANCE TRAINING

Weight loss cannot be maintained without exercise. The same principle can be applied to athletes gaining muscle. For athletes trying to lose weight, aerobic exercise is recommended with anaerobic exercise (i.e., resistance training) for the added development of muscle. The weight-gaining athlete, however, is more likely to focus primarily on resistance training rather than aerobic activities. Although energy is required for both types of exercise, less energy is required for resistance training, commonly known as weight training.[3]

Williams[3] has identified five principles of resistance training that are important for the athlete attempting to increase muscle tissue. The first principle is known as the overload principle and refers to mechanism by which weight training promotes muscle hypertrophy. By lifting weights, muscles are stressed and stimulated to grow to compensate for the increased resistance brought about by the weight training.[63–66]

The second principle is progressive resistance exercise.[3] Because resistance training encourages increased strength through muscle growth, at some point the athlete will be able to lift the current amount of weight without difficulty. When this occurs, the stress initially placed on the muscle will be diminished. Therefore, the amount of resistance placed on the muscle will need to be increased to maintain the stimulus of growth, either by increasing the amount or number of times (repetitions and sets) the weight is lifted.[67] Using the third principle, specificity, an athlete can increase strength and size of muscles by choosing the resistance exercises targeted towards selected muscle groups.

The principle of exercise sequence relates to the practice of conducting resistance training in a manner to avoid muscle fatigue early in the exercise routine.[3] If fatigue occurs early in the exercise routine, the athlete will not be able to lift the weight necessary to stress the muscle, which is required for continued growth.

The fifth principle reflects the muscle's need for rest to recover from the induced stress. Weight training has been shown to rapidly deplete high-energy compounds, when performed correctly. Because the body may require up to three minutes to restore these compounds, Williams[3] has recommended that athletes rest for several minutes between sets of the same exercise. In addition, it is recommended that athletes who are at the beginning stages of weight training rest for 24 hours between workouts to allow time for the repair and synthesis of muscle tissue.[3]

Resistance exercises are typically categorized as isometric, isotonic, or isokinetic, depending on the degree of muscular tension and movement that occurs when resistance is placed on the muscle.[68] The success an athlete has with resistance training depends to an extent on training frequency as well as hormonal factors (androgen to estrogen ratios).[67] It has also been suggested that athletes who have a high percentage of fast-twitch muscles will achieve a greater increase in lean tissue development in comparison to those with lower amounts of this muscle type.[67] Monitoring weight, percentage body fat, and other anthropometric measurements can help evaluate the athlete's progress. Is should be noted that athletes should seek instruction for resistance training from a qualified expert before embarking on this component of the weight gain regime. Furthermore, the American College of Sports Medicine recommends that men and women over the age of 45 and 55, respectively, obtain a physical examination by their physician, before beginning this or any type of exercise program.[69]

15.4 ERGOGENIC SUPPLEMENTS

Ergogenic aids, in addition to the amino acids and minerals previously discussed, are promoted for their ability to enhance an athlete's ability to gain weight. Several ergogenic aids are targeted at athletes who desire to enhance the growth and development of lean tissue beyond what would be expected from diet and resistance training.

Creatine, a nitrogenous compound synthesized from the amino acids arginine, glycine, and methionine, is produced by the liver, kidneys, and pancreas at an estimated rate of 1 g per day.[70] A varied diet that includes meat and fish has been reported to provide an additional gram of creatine daily.[71] Creatine phosphate is formed in the muscle when creatine combines with phosphate and regenerates the ATP required for muscle contractions.[72] As discussed elsewhere in this volume, creatine supplementation has been reported to be beneficial in weight-training athletes and in athletes performing anaerobic activities.[73–75] Endurance athletes have not been reported to benefit from this supplement.[76]

Other ergogenic aids targeted at strength athletes include conjugated linoleic acid (CLA), beta-hydroxy beta-methylbutyrate (HMB), L-carnitine, and yohimbe. Conjugated linoleic acid is an 18-carbon fatty acid that occurs in animal food, primarily dairy products, beef, and lamb.[77] Animal studies have suggested CLA has antitumor[78] and antioxidant[79] effects and may regulate the manner in which body fat is deposited.[80] Published studies demonstrating any ergogenic benefits in humans do not exist.

Beta-hydroxy beta-methylbutyrate (HMB) is produced by the body during the metabolism of leucine, a branched-chain amino acid.[81] Nissen[82] reported that weight-training males supplemented with HMB (1.5 or 3.0 g per day) demonstrated a reduction in the amount of muscle damage, increased the amount of weight lifted, and increased the amount of fat-free mass in comparison to the control group. However, no other human studies confirming these outcomes with HMB supplementation have been published.

These and other supplements marketed as ergogenic aids have not been studied on a long-term basis. In addition, most of the investigations surrounding the potential ergogenic effects of these compounds have been conducted using mostly male subjects. Because the long-term safety and the possibility of interactions between multiple supplements are not yet understood, athletes should proceed with caution in the use of these ergogenic aids.

15.5 CONCLUSIONS AND RECOMMENDATIONS

Weight-gaining athletes are challenged to adopt a diet and exercise program that will allow them to increase their weight through the synthesis of lean body tissue. Although the energy and protein requirements to support muscle growth and development should be increased, there is no scientific reason why the nutritional needs cannot be met through the consumption of a nutrient-dense, well-balanced diet. A general multivitamin and mineral supplement that provides no more than 100% of the RDA may be beneficial for athletes with special dietary restrictions, but the scientific literature does not support the efficacy of excessive dosages. Resistance training is a key component in stimulating muscle synthesis and must be incorporated in the athlete's exercise program. Although some ergogenic supplements, particularly creatine, may have some merit, others are unproven at best and may have adverse side effects. More research, including long-term studies, needs to be conducted before any recommendations regarding their use can be proposed.

REFERENCES

1. Committee on Diet and Health, Food and Nutrition Board, *Diet and Health: Implications for Reducing Chronic Disease Risk*. National Academy Press, Washington, D.C., 1989.
2. Wilmore J. H., Body weight standards and athletic performance, in *Eating, Body Weight, and Performance in Athletes*, Brownell K. D., Rodin J., and Wilmore J. H., Eds., Philadelphia: Lea & Febiger, 1992; 315-329.
3. Williams, M. H., *Nutrition for Fitness & Sport*, 4th ed., Benchmark, Chicago, IL, 1995.
4. Food and Nutrition Board, Commission on Life Sciences, National Research Council. *Recommended Dietary Allowances*, 10th ed., National Academy Press, Washington, D.C., 1989.
5. Manjarrez C. and Birrer R.B. Nutrition and athletic performance. *AFP*, 28, 105, 1983.
6. Pearson, R. L., *Nutrition in Sports, in Sports Medicine for the Primary Care Physician*, Birrer R. B., Ed. CRC Press LLC, Boca Raton, FL, 1994. pp 100-101.
7. Fahey T. and Brown C., The effects of an anabolic steroid on the strength, body composition, and endurance of college males when accompanied by a weight training program, *Med. Sci. Sports Exerc.*, 5, 272, 1973.
8. Grandjean, A.C., Current nutritional beliefs and practices in athletes for weight/strength gains, in *Muscle Development: Nutritional Alternatives to Anabolic Steroids*, Garrett W. E., Jr. and Malone, T.R., Eds., Columbus, Ross Laboratories, 1988, pp. 56-61.
9. Von Liebig, J., Animal Chemistry or Organic Chemistry in Its Application to Physiology and Pathology (translated by W. Gregory). London, Taylor & Walton, 1942.
10. Lemon, P.W.R., Do athletes need more dietary protein and amino acids? *Int. J. Sport Nutr.*, 5, S39, 1995.
11. Durnin, J.V.G.A., Protein requirements and physical activity, in *Nutrition, Physical Fitness and Health*, Parizkova, J. and Rogozkin V.A., Eds., Baltimore, University Park Press, 1978.
12. Hickson, J. F. Jr., Wolinsky, I., Rodriguez, G. P., Pivarnik, J. M., Kent, M.C., and Shier, N. W., Repeated days of body building exercise do not enhance urinary nitrogen excretions from untrained young males. *Nutr. Res.*, 10, 723, 1990.
13. Chesley, A., MacDougall, J. D., Tarnoppolsky, M.A., Atkinson, S. A., and Smith, K., Changes in human muscle protein synthesis after resistance exercise, *J. Appl. Physiol.*, 73, 1383, 1992.
14. Marable, N. L., Hickson, J. F., Korslund, M. K., Herbert, W. G., Desjardins, R. F., and Thye, F. W., Urinary nitrogen excretion as influence by a muscle-building exercise program and protein intake variation, *Nutr. Rep. Int.*, 19, 795, 1979.
15. Fern, E. B., Bielinski, R. N., and Schultz, Y., Effects of exaggerated amino acid and protein supply in man, *Experientia*, 47, 168, 1991.
16. Laritcheva, K. A., Yalovaya, N. I., Shubin, V. I., and Smirnov, P. V., Study of energy expenditure and protein needs of weight lifters, in *Nutrition, Physical Fitness, and Health*, Parizkova J. and Rogozkin V.A., Eds., University Park Press, Baltimore, 1978, pp 155-163.
17. Lemon, P. W. R., Protein and exercise: update 1987, *Med. Sci. Sport Exer.*, 19, S179, 1987.
18. Lemon, P. W. R., Effect of exercise on protein requirements, *J. Sports Sci.*, 9 Spec No., 53, 1991.
19. Lemon, P. W. R., Protein and amino acid needs of the strength athlete, *Int. J. Sport Nutr.*, 1, 127, 1991.
20. Allen, L. H., Oddoye, E. A., and Margen, S., Protein-induced hypercalciuria: A longer term study, *Am. J. Clin. Nutr.*, 32, 741, 1979.

21. Lemon, P. W., Yarasheski, K. E., and Dolny, D. G., The importance of protein for athletes. *Sports Med.*, 1, 474, 1984.

22. Vanhelder, W. P., Radmonski, M. W., and Goode, R. C., Growth hormone responses during intermittent weight lifting exercise in men. *Eur. J. Appl. Physiol.*, 51, 31, 1984.

23. MacDougall, J. D., Ward, G. R., Sale, D. G., and Sutton, J. R., Biochemical adaptation of human skeletal muscle to heavy resistance training and immobilization. *J. Appl. Physiol.*, 43, 700, 1977.

24. Elam, R. P., Morphological changes in adult males from resistance exercise and amino acid supplementation. *J. Sports. Med.*, 28, 35, 1988.

25. Elam, R. P., Hardin, D. H., Sutton, R. A. L., and Hagen, L. O., Effects of arginine and ornithine on strength, lean body mass and urinary hydroxyproline in adult males. *J. Sports Med.*, 29, 52, 1989.

26. Bucci, L. R., Hickson, J. F., Wolinsky, I., and Pivarnik, J. M., Ornithine supplementation and insulin release in bodybuilders. *Int. J. Sport Nutr.*, 2, 287, 1992.

27. Isidori, A., Lo Monaco, A., and Cappa, M., A study of growth hormone release in man after oral administration of amino acids, *Curr. Med. Res. Opin.*, 7, 475, 1981.

28. Suminski, R.R., Robertson, R. J., Goss, F. L., Arslanian, S., Kang, J., DaSilva, S., Utter, A.C., and Metz, K. F., Acute effect of amino acid ingestion and resistance exercise on plasma growth hormone concentration in young men, *Int. J. Sport Nutr.*, 7, 48, 1997.

29. Walberg-Rankin, J., Hawkins, C. E., Fild, D. S., and Sebolt, D. R., The effect of oral arginine during energy restriction in male weight trainers, *J. Strength Cond. Res.*, 8, 170, 1994.

30. Fogelholm, G. M., Naveri, H. K., Kiilavuori, K. T. K and Harkonen, M. H. A., Low-dose amino acid supplementation: No effects on serum human growth hormone and insulin in male weightlifters, *Int. J. Sport Nutr.*, 3, 290, 1993.

31. Lambert, M. I., Hefer, J. A., Millar, R. P., and Macfarlane, P. W., Failure of commercial oral amino acid supplements to increase serum growth hormone concentrations in male body-builders, *Int. J. Sport Nutr.*, 3, 298, 1993.

32. Fry, A. C., Kraemer, W. J., Stone, M. H., Warren, B. J., Kearney, J. T., Maresh, C. M., Weseman, C. A., and Fleck, S. J., Endocrine and performance responses to high volume training and amino acid supplementation in elite junior weightlifters, *Int. J. Sport. Nutr.*, 3, 306, 1993.

33. Hatfield, F.C., Without insulin, muscles don't grow! *Muscle & Fitness*, 5, 70, 1990.

34. Bucci, L., Hickson, J. F., Pivarnik, J. M., Wolinsky, I., McMahon, J. C., and Turner, S. D., Ornithine ingestion and growth hormone release in bodybuilders, *Nutr. Res.*, 10, 239, 1990.

35. Cynober, L., Coudray-Lucas, C., de Bandt, J. P., Guechot, J., Aussel, C., Salvucci, M., and Giboudeau, J., Action of ornithine alpha-ketoglutarate, ornithine hydroxholoride and calcium alpha-ketoglutarate on plasma amino acid and hormonal patterns in healthy subjects, *J. Am. Coll. Nutr.*, 9, 2, 1990.

36. Cynober, L., Vaubourdolle, M., Dore, A., and Giboudeau, J., Kinetics and metabolic effects of orally administered ornithine-alpha-ketoglutarate in healthy subjects with a standardized regimen, *Am. J. Clin. Nutr.*, 39, 514, 1984.

37. Harper, A. E., Benevenga, N. J., and Wohlheuter, R. M., Effects of ingestion of disproportionate amounts of amino acids, *Physiol. Rev.*, 50, 428, 1970.

38. Benevenga, N. J. and Steele, R. D., Adverse effects of excessive consumption of amino acids, *Ann. Rev. Nutr.*, 4, 157, 1984.

39. Hargrove, D. M., Rogers, Q. R., Calvert, C. C., and Moris, J. G., Effects of dietary excesses of branched-chain amino acids on growth, food intake, and plasma amino acid concentrations in kittens, *J. Nutr.*, 118, 311, 1988.

40. Volek, J., Draemer, W., Bush, J., Incledon, T., and Boetes, M., Testosterone and cortisol in relationship to dietary nutrients and resistance exercise, *J. Appl. Physiol.*, 82, 49, 1997.

41. Hawley, J. A., Dennis, S. C., Lindsay, F. H., and Noakes, T. D., Nutritional practices of athletes: Are they sub-optimal?, *J. Sport Sci.*, 13, S75, 1995.

42. Lambert, E. V., Speechly, D. P., Dennis, S. C., and Noakes, T. D., Enhanced endurance in trained cyclists during moderate intensity exercise following 2 weeks adaptation to a high fat diet, *Eur. J. Appl. Physiol.*, 69, 287, 1994.

43. Belko, A. Z., Vitamins and exercise — an update, *Med. Sci. Sport Exer.*, 19, S191, 1987.

44. Burke, L. M. and Read, R. S. D., Sports Nutrition: Approaching the Nineties, *Sports Med.*, 8, 80, 1989.

45. Nielsen, F. H., Hunt, C. D., Mullen, L. M., and Hunt, J.R. Effect of dietary boron on mineral estrogen, and testosterone metabolism in postmenopausal women, *FASEB J.*, 1, 394, 1987.

46. Ferrando, A. A. and Green, N. R., The effect of boron supplementation on lean body mass, plasma testosterone levels, and strength in male body builders, *Int. J. Sport. Nutr.*, 3, 140, 1993.

47. Nielsen, F., Facts and Fallacies about boron, *Nutr. Today*, 27, 6, 1992.

48. Mertz, W. and Roginski, E.E., The effect of trivalent chromium on galactose entry in rat epididymal fat tisue, *J. Biol. Chem.*, 238, 868, 1963.

49. Moore. R. J. and Friedl. K. E., Physiology of nutritional supplements: chromium picolinate and vanadyl sulfate, *Nat. Strength Cond. Assoc. J.*, 14, 47, 1992.

50. Evans, G. W., The effect of chromium picolinate on insulin controlled parameters in humans, *Int. J. Biosocial. Res.*, 11, 163, 1989.

51. Hasten, D. L., Rome, E. P., Franks, B. D., and Hegsted, M., Effects of chromium picolinate on beginning weight training students, *Int. J. Sport. Nutr.*, 2, 343, 1992.

52. Clancy, S. P., Clarkson, P. M., DeCheke, M. E., Nosaka, K., Freedson, P. S., Cunningham, J. J., and Valentine, J. J., Effects of chromium picolinate supplementation on body composition, strength, and urinary chromium loss in football players, *Int. J. Sport. Nutr.*, 4, 142, 1994.

53. Lukaski, H. C., Bolonchuk, W. W., Siders, W. A., and Milne, D.B., Chromium supplementation and resistance training: effects on body composition, strength and trace element status in men, *Am. J. Clin. Nutr.*, 63, 954, 1996.

54. Hallmark, M. A., Reynolds, T. H., DeSouza, C. A., Dotson, C. O., Anderson, R. A., and Rogers, M. A., Effects of chromium and resistive training on muscle strength and body composition, *Med. Sci. Sports Exerc.*, 28, 139, 1996.

55. Clarkson, P. M., Effects of exercise on chromium levels. Is supplementation required?, *Sports Med.*, 23, 341, 1997.

56. Brilla, L. R. and Haley, T. F., Effect of magnesium supplementation on strength training in humans, *J. Am. Coll. Nutr.*, 1992; 11:326-329.

57. Terblance, S., Noakes, T., Dennis, S., Marais, D., and Eckert, M., Failure of magnesium supplementation to influence marathon running performance or recovery in magnesium-replete subjects, *Int. J. Sport. Nutr.*. 1992; 2:154-164.

58. McDonald, R. and Keen, C.. Iron, zinc and magnesium nutrition and athletic performance, *Sports Med.*, 1988; 5:171-184.

59. Halberstam, M., Cohen, N., Shlimovich, P., Rossetti, L., and Shamoon, H., Oral vanadyl sulfate improves insulin sensitivity in NIDDM but not in obese nondiabetic subjects, *Diabetes*, 45, 659, 1996.

60. Boden, G., Chen, X., Ruiz, J., van Rossum, G. D., and Turco, S., Effects of vanadyl sulfate on carbohydrate and lipid metabolism in patients with non-insulin dependent diabetes mellitus, *Metabolism*, 45, 1130, 1996.

61. Fawcett, J. P., Farquhar, S. J., Walker, R. J., Thou, T., Lowe, G., and Goulding, A., The effect of oral vanadyl sulfate on body composition and performance in weight-training athletes, *Int. J. Sport. Nutr.*, 6, 382, 1996.

62. Nielsen, F. H., Other trace elements, in *Present Knowledge in Nutrition* 7th ed. Ziegler, E.E. and Filer, L.H., Jr. Eds., Washington, D.C.: International Life Sciences Institute, 1998 pp. 353-377.

63. Cullinen, K. and Caldwell, M., Weight training increases fat-free mass and strength in untrained young women, *J. Am. Diet. Assoc.*, 98, 414, 1998.

64. Chilibeck, P.D., Calder, A. W., Sale, D. G., and Webber, C. E., A comparison of strength and muscle mass increase during resistance training in young women, *Eur. J. Appl. Physiol.*, 77, 170, 1998.

65. McCall, G. E., Byrnes, W. C., Dickinson, A., Pattany, P. M., and Fleck, S. J., Muscle fiber hypertrophy, hyperplasia, and capillary density in college men after resistance training, *J. Appl. Physiol.*, 81, 2004, 1996.

66. O'Hagan, F. T., Sale, D. G., MacDougall, J. D., and Garner, S. H., Response to resistance training in young women and men, *Int. J. Sports Med.*, 16, 314, 1995.

67. McArdle, W. D., Katch, F. I., and Katch, V. L., *Exercise Physiology: Energy, Nutrition, and Human Performance*, 4th ed. Williams & Wilkins, Baltimore, 1996, pp 427.

68. Kendrick, Z. V., Exercise Physiology: Implications for Sports Nutrition, in *Nutrition for Sport & Exercise*, 2nd ed. Bering, J. R., Steen, S. N. Eds., Aspen, Gaithersburg, 1998.

69. American College of Sport Medicine. *ACSM's Guidelines for Exercise Testing and Prescription*. 5th ed. Baltimore, Williams and Wilkins; 1995.

70. Balsom, P. D., Soderlund, K., and Ekblom, B., Creatine in humans with special reference to creatine supplementation, *Sports Med.*, 18, 268, 1994.
71. Hoogwerf, B. F., Laine, D. C., and Greene, E., Urine C-peptide and creatine (Jaffe method) excretion in healthy, young adults on varied diets: sustained effects of varied carbohydrate, protein, and meat content, *Am. J. Clin. Nutr.*, 43, 350, 986.
72. Eichner, E. R., Ergogenic Aids. What athletes are using — and why, *Phys. Sportsmed.*, 25, 70, 1997.
73. Kreider, R. B., Ferreira, M., Wilson, M., Grindstaff, P., Plisk, S., Reinardy, J., Cantler, E., and Almada, A. L., Effects of creatine supplementation on body composition, strength, and sprint performance, *Med. Sci. Sports Exerc.*, 30,73,1988.
74. Jacobs, I., Bleue, S., and Goodman, J., Creatine ingestion increases anaerobic capacity and maximum accumulated oxygen deficit, *Can. J. Appl. Physiol.*, 22, 231,1997.
75. Soderlund, K., Balsom, P. D., and Ekblom, B., Creatine supplementation and high-intensity exercise; influence on performance and muscle metabolism, *Clin. Sci.*, 87, (suppl), 120, 1994.
76. Balsom, P. D., Harridge, S. D. R., Soderlund, K., Sjodin, B., and Ekblom, B., Creatine supplementation per se does not enhance endurance exercise performance, *Acta. Physiol. Scand.*, 149, 521, 1993.
77. Kohlmeier, L., Simonsen, N., and Mottus, K., Dietary modifiers of carcinogenesis, *Environ. Health Perspec.*, 103, 177, 1995.
78. Belury, M. A., Nickel, K. P., Bird, C. E., and Wu, Y., Dietary conjugated linoleic acid modulation of phorbol ester skin tumor promotion, *Nutr. Cancer.*, 26, 149, 1996.
79. Decker, E. A., The role of phenolics, conjugated linoleic acid, carnosine, and pyrroloquinoline quinone as nonessential dietary antioxidants, *Nutr. Rev.*, 53, 49, 1995.
80. Park, Y., Albright, K. J., Liu, W., Storkson, J. M., Cook, M. E., and Pariza, M. W., Effect of conjugated linoleic acid on body composition in mice, *Lipids*, 32, 853, 1997.
81. Nonnecke, B., Franklin, S. T., and Nissen S., Leucine and its capabilities alter mitogen-stimulated DNA synthesis by bovine lymphocites, *J. Nutr.*, 121, 1665, 1991.
82. Nissen, S., Sharp, R., Ray, M., Rathmacher, J. A., Rice, D., Fuller, J. C., Jr, Connelly, A. S., and Abumrad, N., Effect of leucine metabolite beta-hydroxy-beta-methylbutyrate on muscle metabolism during resistance-exercise training, *J. Appl. Physiol.*, 81, 2095, 1996.

Summary

CHAPTER 16

Summary—Energy-Yielding Macronutrients and Energy Metabolism in Sports Nutrition

Ira Wolinsky and Judy A. Driskell

CONTENTS

16.1 INTRODUCTION

After water, the most important requirement to sustain life is a source of endogenous energy. And the most important fuel is, of course, food. Without sufficient energy, the supply of other required nutrients is without effect. Athletes, both recreational and professional, have used a wide variety of aids to enhance performance and give them the competitive edge. Of all possible performance aids (nutritional, biomechanical, mechanical, physical, physiological, psychological, pharmacological), nutritional aids, and nutritional practices have been very popular. Ergogenics (from the Greek word ergon meaning work) is the production of energy, and ergogenic aids are nutrients employed to improve energy production, energy control, or energy efficiencies during exercise or sport and, therefore heighten performance. Foodstuffs, then, can be manipulated in an effort to improve performance. Although scientists and laymen alike may wish to distill our diets to some specific common denominator, a panacea or formula for success, we must remember that there must be a range of diets that will support health and excellent physical performance.

This volume reviewed the roles, including the speculative or hypothetical, of energy and energy-yielding macronutrients and derivatives in sports nutrition and performance.

16.2 ENERGY-YIELDING NUTRIENTS

Within the human cell is the ability to convert potential chemical energy derived from food macronutrients into high-energy compounds that can provide useable chemical energy for mechanical energy and work. The cell interconverts energy forms through different metabolic channels to form adenosine triphosphate (ATP), both a universal energy receiver and donor. The dietary sources of energy are carbohydrates, lipid and protein. At rest and during normal daily activities, lipids are the primary energy source, providing 80–90% of the energy, while carbohydrates and protein may provide 5–18% and 2–5%, respectively. Individuals who exercise need to understand how energy is transferred within the body and choose modes of conditioning, training, and dietary practices that complement each other.

To meet the caloric demands of daily exercise, the athlete must digest and absorb large, often tremendous, amounts of the major energy-yielding nutrients, i.e., carbohydrates, proteins and fats. Very few studies describe the effects of exercise on digestion and absorption of fats and proteins, but there is a lot of information on gastric emptying and absorption of carbohydrates during exercise. Strenuous exercise can probably adversely affect gastrointestinal function, although there is a paucity of evidence on the subject. Many endurance athletes report vomiting, bloating, abdominal cramps, and diarrhea during strenuous training and exercise. Most evidence indicates that gastric emptying of water or up to 8% carbohydrate solutions is not a limiting factor for fluids or energy replenishment during exercise and recovery. Little is known about the emptying of solid foods during exercise. Exercise intensity has no, or little, effect on carbohydrate absorption. During prolonged moderate intensity exercise, the intestines of healthy subjects are capable of absorbing carbohydrate at high rates. There is some evidence to suggest the athlete's gastrointestinal tract may show structural and functional adaptations in response to high daily intakes of calories and carbohydrates. These adaptations may enhance absorptive capacity and may provide benefits for athletes with high-energy needs.

The energy demands of competitive endurance training and events generally exceed the rate at which fat can be oxidized, so carbohydrates are the predominant fuel sources for these activities. Severely reduced carbohydrate stores are closely associated with fatigue and impaired performance. Athletes must make appropriate dietary decisions concerning carbohydrate intake. They must consider the effect of carbohydrate intake on short-term training and competition, keeping in mind the potential effect of their choices on long-term health and fitness. A relatively recent approach in sports nutrition research has been to study carbohydrates by the physiological response they provide, especially the blood glucose and insulin response resulting from their consumption. This categorization by glycemic response (the glycemic index) may be a more appropriate way to look at carbohydrates, since not all simple carbohydrates provide the same glycemic response and there is a wide range of responses among complex carbohydrates. Athletes may also benefit from considering the Glycemic Index of the carbohydrates they consume, as well as whether they are simple or complex carbohydrates. Concerning carbohydrate intake, the athlete must consider two major determinants when making dietary plans—carbohydrate must make up the majority of energy intake for maintenance of long-term health, and athletes must consider the demands of their sport or activity.

Fiber, though virtually unavailable for energy production, does affect carbohydrate and lipid absorption and carbohydrate oxidation rates. The possibility that dietary fiber may help improve athletic performance is a relatively new concept. Studies have established that certain dietary fibers flatten the postprandial blood glucose and insulin curves due to a delayed rate of glucose absorption, possibly because of the viscosity characteristic of fiber, which would slow the rate of entry of a meal from the stomach into the small intestine. Decreased lipid absorption by viscous dietary fiber has also been demonstrated, but the physiological significance is not certain. Slowing glucose absorption by viscous dietary fiber appears to be a means to attenuate the hyperinsulinemia normally occurring with exercise onset. This slowed glucose absorption may help by increasing glucose availability later in exercise to meet the need for carbohydrate oxidation. The evidence that a slowed rate of glucose absorption, mediated by either viscous fiber or low Glycemic Index foods, increases athletic endurance is intriguing but not yet compelling. Thus, there is no strong basis for recommending consumption of viscous fibers or low Glycemic Index foods prior to endurance exercise in order to enhance performance.

Knowledge of the beneficial effects of physical activity on plasma lipid and lipoprotein metabolism has been greatly expanded in recent years. Additionally, the role of lipids as an aid to enhanced physical performance has received increasing attention. Athletes and the noncompetitive recreational exerciser have tried many ways to increase fat utilization and reduce carbohydrate oxidation during exercise, the rationale being to increase endurance performance or to reduce total body adiposity or improve blood lipid profiles. While fats may be the preferred substrate during rest and during exercise up to 50% of $\dot{V}O_{2\,max}$, most athletic events occur between 75–100% of $\dot{V}O_{2\,max}$. At these intensities, a greater reliance on carbohydrates is found typically because of their greater ATP yield. Thus, athletes are at a quandary how to increase fatty acid oxidation during training and sport. Some studies suggest a high-fat diet will mandate increased fatty acid oxidation during exercise, especially in trained athletes at moderate work intensities. Other studies indicate diets supplemented with carnitine and caffeine will enhance fatty acid oxidation. Muscle oxidative potential has also been implicated.

Not only do athletes need more protein than others but there is also a vast body of research on the profound effects of protein and individual amino acids on athletic performance, primarily on muscle size and strength, energy metabolism, and immune function. Some researchers believe that current dietary protein recommendations for athletes are insufficient, one reason being that they are based primarily on data obtained from sedentary subjects. Others disagree and point out that protein overconsumption in athletes may be detrimental because of increased load in the kidneys in disposing of catabolic products. The effect of exercise on protein/amino acid needs must be taken into account. With exercise, amino acid catabolism can rise substantially, protein balance becomes positive through a rise in the net rate of whole body synthesis, and the fractional rate of myofibrillar protein breakdown may decrease. Just what factors control protein synthesis during exercise remain largely unknown. The use of specific protein and amino acid supplements can have anabolic and anticatabolic effects (partly by stimulating anabolic hormones and decreasing the effect of catabolic hormones).

16.3 SUPPLEMENTS CONTAINING MACRONUTRIENT DERIVATIVES

Supplement usage among athletes is widespread. The type of supplements can vary from vitamins and mineral supplements to carbohydrate-electrolyte sports beverages to that of bran supplements. The use of these supplements will vary depending on the sport. As a group, athletes have a significantly higher prevalence of usage than the general public. One of the main reasons for the athlete to use supplements is as ergogenic aids to enhance performance. Two methods of carbohydrate supplementation have been commonly used to increase exercise or athletic performance—increasing glycogen storage in muscle via carbohydrate loading and consuming carbohydrates during exercise. Carbohydrate loading (glycogen supercompensation) produces supranormal levels of muscle glycogen, which can improve athletic performance. Carbohydrate ingestion during exercise can improve long-term (>90 min.) endurance performance and delay fatigue up to one hour. Carbohydrate supplements used by athletes are generally readily digested and absorbed, and they increase and/or maintain blood glucose levels during prolonged exercise. The main carbohydrate component in most supplements is glucose, serving as energy substrate for exercising skeletal muscle. Glucose, sucrose, and maltodextrins appear to be equally effective in maintaining blood glucose concentration, carbohydrate oxidation, and in improving performance. Ingestion of fructose during prolonged exertion has not been shown to improve performance and may cause gastric distress. The major limiting factors for prolonged heavy exercise are dehydration and carbohydrate depletion. Therefore, replenishing body fluids with carbohydrate-containing beverages should minimize dehydration and benefit prolonged exercise. The amount of carbohydrate-containing fluids depends on the pace of the exercise, rate of dehydration due to sweating, environmental conditions, and gastrointestinal comfort. Based on some studies, it has been suggested that carbohydrate ingestion during exercise delays fatigue onset by maintaining euglycemia and blood glucose oxidation at high rates late in exercise, rather than reducing the rate of muscle glycogen utilization. A dose-response relationship between carbohydrate supplement intake and improvement in exercise capacity does not seem to exist.

Lipid supplementation as a means of enhancing exercise performance has received only limited attention. Information as to consumption of lipid dietary supplements is sparse and inconclusive. To date, the majority of studies have focused on the use of medium-chain triglycerides as an ergogenic acid. Due to their solubility in biological fluids, the digestion, absorption and oxidation of medium-chain carbohydrates are more reflective of carbohydrates than naturally occurring triglycerides, and experimental evidence suggests that they are at best equal to dietary carbohydrate in the ability to be utilized as an energy source. Both medium-chain triglyceride supplements and exogenous carbohydrate are about 50% oxidized during exercise and appear to contribute up to 10% of the total energy used. Whether medium-chain triglycerides can spare muscle glycogen during prolonged exercise is not certain. The effectiveness of lipid supplementation in the form of medium-chain triglycerides to enhance exercise performance is in question. The same can be said for omega-3 fatty acids, which have also received some scientific attention.

It is generally agreed that exercising individuals, in both endurance and strength exercise, require protein intakes past the current recommended dietary allowances to maintain nitrogen balance and prevent a predominance of amino acid oxidation. The current recommendation of 0.8 g/kg/d was based on needs of sedentary subjects. Strength athletes and weight lifters have traditionally focused on high dietary intakes of protein, including protein supplements. Protein supplements have proliferated because they fill a need for consumers. Reasons for the use of protein supplements instead of eating more protein-rich foods are simplicity, convenience, and lack of concomitant fat intake. Protein supplements also make possible the manufacture of meal replacements with specific macronutrient and micronutrient compositions to facilitate muscle gain, maintenance, and body fat loss. Recent advances in extraction and purification of proteins from various sources have made relatively pure proteins available at affordable prices. The major protein sources used in protein supplements are milk, egg, and soy products. Most of the human clinical trials of protein supplementation and exercise have used milk proteins. At present, whey protein is the preferred protein for strength athletes and forms the majority of protein powder products. Supplementation trials with soy protein in human athletes have been associated with improvements in training and recovery. Protein hydrolysates produced from protein sources include milk protein, collagen, glutamine peptides, peptide FM, and other sources (fish, soy, egg, vegetable) and have been employed as supplements. Since the 1989 ban on tryptophan for supplements in the U.S.A., amino acid mixtures as dietary supplements have been greatly reduced in number. Amino acids most commonly used to fortify protein supplements are glutamine, branched-chain amino acids, taurine, methionine, arginine, and ornithine. If supplemental protein intake is desired, it is important for each person to try various protein supplement sources because of the tremendous variation in taste, mixability, cost, and overall acceptance. There is compelling evidence to indicate that individuals engaged in strenuous exercise should consider protein supplements to maintain or increase muscle mass, especially if there is a desire to lower or prevent an increase of body fat.

The importance of creatine for muscle metabolism has been long appreciated, and recently it has catapulted to become one of the most popular nutritional supplements for athletes on the market. Although not all studies report ergogenic benefits, most indicate that it is probably an effective and safe supplement. Creatine phosphate serves as a reservoir of high-energy phosphate levels in muscle for maintenance and replenishment of ATP levels during muscular activity. Thus, creatine phosphate supplementations should theoretically delay fatigue in repetitive, exhaustive, short-term exercise.

Although not all studies concur, short-term creatine supplementation may improve maximal strength/power by 5–15%, work performed during sets of maximal effort muscle contractions by 5–15%, single effort spring performance by 1–5%, and work performed during repetitive sprint performance by 5–15%. Long-term supplementation may promote greater gains in strength, sprint performance, and lean body mass during training.

16.4 PHYSIOLOGICAL ASPECTS OF ENERGY METABOLISM

Because most research in the area of nutrition, muscle metabolism, and exercise physiology has been conducted using male participants, the conclusions and recommendations may have an inherent gender bias. Therefore, the applicability of some conclusions to females lacks scientific validation. Some studies have concluded that there are no gender differences in energy metabolism; others have found significant differences. Only past and future studies where there has been careful gender matching can resolve this controversy. Such studies employing appropriate matching have found that females oxidize more lipid and less protein and carbohydrate during endurance exercise than equally trained males. The potential mechanism(s) to explain possible gender differences in metabolism is still hypothetical. It may relate to the presence of the female hormone, 17-β-estradiol, a restricted energy intake in females, or the propensity of females to have a higher body fat (arising out of evolutionary pressures for energy conservation in times of shortage).

Changes in body composition and functioning occur with age. Age-related decreases in basal metabolic rate and physical activity and changes in energy metabolism are doubtless responsible, at least in part. Daily energy expenditure declines progressively throughout life. Body composition and energy balance exist in a simple relationship. Energy metabolism is a strong modulator on muscle mass, fat-free mass, and fat mass. Energy imbalance results in overnutrition (obesity) or undernutrition (wasting), which can be seen at any stage of life. There may be gender and ethnic differences manifest in energy metabolism as the human organism ages.

For many athletes, weight loss is a common goal, a necessity for ensuring successful performance. Weight loss is generally brought about by an imbalance between energy intake and energy expenditure. Several factors affect an individual's ability to lose weight, including changes in the components of the energy balance equation (energy intake = energy expenditures when body mass is constant) and the manipulation of fuel oxidation through alterations in nutrient composition. The latter includes the use of high-carbohydrate/low-fat diets and low-carbohydrate/high-protein diets. Numerous studies have demonstrated a negative relationship between body fat and performance. Percentage of body fat appears to be a better predictor of performance than body weight. Weight loss strategies include safe weight loss procedures (for example, exercise, and appropriate dietary manipulations) and pathogenic strategies, which are potentially harmful (such as dehydration, binging and purging, skipping meals, excessive exercise, and chronic dieting).

Some athletes may wish to gain weight to improve their appearance or their athletic performance. For these, the goal is to increase body weight by building lean body mass, not adding body fat. Energy intake and expenditure play a role in weight gain just as in weight loss. Ingesting sufficient extra energy to promote lean body tissue synthesis may be a challenge to athletes because their energy requirements are typically higher than matched non-athletes. They are encouraged to consume the majority of their energy requirements from carbohydrates. Weight resistance training is a vital component in stimulating muscle synthesis and should be incorporated in the athlete's exercise program during weight gain.

REFERENCES

1. Bucci, L., *Nutrients as Ergogenic Aids for Sports and Exercise*, CRC, Boca Raton, FL, 1993.
2. Watson, R.R. (Ed.), *Handbook of Nutrition in the Aged*, CRC, Boca Raton, FL, 1994.
3. Jackson, C.G.R., *Nutrition for the Recreational Athlete*, CRC, Boca Raton, FL, 1995.
4. Ruud, J.S., *Nutrition and the Female Athlete*, CRC, Boca Raton, FL, 1996.
5. Wolinsky, I. (Ed.), *Nutrition in Exercise and Sport,* third edition, CRC, Boca Raton, FL, 1998.
6. Tarnopolsky, M., *Gender Differences in Metabolism. Practical and Nutritional Implications*, CRC, Boca Raton, FL, 1998.
7. Driskell, J.A., Wolinsky, I. (Eds.), *Macroelements, Water, and Electrolytes*, CRC, Boca Raton, FL, 1999.

INDEX

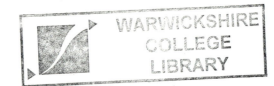